USING
AND
CONDUCTING
NURSING
RESEARCH
IN THE
CLINICAL
SETTING

USING
AND
CONDUCTING
NURSING
RESEARCH
IN THE
CLINICAL
SETTING

Magdalena A. Mateo, PhD, RN, FAAN
Formerly Director, Education and
   Professional Development
Department of Nursing
Mayo Clinic and Mayo Foundation
Rochester, Minnesota

Karin T. Kirchhoff, PhD, RN, FAAN
Professor
College of Nursing
University of Utah
Salt Lake City, Utah

SECOND EDITION

W.B. SAUNDERS COMPANY
A Division of Harcourt Brace & Company
Philadelphia   Montreal   London   Sydney   Toronto   Tokyo

W.B. SAUNDERS COMPANY
A Division of Harcourt Brace & Company

The Curtis Center
Independence Square West
Philadelphia, Pennsylvania 19106

Library of Congress Cataloging-in-Publication Data

Using and conducting nursing research in the clinical setting / [edited by] Magdalena A. Mateo, Karin T. Kirchhoff—2nd ed.

p.   cm.

Rev. ed. of: Conducting and using nursing research in the clinical setting. c1991.

Includes bibliographical references and index.

ISBN 0–7216–7165–9

1. Nursing—Research.   2. Medicine, Clinical—Research.   I. Mateo, Magdalena A.   II. Kirchhoff, Karin T.   III. Conducting and using nursing research in the clinical setting.

RT81.5 .M3 1999

610.73'072—ddc21   98-4260
                                                       Rev

USING AND CONDUCTING NURSING RESEARCH IN THE CLINICAL SETTING   ISBN 0–7216–7165–9

Printed in the United States of America.

Last digit is the print number: 9   8   7   6   5   4   3   2   1

Contributors

Susan L. Beck, PhD, RN, AOCN
Associate Professor, University of Utah, College of Nursing, Salt Lake City, Utah
Selecting a Design for the Study

Robert J. Caswell, PhD
Associate Professor of Health Services Management and Policy, College of Medicine and Public Health, The Ohio State University, Columbus, Ohio
Cost as a Dimension of Outcomes

Dominick L. Flarey, PhD, MBA, RN, CS, FACHE
Faculty, Department of Nursing, Learning Tree University, Chatsworth, California; President and Medical-Legal Consultant, The Center for Medical-Legal Consulting; Editor-in-Chief, JONA Health Care Law, Ethics & Regulation
Disseminating Research: The Medium and The Message

Marquis D. Foreman, PhD, RN, FAAN
Department of Medical-Surgical Nursing, College of Nursing, University of Illinois at Chicago; Clinical Scientist, University of Illinois at Chicago Medical Center, Chicago, Illinois
Gaining Support for the Study

Susan K. Frazier, PhD, MS, BS, RN
Assistant Professor, College of Nursing, The Ohio State University, Columbus, Ohio
Biomedical Instrumentation

Marguerite R. Kinney, DNSc, RN, FAAN
Professor Emerita, University of Alabama at Birmingham; Research Nurse, Birmingham Veterans Affairs Medical Center, Birmingham, Alabama
Seeking Funding for Clinical Research

Karin T. Kirchhoff, PhD, RN, FAAN
Professor, College of Nursing, University of Utah, Salt Lake City, Utah
Strategies in Research Utilization, One Form of Evidence-Based Practice; Research Skill Development; Outcomes Evaluation; Research Facilitation; Design of Questionnaires and Structured Interviews

Dorothy M. Lanuza, PhD, RN, FAAN
Professor, Department of Medical-Surgical Nursing, Loyola University of Chicago, Niehoff School of Nursing, Chicago, Illinois
Research and Practice

Heidi S. Lepper, PhD
Adjunct Faculty, University of California, Riverside, Department of Psychology, Riverside, California
Program Evaluation

Ada M. Lindsey, PhD, RN, FAAN
Dean and Professor, College of Nursing, University of Nebraska Medical Center, Omaha, Nebraska
Integrating Research and Practice

Mary R. Lynn, PhD
Associate Professor, School of Nursing, University of North Carolina at Chapel Hill, Chapel Hill, North Carolina
Data Analysis

Susan L. MacLean, PhD, RN
Director of Research Services, Emergency Nurses Association, Park Ridge, Illinois
Writing the Research Report

Magdalena A. Mateo, PhD, RN, FAAN
Formerly, Director, Education and Professional Development, Department of Nursing, Mayo Clinic and Mayo Foundation, Rochester, Minnesota

Exploring Innovative Ways of Giving Nursing Care; Research Skill Development; Managing Variances of Care; Research Facilitation; Progressing from an Idea to a Research Question; Psychosocial Measurement; Disseminating Research: The Medium and the Message

Deborah B. McGuire, PhD, BSN, MS
Associate Professor; Coordinator, Adult Immunology/Oncology Graduate Specialty, Department of Adult and Elder Health Nursing, Nell Hodgson Woodruff School of Nursing, Emory University, Atlanta, Georgia

Implementing the Study

Eileen McMyler, BSN, BS, MS
Nursing Education Specialist, Mayo Clinic and Mayo Foundation, Rochester, Minnesota

Managing Variances of Care

Cheryl Newton, BSN, MSN, CCRN, CNRN
Case Manager, Ohio Health Home Reach, Columbus, Ohio

Managing Variances of Care; Progressing from an Idea to a Research Question

Jennie T. Nickel, PhD, RN
Associate Professor, Community Health Nursing, College of Nursing, The Ohio State University, Columbus, Ohio

Case Management Outcomes in the Community Setting

Kathy J. Oleson, MS, RN, CPHQ
Auxiliary Faculty as Clinical Instructor, University of Utah College of Nursing; Quality Management Coordinator, Office of Performance Monitoring and Improvement, University of Utah Hospitals and Clinics, Salt Lake City, Utah

Continuous Quality Improvement/Total Quality Management, and the Relationship to Research

Geraldine V. Padilla, PhD
Professor and Associate Dean for Research, School of Nursing, University of California at Los Angeles, Los Angeles, California

Writing the Research Proposal

Barbara A. Rakel, MA, RN
Advance Practice Nurse in Clinical Outcomes and Resource Management, University of Iowa Hospitals and Clinics, Iowa City, Iowa

Outcomes Evaluation

Mary G. Schira, PhD, RN, ACNP
Director, Acute Care Nurse Practitioner Program, University of Texas at Arlington, Arlington, Texas

Research Skill Development; Exploring Innovative Ways of Giving Nursing Care; Looking in the Literature

Madeline H. Schmitt, PhD, MS, RN
Professor and Independence Foundation Professor of Nursing and Interprofessional Education and Coordinator, Doctoral Program, University of Rochester School of Nursing, Rochester, New York

The Conceptual Framework

Suzanne Smith, EdD, RN, FAAN
Courtesy Honorary Professor, College of Nursing, University of South Florida, Tampa, Florida; Editor-in-Chief, Journal of Nursing Administration and Nurse Educator, Bradenton, Florida

Disseminating Research: The Medium and the Message

Kathleen S. Stone, PhD, RN, FAAN
Professor, College of Nursing, The Ohio State University, Columbus, Ohio

Collaboration; Biomedical Instrumentation

Marita G. Titler, PhD, RN, FAAN
Director, Research and Quality Management, University of Iowa Hospitals and Clinics, Iowa City, Iowa

Program Evaluation

B. Lee Walker, PhD, RN
Associate Professor, College of Nursing, University of Utah, Salt Lake City, Utah

Qualitative Methods

Katherine A. Yeager, MS, RN
Adjunct Faculty and Research Project Manager, Nell Hodgson Woodruff School of Nursing, Emory University, Atlanta, Georgia

Implementing the Study

Foreword

Using nursing research . . . conducting nursing research—the sum of these two concepts is professional nursing practice that is based on evidence to achieve optimal outcomes.

Today professional nurses strive for more than high-quality nursing care. The rapidly changing health care environment—characterized by cost reduction, resizing, and restructuring—demands that we also steward our resources. We have the responsibility to provide the highest quality nursing care in the most cost-efficient manner.

To meet our responsibilities we must identify proven methods that produce better results more efficiently. We must seize those methods and apply them. Once we know that our actions benefit our patients, we can allocate our resources accordingly.

Whatever our nursing roles, each of us is accountable for using and conducting nursing research in the clinical setting. Administrators and faculty must include research methods and utilization into the education curricula and must integrate the concepts into practice arenas. Practitioners must raise questions, stimulate inquiry, engage in studies, analyze results, and apply results to practice. We must change our practices based on compelling evidence that the changes will benefit patients. As we conduct nursing research and use the results to make changes, we will rely on the type of guidance found in this second edition of *Using and Conducting Nursing Research in the Clinical Setting*. The book will serve as a reference to provide expertise, stimulate inquiries, and guide future tasks. Drs. Mateo and Kirchhoff and the contributors present practical approaches to a complex topic.

These practical approaches are the tools we need because changes in health care delivery are inevitable. If we are going to provide high quality, cost-effective care to our patients, then we must build professional practices based on strong evidence. We must conduct nursing research, and we must apply the results of that research to benefit our patients.

DOREEN K. FRUSTI, MSN, MS, RN
Chair, Department of Nursing
Mayo Clinic and Mayo Foundation
Rochester, Minnesota

Preface

Nurses provide care for patients in clinical settings. These settings include but are not limited to hospitals, clinics, homes, physicians' offices, and even the street, in cases of trauma. To give the best possible care in all of these places, nurses need to conduct studies and use research in their practice. This book represents our commitment to the belief that all nurses play an essential role in the conduct and use of research.

We have developed this research book so nurses can learn pragmatic considerations of scientific inquiry in the use and conduct of research in practice. In the late 1980s, members of the research committee at The Ohio State University Hospitals Department of Nursing developed a unit-based research manual. Since the staff nurses found the unit-based research manual helpful, we examined the material covered to assess sections that needed more depth and sections that needed to be added. Because the manual was from only one hospital and because enactment of research roles and responsibilities differs across institutions, we invited nurse researchers from across the country to serve as chapter contributors, and the manual became *Conducting and Using Nursing Research in the Clinical Setting,* published in 1991. One valuable source of input was comments from staff nurses who reviewed final drafts. We believe this book is a "second-generation" product that nurses from many institutions will find useful in enacting their research roles and responsibilities.

In this second edition, *Using and Conducting Nursing Research in the Clinical Setting,* we have added chapters on outcomes, evaluation, the use of conceptual frameworks to guide research, and qualitative research methods. Although the intended audience of the first edition was nurses in clinical settings, some schools of nursing have adopted it as a nursing research textbook for their students. The addition of these new chapters may benefit such usage.

Unit 1, Using Research in Clinical Practice, introduces the reader to ways in which research could be used in practice. The importance of research to practice is addressed in Chapter 1. The goal of Chapters 2 and 3 is to present ways of applying research to continuous quality improvement and clinical problem solving. Chapter 4 includes clinical studies and the application of findings to clinical practice. Various strategies for using research in practice are the focus of Chapter 5. Finally, experiences that facilitate the acquisition of research skills are presented in Chapter 6. Unit 2 is Using Research to Evaluate Practice. Chapter 7 presents an overview of outcomes and evaluation, including the forces influencing the emphasis on outcomes. Guidelines for evaluating programs are presented in Chapter 8. Defining case management, assessing research related to the effectiveness of case management in community settings, and evaluating case management are addressed in Chapter 9. Chapter 10 addresses steps to consider in timely management of variances of care. Chapter 11 includes the concepts related to cost, evaluating costs as a dimension of outcomes, and issues and concerns in measurement and analysis. Unit 3, Conducting Research, consists of strategies for research facilitation (Chaper 12), gaining access to a clinical setting (Chapter 13), acquiring funding (Chapter 14), collaboration (Chapter 15) and steps in conducting a study (Chapters 16 through 26). It concludes with chapters on writing the research report (Chapter 27) and disseminating research through presentation and publication (Chapter 28).

MAGDALENA A. MATEO
KARIN T. KIRCHHOFF

Acknowledgments

We wish to thank our colleagues who have shared their knowledge and experience with us. A special appreciation goes to nurses who have given us suggestions at various stages of the book's development and reviewed chapter manuscripts. Finally, we would like to thank the chapter authors for their dedication and commitment that have made the publication of this book possible.

MAGDALENA A. MATEO
KARIN T. KIRCHHOFF

Contents

Using Research in Clinical Practice

Research and Practice

Dorothy M. Lanuza

The impact that the profession of nursing has on the health care of the society depends upon the competence of its practitioners; their ability to achieve positive, cost-effective client outcomes; and their ability to develop, evaluate, and expand nursing knowledge. Many of the challenges facing nursing, such as high patient acuity levels, shortened hospital stays, earlier discharges to community settings, and changes in staff ratio mix, require new and innovative solutions. Research is an inherent aspect of the strategies aimed at meeting these challenges.

> Research can improve practice by providing a process that can
>
> • Provide answers to clinical questions
> • Evaluate the effectiveness of nursing actions
> • Test theories relevant to practice
> • Expand nursing knowledge

WAYS THAT RESEARCH IMPROVES PRACTICE

During the past several decades, it has become clear that research is essential to provide a scientific basis for the practice of nursing and to ensure that nursing actions are based on more than just tradition and intuition.

The purpose of this chapter is to emphasize the important reciprocal relationship between research and practice. Examples demonstrate how clinical questions can be an impetus for research, as well as how research can be used to evaluate the effectiveness of nursing interventions and to test theories that guide nursing actions. In addi-

tion, the important role that all nurses can play in supporting and participating in research is addressed.

Provide Answers to Clinical Questions

During clinical practice, it is not uncommon for questions to arise that challenge the way care is being provided. Research provides a systematic process for seeking answers to those clinical questions. For example, several decades ago, prolonged bedrest was thought to be therapeutic. In fact, enforced bedrest was thought to be an essential component of treatment of myocardial infarction (MI). It has come to be known, however, that there are many serious adverse effects associated with prolonged immobilization, such as impairments of the vascular system (for example, venous stasis, thrombus formation), respiratory system (for example, pneumonia), renal system (for example, kidney stone formation), and musculoskeletal system (for example, osteoporosis, muscle atrophy). Thus, when Levine and Lown introduced the idea of "armchair" treatment for MI patients in 1951, they caused a great controversy (Schmitt, Hood, & Lown, 1969). Levine and Lown believed that the physiological effects associated with allowing MI patients to sit up in a chair were less taxing than enforced bedrest. Therefore, over a 2½-year period, these physicians, with the assistance of the unit nurses, studied the effects on heart rate (HR) and blood pressure (BP) of getting patients (N = 184) up in a chair, as tolerated. Patients were not gotten up if they were experiencing chest pain, cardiogenic shock, or unconsciousness resulting from cerebral insufficiency. During the study period, approximately 75% of the MI patients were assisted into a chair at their bedside (71% of the patients within 24 hours after admission). Blood pressure and HR were measured before (lying position) and 5 minutes after the patients were assisted into a sitting position in an armchair.

Findings: The investigators reported that clinically important changes in the patients' HR and BP were rarely observed and the patients tolerated armchair treatment very well.

Impact: Despite several design weaknesses (for example, no control group was used for comparison), the findings of the study were clinically significant because they supported the trend toward early ambulation of MI patients. In addition, the unit nurses had an opportunity to be involved with the implementation and evaluation of this new form of treatment (that is, armchair treatment).

Schmitt, Hood, & Lown, 1969

Nurses often pose clinical questions about different methods of carrying out assessments or providing care that can be answered through clinical research. For example, several staff nurses in a coronary care unit at a university medical center wondered whether it made a difference which site (right atria or catheter) was used as a reference point to measure mean arterial pressure (MAP). They also questioned whether it was really necessary to lower the patient's position from a semi-Fowler position to a supine position in order to obtain an accurate measurement.

One of the staff nurses sought the assistance of the nurse research scientist at the hospital for help in investigating the answers to these questions. In their subsequent study, four MAP readings (two positions: supine and semi-Fowler; two sites: right atrium and catheter) were obtained in 29 hemodynamically stable coronary care unit patients (Kirchhoff, Rebenson-Piano, & Patel, 1984).

Findings: The measurements for each site and position were as follows:

1. Supine—82.6 mmHg (right atrium) and 84.0 mmHg (catheter site)
2. Semi-Fowler—82.2 mmHg (right atrium) and 90.3 mmHg (catheter site)

Measurements for the various positions and sites were highly correlated ($r = .90$). The investigators, however, recommended that the right atrium site (that is, the phlebostatic level) be used in stable patients because the values were very similar and changed very little whether the patient was in the supine or semi-Fowler position.

Impact: The findings answered the clinical questions the staff nurses asked, that is, in hemodynamically stable coronary care unit patients, the right atrium would be the best site for measurement and it would not matter whether the patient was in a supine or semi-Fowler position at the time of the measurement.

Kirchhoff et al., 1984

In another example, a maternal-child clinical nurse specialist at a university medical center was concerned that postoperative pain management for mothers who underwent cesarean sections may not be adequate. She wondered whether there might be a better way of providing pain management than the method that was being used (that is, parenteral analgesic given as needed), so she collaborated with a doctorally prepared faculty member from the university's School of Nursing and several medical center nurses and physicians. After reviewing the literature on pain management, the research team decided to investigate whether patient-controlled analgesia (PCA) was more effective in relieving postoperative pain than the current method that was being used.

Forty-two women (PCA group, N = 25; control group, N = 17) who underwent cesarean sections participated in this study (Perez-Woods et al., 1991). Initially, this study met with some resistance from the unit nurses because it meant additional paperwork. As the study progressed, however, the staff began to appreciate the value of the study and were impressed by the study results.

Findings: The findings of the study indicated that PCA patients

1. Used *more* analgesia
2. Were *less* sedated (that is, more alert)
3. Were *more* satisfied with their pain relief
4. Ambulated *earlier* and more frequently
5. Did *not* differ from the control group in relation to length of hospital stay

Impact: Although the subjects in the PCA group received more analgesia, they ambulated earlier and more frequently and were more satisfied with their pain management than the control group who received parenteral analgesic (that is, morphine via intramuscular route as needed). At the study institution, these findings resulted in PCA's being instituted as an option for all cesarean mothers for whom it is not contraindicated. The findings also helped to pave the way for PCAs to be used more extensively throughout the hospital and promoted greater interest in research by staff nurses. On a more general basis, the findings added to the growing body of knowledge on the value of using PCAs as a pain management strategy.

Perez-Woods et al., 1991

Sometimes questions arise related to products used in providing clinical care. Product evaluation provides a process for answering those questions. It is undertaken for a variety of reasons, such as (1) finding a replacement for a product currently being used that is considered unsatisfactory, (2) determining which of several available products is the most cost-effective while still achieving desired outcomes, and (3) evaluating the safety and efficacy of new products or devices (Mateo, 1993). Because nurses often are the individuals who will be using or supervising the use of many of these products, they play a very important role in product evaluation research.

In the following example of product evaluation research, a representative for a company that manufactured a brand of urine collection bags used with infants asked neonatal clinical nurse specialists from two hospitals whether they or their neonatal nurse colleagues were dissatisfied with any of the company's products. The nurses responded that they were dissatisfied with the urine collection bags being used with low birth weight (LBW), premature infants. The bags were designed for a normal size newborn infant and were too big and inappropriate for LBW (<2.27 kg), premature infants.

Comments were similar to those made by staff at other neonatal settings, and the company responded by developing a urine collection bag designed for LBW, premature infants. Two neonatal clinical nurse specialists were then asked to conduct research to evaluate the new Premie U-Bag. They and the nurses on their units participated in the company-sponsored product evaluation study that compared the newly designed Premie U-Bag with the urine collection bag designed for full-term infants (Fig. 1–1).

Findings: The nurses reported that the Premie U-Bag was easier to apply and more effective for collecting urine because it fit better, it adhered better, and it was not associated with adverse skin responses.

Impact: The impact of this endeavor was the introduction of a new product

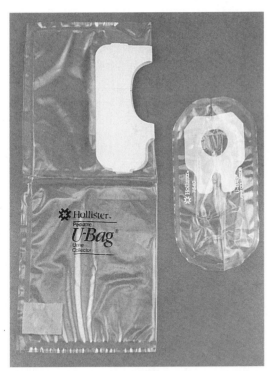

Figure 1–1
Left, The pediatric urine collection bag (U-Bag) designed for normal term infants. *Right,* The urine collection bag (Premie U-Bag) designed for low birth weight premature infants. (Courtesy of Hollister Inc., Libertyville, IL.)

that was an effective urine collection bag for LBW, premature infants. In addition, the nursing units were reimbursed for the extra work associated with their nurses' participation in the product evaluation study. At one of the study sites, these funds were used by the unit nurses to buy a couch for the "grieving" room that was located near the neonatal intensive care unit.

Lawrence, Malloy, & Balis, 1990

Evaluate the Effectiveness of Nursing Actions

Nursing research also provides a method for evaluating nursing interventions and patient care protocols, such as for endotracheal suctioning (ETS), which is a common intervention performed to remove secretions and maintain a patent airway in patients who are connected to ventilators. It may seem like a fairly simple, straightforward procedure, but it has been the source of many research investigations to assess the safety and efficacy of different methods and procedures related to ETS. Nurses usually administer several hyperinflation and hyperoxygenation breaths before and after ETS in order to briefly increase alveolar oxygen and thus prevent or minimize a decrease in oxygenation resulting from suctioning. Some nurses also instill a small amount of sterile normal saline before ETS. In the past, it was common practice to use manual resuscitation bags (with reservoir) to deliver the hyperinflation (increase tidal volume $1\frac{1}{2}$ times) and hyperoxygenation (increase inspired oxygen content [FIO_2]). Are these interventions safe and effective? During the past few years, there has been a strong effort to build a research base in the area of ETS. The following is a discussion on how research can be used to evaluate the effectiveness of nursing actions, build nursing practice knowledge, and improve patient care.

Table 1–1 lists a number of questions related to ETS that nurse clinicians have asked and that have stimulated subsequent investigations. Many studies have addressed ETS-related questions. Five literature reviews are available for further information on this topic (Riegel, 1985; Barnes & Kirchhoff, 1986; Stone & Turner, 1989; Manicelli-Van Atta & Beck, 1992; Wainwright & Gould, 1996).

Chulay (1988) studied the effect on arterial blood gases of hyperinflation and hyperoxygenation before and after two ETS passes in 32 postoperative coronary artery bypass graft patients within 24 hours of admission to an intensive care unit. Five hyperinflation breaths were given with a resuscitation bag before each of two suction passes.

Findings: The findings supported the efficacy of this protocol, that is, hyperinflation and hyperoxygenation with a resuscitation bag before suctioning significantly increased oxygenation.

Chulay, 1988

Anderson (1989) compared manual bagging to mechanical ventilatory sighing during suctioning of 28 patients who under-

Table 1–1 ·····································

Clinical Questions Related to Endotracheal Suctioning

1. Would hyperinflation and/or hyperoxygenation provided prior to suctioning prevent marked declines in oxygen saturation?
2. Are manual resuscitation bagging and ventilatory sighing effective in producing hyperinflation prior to suctioning? If so, how many hyperinflation breaths should be given?
3. Are both methods comparable in providing hyperinflation and hyperoxygenation prior to suctioning? Do they have similar cardiovascular effects?
4. Is hyperoxygenation at less than 100% oxygen as effective as 100% oxygen prior to suctioning?
5. Should the cuff of the endotracheal tube be deflated during endotracheal suctioning (ETS)?
6. Does instillation of sterile normal saline into the endotracheal tube prior to ETS improve the effectiveness of suctioning? Does it matter whether the volume of normal saline instilled is 5 mL or 10 mL? Are there any adverse effects to instilling normal saline?
7. Is oxygen insufflation as effective as preoxygenation and/or hyperinflation in preventing decreases in oxygen saturation?
8. Does the use of a closed endotracheal system with an adaptor for suctioning prevent or minimize hypoxemia resulting from suctioning?
9. Should ETS be done continuously or intermittently?
10. Should ETS be done routinely or only as needed?
11. When examining the effects of ETS on oxygen levels, what laboratory method is the best indication of tissue oxygenation, arterial oxygen tension or mixed venous oxygen saturation?

went coronary artery bypass graft surgery in order to determine the best method for providing oxygenation.

Findings: Ventilatory sighing was shown to produce a greater increase in arterial oxygen saturation and the investigator recommended that, when possible, ventilatory sighing be used (instead of manual resuscitation bagging) during suc-

tioning in stable coronary artery bypass graft patients.

Anderson, 1989

Investigators were also interested in comparing the effects of continuous versus intermittent ETS on tracheal tissue. Czarnik, Stone, Everhart, and Preusser (1991) used an animal model to compare these two suctioning methods.

Findings: The investigators found that both methods caused tracheal tissue damage and concluded that there were no significant differences between the methods. They recommended that routine suctioning should be avoided and the number of suction passes should be kept to a minimum to avoid injury.

Czarnik et al., 1991

As research strategies to prevent or limit hypoxemia during ETS progressed, it became clear that there were many factors that needed to be considered when investigating this topic. Reviews of ETS studies also indicated there were many variations in the research protocols used, for example, in the methods used for providing oxygenation or hyperinflation, in the percent of oxygenation provided, in the ratio of the suction catheter to the endotracheal tube, in the use of intermittent or continuous suctioning, in the use of different methods (for example, a closed system with an adaptor for suctioning, oxygen insufflation, or disconnecting the patient from the ventilator to perform ETS), and in instillation versus no instillation of sterile normal saline before suctioning. The lack of common conceptual definitions of terms, protocols, instruments, or types of subjects make it difficult to compare findings across studies. In order to build clinical knowledge and develop research-based, clinical ETS protocols, it became clear that well-controlled, multisite studies or replication of studies in which similar definitions of terms, protocols, and samples are used was needed.

In 1984, American Association of Critical Care Nurses (AACN) funded a National Study Group of nurse physiologists to investigate issues related to ETS. Many studies resulted from this multisite project.

In one study, Stone, Vorst, Lanham, and Zahn (1989) found that manual bagging done to induce hyperinflation caused greater changes in MAP and HR than using ventilatory sighing. They concluded that, in critically ill patients, the changes induced by bagging may not be tolerated well.

In another study, Stone, Preusser, Groch, Karl, and Gonyon (1991) examined the effects of hyperinflation on MAP and postsuctioning hypoxemia. They used ventilatory sighing for two reasons: (1) because manual bagging caused greater changes in MAP and HR and (2) because hyperinflation volumes produced via manual bagging varied too much and they wanted to examine the effects of using four different hyperinflation volumes, ranging from 12 to 18 mL/kg.

Findings: 1. The investigators found that all the volumes of hyperinflation that they tested provided adequate postsuctioning oxygenation, thus a volume of 12 mL/kg was just as effective as 18 mL/kg.

2. They also found, however, that hyperinflation of the lung using ventilatory sighing resulted in a significant 15-mmHg increase in MAP, with the greatest increase occurring at the beginning and end of the second hyperinflation sequence. The investigators recommended that lung hyperinflation and suction sequences be limited to two per session.

This project was a fine example of several nurse scientists independently, yet collaboratively, investigating a clinical problem using similar methods and approaches (Stone et al., 1991).

As the reviews (Riegel, 1985; Barnes & Kirchhoff, 1986; Stone & Turner, 1989; Manicelli-Van Atta & Beck, 1992; Wainwright & Gould, 1996) on ETS suggest, there are still many issues that need investigation. With each new study, information is obtained that helps to build the state-of-the-art knowledge base related to ETS and to develop and refine research-based ETS guidelines for practice. A summary of findings from selected studies and gleaned from five published ETS review articles is presented in Table 1–2. Whenever ETS guidelines are developed, they must be flexible and their use individualized to the needs of the patient.

Research can contribute to nursing knowledge by

- Testing theories relevant to practice
- Providing a link between education and practice

Expand Nursing Knowledge

Research contributes to improving nursing practice and provides the information and knowledge needed to link education and practice. Clinical practice provides a rich source of ideas for research. Theories about phenomena of interest to nursing and health care are another source for research ideas. In addition, conceptual frameworks and theories can guide the study of clinical problems by providing a blueprint or structure for viewing phenomena. Kerlinger (1986) defines a theory as

. . . a set of interrelated constructs (concepts), definitions, and propositions that present a systematic view of phenomena by specifying relations among variables, with the purpose of explaining and predicting the phenomena (p. 9).

Conceptual frameworks and theories direct the focus of the inquiry by identifying the variables and concepts that are of interest and suggesting the potential relationships among the variables and concepts. When a relationship among variables is specified, then it is usually possible to test the relationship. Even if the theory or the specified relationships between or among variables and concepts do not hold up under testing, knowledge about the phenomenon is gained (Newman, 1979). The testing of theories is an important aspect of expanding knowledge.

An example of a theory that has been used to guide clinical research is the gate control theory, which views pain as a multidimensional concept with physical (that is, sensory-discriminative) and psychological (that is, affective-motivational) components. The gate control theory was proposed by Melzack and Wall in 1965 and it continues to play an important and influential role in guiding pain research and pain manage-

Table 1–2 ....

Summary of Findings from Selected Studies and from Published Literature Reviews of ETS Research in Adult Patients

1. Suctioning alone leads to a decrease in oxygenation (Barnes & Kirchhoff, 1986; Manicelli-Van Atta & Beck, 1992; Riegel, 1985; Stone & Turner, 1989; Wainwright & Gould, 1996).
2. Preoxygenation should be used before and after suctioning (the preferred method of delivery, the percentage of oxygen [Rogge et al., 1989], and the timing need further research [Barnes & Kirchhoff, 1986; Manicelli-Van Atta & Beck, 1992; Riegel, 1985]).
3. The use of hyperinflation combined with hyperoxygenation prevents or minimizes hypoxemia (Barnes & Kirchhoff, 1986; Manicelli-Van Atta & Beck, 1992; Goodnough, 1985); the effects of hyperinflation alone on hypoxemia varies (Manicelli-Van Atta & Beck, 1992).
4. Manual resuscitation bagging (MRB) and ventilatory sighing both produce hyperinflation and combined with preoxygenation prevent or minimize ETS induced hypoxemia (Barnes & Kirchhoff, 1986; Wainwright & Gould, 1996; Anderson, 1989; Chulay & Graeber, 1988).
5. MRB, however, causes greater changes in HR and MAP (Manicelli-Van Atta & Beck, 1992; Stone & Turner, 1989). In addition, the hyperinflation volumes vary from one instance to the next (Stone & Turner, 1989; Wainwright & Gould, 1996; Stone et al., 1989, 1991).
6. Ventilatory sighing produces a more consistent increase in oxygenation and volume and less change in HR and MAP than MRB (Manicelli-Van Atta & Beck, 1992; Riegel, 1985; Stone & Turner, 1989; Chase et al., 1989; Stone et al., 1989) but it still produces a marked increase in MAP (Stone & Turner, 1989; Stone et al., 1989).
7. PEEP ($\geq$10 cm) may have a protective effect during ETS (Barnes & Kirchhoff, 1986).
8. Closed system ETS using adapters to maintain ventilation and PEEP prevented significant decreases in PaO_2 (Gonzalez et al., 1983; Brown et al., 1983).
9. Czarnick et al.'s (1991) work with animal models showed that both intermittent and continuous suctioning damages tracheal tissue, and no significant differences were found between the two methods.
10. Suction catheters should not occlude more than 50% of the endotracheal tube (Riegel, 1985; Stone & Turner, 1989).
11. There is insufficient research to support the proposal that instillation of sterile normal saline prior to ETS is beneficial (Gray, MacIntyre, & Kronenberger, 1990) and, in fact, findings from several studies have suggested it may have deleterious effects because it may interfere with gas exchange (Ackerman, Ecklund & Abu-Jumah, 1996; Haglar & Traver, 1994; Raymond, 1995).
12. Oxygen insufflation has been reported to be as effective as preoxygenation and hyperinflation in preventing a significant decrease in PaO_2 levels (Bodai et al., 1987; Dam, Wild, & Baun, 1994; Langrehr et al., 1981; Taft et al., 1991).
13. The endotracheal cuff should *not* be deflated during ETS because it increases the risk of aspiration pneumonia (Thelan et al. cited in Wainwright & Gould, 1996).
14. The McIntosh et al. (1993) investigation of tissue oxygenation, using animal models, found that SvO_2 provided a better estimation of tissue oxygenation than arterial oxygen tension alone, because it allows the calculation of oxygen delivery and extraction ratio.

  The general conclusions were: suctioning should **NOT BE DONE ROUTINELY,** but only as needed, with preoxygenation and hyperinflation induced by ventilatory sighing and a minimal number of passes—if possible, only two suctioning passes per session. Oxygen insufflation, as well as a closed system with an adaptor to maintain ventilation, has also been shown to be beneficial for preventing or minimizing hypoxemia associated with ETS (Wainwright & Gould, 1996).

PEEP, positive end-expiratory pressure; HR, heart rate; MAP, mean arterial pressure.

ment interventions. According to this theory, when noxious stimuli cause damage or injury, substances are released that activate the transmission of pain impulses to the substantia gelatinosa (SG) in the dorsal horn of the spinal cord. Pain impulses are transmitted via small fiber A-delta or c fibers. Other nociceptive (for example, temperature, vibration) impulses are also transmitted to the SG in the spinal cord via large fibers. Impulse transmission can be modified by intraspinal and descending neuromodulation (that is, impulses can be inhibited or facilitated). In other words, pain impulses must be transmitted via neural spinal pathways to the brain before pain is perceived (Davis, 1995). Thus, inhibition of pain impulse transmission can eliminate or decrease the experience of pain.

The intraspinal gate control mechanism involves a relative balance between small fiber and large fiber activity. If small fiber activity exceeds large fiber activity, then pain impulse transmission is facilitated (that is, gate opens). On the other hand, if the large fiber activity is greater, pain impulse transmission is inhibited (that is, gate closes). Because large fibers transmit impulses to both the SG and the control system in the brain (Fig. 1–2), the brain also plays a role in neuromodulation. In response to large fiber input, impulses from the control (cognitive-evaluative) system of the brain are sent via efferent (descending) pathways to the SG, influencing impulse inhibition (that is, gate closes). When the transmission of impulses from the SG to T cells exceed a critical level, the action system is activated (Fig. 1–3). The action system consists of three interacting systems in the brain (cognitive-evaluative, affective-motivational, and sensory-discriminative), which are responsible for pain perception, evaluation, selective modulation, and re-sponse (Melzack & Wall, 1965; Melzack & Casey, 1965; Kim, 1980; Puntillo & Tesler, 1993; National Institute of Nursing Research, 1994).

Although there are limitations to the accuracy and completeness of the gate control theory (Hoffert, 1986), it has proved invaluable because it introduced the concept of neuromodulation and suggested that pain was a multidimensional concept. Using the gate control theory as a framework, research findings have contributed to a growing knowledge about pain and pain management. Thus, a multimodal pain management approach is recommended involving both pharmacological and nonpharmacological interventions to inhibit pain impulse transmission or activation of the action system (that is, cognitive-evaluative, affective-motivational, and sensory-discriminative). For example, peripheral interventions such as rubbing, massage, or applying pressure to pressure points are based on the stimulation of large, nonpain fibers, which are postulated to close the spinal cord "gate" to transmission of pain impulses. Similarly, application of cold to painful areas is postulated to relieve pain because it decreases

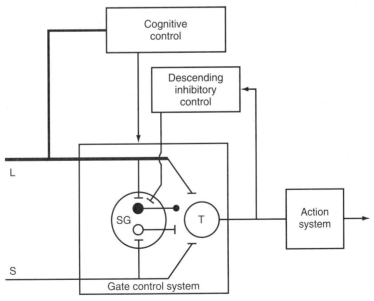

Figure 1–2
The gate control theory model includes excitatory (*white circles*) and inhibitory (*black circles*) links from the substantia gelatinosa (SG) to the transmission (T) cells, as well as descending inhibitory control from brain stem systems. The round knob at the end of the inhibitory link implies that its action may be presynaptic, postsynaptic, or both. All connections are excitatory, except the inhibitory link from the SG to the T cell. (From Jeans, M. E., & Melzack, R. [1992]. Conceptual basis of nursing practice: Theoretical foundations of pain. In J. H. Watt-Watson & M. I. Donovan, [Eds.], *Pain management: Nursing perspective* [p 20]. Philadelphia: Lippincott-Raven.)

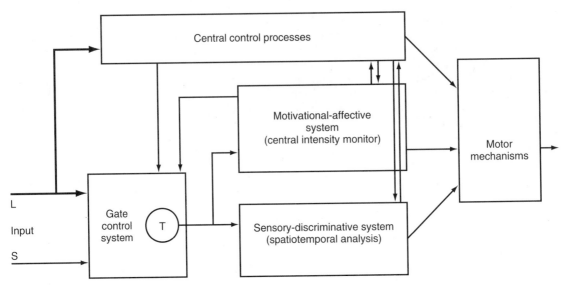

Figure 1–3
Conceptual model of the sensory, motivational, and central control determinants of pain. The output of the T cells of the gate control system projects to the sensory-discriminative system (via neospinothalamic fibers) and the motivational-affective system (via the paramedial ascending system). The central control trigger is represented by a line running from the larger fiber system to central control processes; these in turn project back to the gate control system and to the sensory-discriminative and motivational-affective systems. All three systems interact with one another and project to the motor system. (From Jeans, M. E., & Melzack, R. [1992]. Conceptual basis of nursing practice: Theoretical foundations of pain. In J. H. Watt-Watson & M. I. Donovan [Eds.], *Pain management: Nursing perspective* [p. 26]. Philadelphia: Lippincott-Raven.)

the conduction velocity of "pain" fibers and reduces swelling. Other nonpharmacological interventions such as distraction, relaxation, and providing information are thought to decrease pain by their influence on central nervous center processes (for example, decreasing anxiety, increasing a sense of control), which then may transmit inhibitory impulses to close the gate, prevent amplification of the pain experience caused by fear or anxiety, and help to focus attention away from the pain experience (McCaffery, 1990; McCaffery & Wolff, 1992; Puntillo & Tesler, 1993; National Institute of Nursing Research, 1994).

NURSES' INVOLVEMENT IN RESEARCH

In addition to understanding and appreciating the important role research can play in improving practice and expanding knowledge, it is also important for nurses to be involved in research. Nurses at all levels can and should participate in research; however, their participation will vary according to their knowledge, preparation, skills, and motivation. As Cronenwett (1987) stated,

Even when nurses can understand only problem statements and discussion sections of research reports, their thinking about ways to assess problems or plan nursing care is expanded. They stay abreast of what questions are being asked about nursing practice, what innovations are being tested, and what potential implications for practice are being proposed. With such exposure, nurses often improve the quality of assessment of a problem, analyze an intervention from a new perspective, or gain increased awareness of the link between nursing care and nursing outcomes (p. 9).

Thus, nurses' participation may be as limited as simply being supportive of research or as complex as being the primary investigator of a research project. In addition to being consumers of research, nurses can actively participate in research. When nursing staff have insufficient research knowledge and skills to conduct research, intradisciplinary and interdisciplinary research collaboration with more experienced clinical or faculty researchers can be sought. As many of the clinical examples in this chapter show, collaborative research could be intradisciplinary (for example, service and educational nursing collaboration) or interdisciplinary (for example, collaboration between nurses and members of other disciplines such as physicians).

SUMMARY

The ultimate purpose of nursing is to provide high-quality patient care. Clinical practice without research is practice based on tradition without validation. Research is needed to evaluate the effectiveness of nursing treatment modalities, to determine the impact of nursing care on the health of patients, or to test out theory. Nursing practice is undergoing tremendous changes and challenges. In order to meet societal challenges and needs, nursing practice must be research based.

REFERENCES

Anderson, K. M. (1989). The effects of manual bagging versus mechanical ventilatory sighing on oxygenation during the suctioning procedure. *Heart & Lung, 18,* 301–302. (Abstract).

Ackerman, M. H., Ecklund, M. M., & Abu-Jumah, M. (1996). A review of normal saline instillation: Implications for practice. *DCCN-Dimensions of Critical Care Nursing, 15,* 31–38.

Barnes, C. A., & Kirchhoff, K. T. (1986). Minimizing hypoxemia due to endotracheal suctioning: A review of the literature. *Heart & Lung, 15*(2), 164–176.

Bodai, B. I., Walton, C. B., Briggs, S., & Goldstein, M. (1987). A clinical evaluation of an oxygen insufflation/suction catheter. *Heart & Lung, 16,* 39–46.

Brown, S. E., Standbury, D. W., Merrill, R. J., Linden, G. S., & Light, R. W. (1983). Prevention of suctioning related arterial oxygen desaturation: comparison off-ventilator and on-ventilator suctioning. *Chest, 83,* 621–627.

Chase, D. Z., Campbell, G., Byram, D., Tribett, D., Ananian, L., & Chulay, M. (1989). Hemodynamic changes associated with endotracheal suctioning. *Heart & Lung, 18,* 292–293.

Chulay, M. (1988). Arterial blood gas changes with a hyperinflation and hyperoxygenation suctioning intervention in critically ill patients. *Heart & Lung, 17*(6), 654–661.

Chulay, M., & Graeber, G. M. (1988). Efficacy of a hyperinflation and hyperoxygenation suctioning intervention. *Heart & Lung, 17*(1), 15–22.

Cronenwett, L. R. (1987). Research utilization in a practice setting. *Journal of Nursing Administration, 17*(7–8), 9–10.

Czarnik, R. E., Stone, K. S., Everhart, C. C., Jr., & Preusser, B. A. (1991). Differential effects of continuous versus intermittent suction on tracheal tissue. *Heart & Lung, 20*(2), 144–151.

Dam, V., Wild, M. C., & Baun, M. M. (1994). Effect of oxygen insufflation during endotracheal suctioning on arterial pressure and oxygenation in coronary artery bypass graft patients. *American Journal of Critical Care, 3,* 191–197.

Davis, P. (1995). Opening up the gate control theory. *Nursing Standard, 7,* 25–27.

Gonzalez, H. F., Erchowsky, P., & Ahmed, T. (1983). Endotracheal suctioning in patients on mechanical ventilation. *American Review of Respiratory Disease, 127,* 151–154.

Goodnough, S. K. C. (1985). The effects of oxygen and hyperinflation on arterial oxygen tension after endotracheal suctioning. *Heart & Lung, 14,* 11–17.

Gray, J. E., MacIntyre, N. R., & Kronenberger, W. G. (1990). The effects of bolus normal saline instillation in conjunction with endotracheal suctioning. *Respiratory Care, 35,* 785–790.

Hagler, D. A., & Traver, G. A. (1994). Endotracheal saline and suction catheters: Sources of lower airway contamination. *American Journal of Critical Care, 3,* 444–447.

Hoffert, M. (1986). The gate control theory re-visited. *Journal of Pain and Symptom Management, 1*(1), 39–41.

International Association for the Study of Pain Subcommittee on Taxonomy. (1979). Pain terms: A list with definitions and usage. *Pain, 6,* 249.

Jeans, M.E., & Melzack, R. (1992). Conceptual basis of nursing practice: Theoretical foundations of pain. In J. H. Watt-Watson & M. I. Donovan (Eds.), *Pain management: Nursing perspective* (pp. 11–35). St. Louis: Mosby–Year Book.

Kerlinger, F. N. (1986). *Foundations of behavioral research* (3rd ed.). Fort Worth: Harcourt Brace Jovanovich College Publishers.

Kim, S. (1980). Pain: Theory, research, and nursing practice. *Advances in Nursing Sciences, 2,* 43–59.

Kirchhoff, K. T., Rebenson-Piano, M., & Patel, M. (1984). Mean arterial pressure readings: Variations with positions and transducer level. *Nursing Research, 33*(6), 343–345.

Langrehr, E. A., Washburn, S. C., & Guthrie, M. P. (1981). Oxygen insufflation during endotracheal suctioning. *Heart & Lung, 10,* 1028–1036.

Lawrence, P., Malloy, M. B., & Balis, N. (1990). Product evaluation study comparing a newly developed premature urine collection bag versus the urine bag currently in use. Unpublished data presented at Loyola University of Chicago Medical Center, Nursing Research Forum, 1990.

Manicelli-Van Atta, J., & Beck, S. L. (1992). Preventing hypoxemia and hemodynamic compromise related to endotracheal suctioning. *American Journal of Critical Care, 1*(3), 62–79.

Mateo, M. A. (1993). Unit-based product evaluation. Part 2: Planning product evaluation studies. *Dimensions of Critical Care Nursing, 12*(2), 88–91.

McIntosh, D., Baun, M. M., & Rogge, J. (1993). Effects of lung hyperinflation and presence of positive end-expiratory pressure on arterial and tissue oxygenation during endotracheal suctioning. *American Journal of Critical Care, 2,* 317–325.

McCaffery, M. (1990). Nursing approaches to nonpharmacological pain control. *International Journal of Nursing Studies, 27,* 1–5.

McCaffery, M., & Wolff, M. (1992). Pain relief using cutaneous modalities, positioning, and movement. *Hospice Journal, 8,* 121–153.

Melzack, R., & Casey, K. L. (1965). Sensory, motivational and central control determinants of pain: A new conceptual model. In D. Kenshale (Ed.), *The skin senses* (pp. 423–443). Springfield, IL: Thomas.

Melzack, R., & Wall, P. D. (1965). Pain mechanisms: A new theory. *Science, 150,* 971–979.

National Institute of Nursing Research. (1994). *6 Symptom Management: Acute Pain* (NIH Publication No. 94241). Washington, DC: National Institute of Nursing Research.

Newman, M. (1979). *Theory development in nursing.* Philadelphia: F. A. Davis Company.

Perez-Woods, R., Grohar, J. C., Skaredoff, M., Rock, S. G., Tse, A. M., Tomih, P., & Polich, S. (1991). Pain control after cesarean birth. Efficacy of patient-controlled analgesia vs traditional therapy (IM morphine). *Journal of Perinatology, 11*, 17–81.

Puntillo, K., & Tesler, M. D. (1993). Pain. In V. Carrieri-Kohlman, A. M. Lindsey, & C. M. West (Eds.), *Pathophysiological phenomena in nursing* (pp. 303–339) (2nd ed.). Philadelphia: W. B. Saunders Co.

Raymond, S. J. (1995). Normal saline instillation before suctioning: Helpful or harmful? A review of the literature. *American Journal of Critical Care, 4*(4), 267–271.

Riegel, B. (1985). A review and critique of the literature on preoxygenation for endotracheal suctioning. *Heart & Lung, 14*, 507–518.

Rogge, J. A., Bunde, L., & Baun, M. M. (1989). Effectiveness of oxygen concentrations of less than 100% before and after endotracheal suction in patients with chronic obstructive pulmonary disease. *Heart & Lung, 18*, 64–71.

Schmitt, Y., Hood, W. B., Jr., & Lown, B. (1969). "Armchair" treatment in the coronary care unit: Effect on blood pressure and pulse. *Nursing Research, 18*(2), 114–118.

Stone, K. S., Preusser, B. A., Groch, K. F., Karl, J. I., & Gonyon, D. S. (1991). The effect of lung hyperinflation and endotracheal suctioning on cardiopulmonary hemodynamics. *Nursing Research, 40*(2), 76–80.

Stone, K. S., & Turner, B. (1989). Endotracheal suctioning. *Annual Review of Nursing Research (Chapter 2), 7*, 27–49.

Stone, K. S., Vorst, E. C., Lanham, B., & Zahn, S. (1989). Effects of lung hyperinflation on mean arterial pressure and postsuctioning hypoxemia. *Heart & Lung, 18*(4), 377–385.

Taft, A. A., Mishoe, S. C., Dennison, F. H., Lain, D. C., & Chaudhary, B. A. (1991). A comparison of two methods of preoxygenation during endotracheal suctioning. *Respiratory Care, 36*, 195–201.

Wainwright, S. P., & Gould, D. (1996). Endotracheal suctioning: An example of problems of relevance and rigour in clinical research. *Journal of Clinical Nursing, 5*, 389–398.

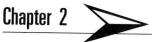
Continuous Quality Improvement/ Total Quality Management, and the Relationship to Research

Kathy J. Oleson

The evolution of the continuous quality improvement (CQI) and total quality management (TQM) movement is presented in this chapter. Essential elements and tools are included as is a discussion of the relationship of quality and research in improving outcomes in patient care delivery. A significant part of the chapter focuses on the management of the quality process.

THE CONTINUOUS QUALITY IMPROVEMENT PROCESS IN ACTION

If a nurse imagines himself or herself participating as a front-line player in a quality improvement (QI) process, he or she may be a member of a CQI team, ready to provide first-hand information about patient care, brainstorm suggestions for improvement, prioritize elements of the improvement plan, and direct communication of this ongoing process between fellow staff nurses and

the CQI team. No longer does the nurse have to "wait and see what changes are being implemented by administration." The nurse is a part of the improvement and change process, bringing vital first-hand information to be used as a basis for revisions and changes. The nurse can provide fellow staff with information about the process developments, and take their ideas and suggestions back to the team. With this process, the entire health care team is involved and works collaboratively toward a common goal of improved patient care.

The team members include a medical director, clinical specialist, fellow staff nurses, respiratory therapist, dietitian, pharmacist, patient care unit clerk, and social worker. A group leader begins the discussion and introduces a person from the human resources department as a team facilitator. The facilitator assists the team in establishing ground rules for the meeting; for example, all members should contribute to each

PATIENT DISCHARGE SURVEY

Unit_____

Person/Position Completing
 Survey (identify optional)_____

Information submitted for which
 shifts (specify approximate time frames)_____

1.   On your unit, when are the majority of patients discharged?
 _____ morning (M)   7 a.m. - 12 noon
 _____ afternoon (A)   12 noon - 5 p.m.
 _____ evening (E)   5 p.m. - 12 midnight

2.   Do you experience problems discharging patients from your unit?
 _____ Yes   _____ No

3.   If yes, what are the problems?_____
 _____
 _____
 _____

4.   Please complete each of the 3 areas below:
 I.   Please check areas that contribute to the difficulties in discharging patients.
 II.   Please specify the time of day on weekday/weekend the problems occur most frequently and check the appropriate column.
 III.   Please add any comments to further explain or give recommendations.

II.

I. Factors Contributing to Problems	Weekday			Weekend			III. Comments
	M	A	E	M	A	E	
___a Communication among departments							
___b Communication from staff to patient/family (Specify discipline or staff position and give details in comments column)							
___c Communication among disciplines (Specify disciplines or staff positions and give details in comments section)							
___d Communication among patient/family members							
___e Timeliness of staff availability to process discharge (specify RN, HUC, MD, etc.)							
___f Timeliness of written orders							
___g Timeliness of orders being taken off							
___h Timeliness of orders being signed off by attending MD							
___i Timeliness of final diagnostic tests and labs being completed							
___j Timeliness of receiving tests and lab results							
___k Timeliness of transportation							

Figure 2–1 *(See legend on opposite page)*

___l Timeliness of external service availability

___m Timeliness of external equipment availability

___n Timeliness of room cleaning (if applicable)

___o Timeliness of bed/room available (if applicable)

___p Other_____

_____

Figure 2–1 *Continued*
Patient discharge communication survey tool. A nurse manager and a staff nurse from each unit were requested to complete the survey.

meeting and meetings should end on time. The facilitator moves the team forward to generate the best results. The individuals in the group have volunteered to be a part of a CQI team to improve the discharge communication process.

First, the outcome for the discharge communication process is identified: "to improve the communication and timeliness of patient discharge and to ensure that the focus of the discharge planning process is the patient and family." This goal is noted in a box at the front end of a fishbone-like diagram. After the group agrees on the goal, the elements in the system that contribute to the outcome are identified. The leader begins to write these as headers on the various branches of the fishbone and moves the group ahead with identifying more detailed items that contribute to the headers. When the process is sidetracked, the facilitator

brings the discussion toward activities required for the goal.

Over the next few months, the group meets for 1 hour twice a month. During this period the group identifies data currently available that they may use for this process improvement, determines what further data are necessary to identify root causes of discharge communication breakdown, designs a survey to collect the data (Fig. 2–1), and collects and assimilates all data (Fig. 2–2). The data are scrutinized closely over several discussions, with analysis and trending. The group develops a flow diagram that charts the ideal discharge communication process that should occur with each patient upon entry into the system through discharge, including points of contact with the various disciplines (Fig. 2–3). The group also develops, in collaboration with the managed care office, a discharge communi-

Figure 2–2
Simple pareto chart depicting survey results of the major factors noted to cause problems during the afternoon. The X-axis legend corresponds to the factors listed by those letters on the survey tool in Figure 2–1.

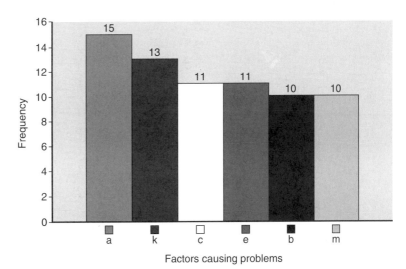

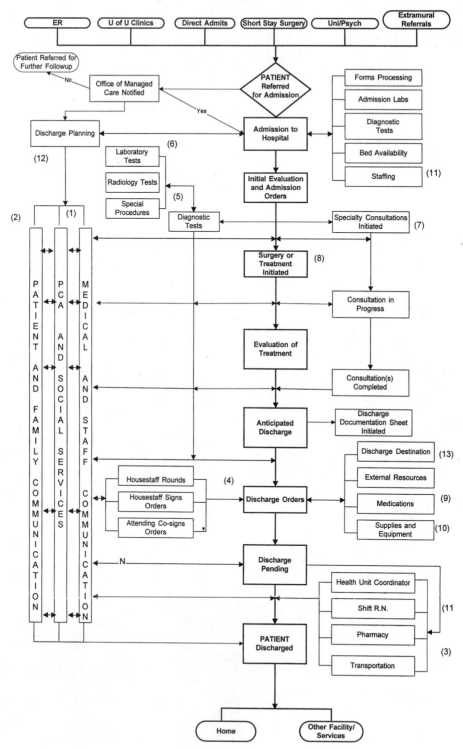

Figure 2–3
University Hospital Discharge Process flowchart.

cation flowsheet to be placed in front of the patient medical record. Staff who make up the discharge communication teams for the patient care units are the intended users of the flowsheet. A policy is drafted to guide the use of the form, and existing policies are revised to meet the other recommendations from the QI team.

The team presents a summary of the findings and recommendations to the quality council, including a cost analysis of implementation of the plan, and recommends a pilot of the plan on selected units. The council, in turn, makes recommendations to the team for further data gathering. The team proceeds with the additional data gathering and assimilates the analysis into a revised plan. After presenting and receiving approval for the revised plan, the team moves into the implementation phase of this improvement process, again collaborating with the managed care team who are to implement the process.

The improvement process is piloted for a month, after which assessment data for the new program are collected and evaluated by the team. Revisions are made in the process, and then the plan is implemented across all patient care units. The process does not end with the implementation of the plan across the hospital; rather, it is an ongoing process of periodic reevaluation, revision, and reimplementation of the improved processes to continually achieve identified outcomes.

THE QUALITY REVOLUTION

In the current turbulence and change occurring in the health care environment, all the buzz about quality activities and the quality terms can be overwhelming, causing staff nurses to withdraw from participation in QI activities. Yet, CQI teams with front-line staff involvement are critical to achieving optimal health outcomes, customer satisfaction, and financial viability—key goals of all health care institutions. Over the past decade, health care organizations have embraced various programs to improve quality and performance. These programs almost always had the quality assurance (QA) title

in the past, but currently they are given a variety of labels including TQM, CQI, outcomes management, reengineering, and process improvement.

From Quality Assurance to Continuous Quality Improvement

QA focuses on the search for standard of care, which usually implies minimal thresholds of structure, process, or outcome above which one is safe from being labeled a "bad apple" in the inspection process. W. Edwards Deming and Joseph M. Juran were two Americans who first theorized a new focus on quality with the CQI approach. They postulated that real improvement in quality depends on understanding and revising processes on the basis of data about the processes themselves (Williams & Howe, 1992). When this occurs throughout the organization as a constant purpose of improvement, results can only improve overall organizational outcomes (Leebov & Ersoz, 1991).

QA was and is primarily accreditation motivated, driven by Joint Commission on Accreditation of Healthcare Organizations and other external regulatory agencies. QA is reactive to problems retrospectively within a specific department. The traditional QA approach focused on staff and practitioners as causes of the problem and directed results of QA studies to them to "fix-it" or to follow policy and standard accurately (Fig. 2–4).

The CQI movement in health care stemmed from an internal motivation within institutions to provide better care and services at same or reduced costs. Regulatory agencies have come to follow that movement by incorporating the CQI concepts within their standard requirements. Even though the CQI process may emerge from a problem identified in the QA process, it generally takes a more proactive approach to "weeding out" problems before they occur by making improvements in the processes and systems across the organization. The focus of CQI is on the processes of care rather than the performance of individ-

Figure 2–4
Graphic depiction of the quality assurance process.

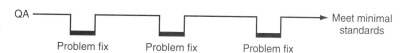

QA ———————————————————→ Meet minimal standards

Problem fix   Problem fix   Problem fix

uals and on improving processes so that care can be provided accurately. It emphasizes the role of leadership in setting the environment, improving systems, and providing resources such as education and time for all staff to be involved in QI efforts (Davis, 1993).

The emphasis in CQI is interdepartmental/interdisciplinary so that improvement can occur with the integration of efforts from all providers and involving all customers being affected by the initiative being addressed. Involving other departments with similar patient populations and product needs from the beginning of the QI process breaks down departmental barriers that have created fragmentation in patient care for so long in health care institutions. Staff members from various departments usually provide patient care; therefore, products are rarely chosen for use by one department of an institution. Similarly, a product may be used by more than one discipline, such as physicians and respiratory therapists; therefore, their involvement in the improvement process is crucial.

The solution to problems identified in the QA process usually ended with a subjective analysis of the data and the "practitioner fix-it implementation plan." CQI, however, uses analytical tools from the beginning of the process (with statistical analysis tools used on data to determine results) and continues with benchmarking or comparison of results against other health care institutions internally, locally, regionally, and nationally. QA activities rarely involved the cost issues related to improvement. CQI, however, relates cost issues to the improvement process, thereby evaluating all factors to achieve the best possible outcomes for all involved. QA was institution-goal-driven to fix problems. CQI, however, introduced the "customer" concept. *Customer* is a broad term that includes not only the patient but also the patient's family, physicians, nurses, other health care professionals, professional associates, and third-party payers. There are many overlapping relationships of customers to each other. The QA approach was to remonitor until results improved, with the hope that practitioners improved the data. The process used in CQI is to first develop a plan for improvement, with input from the staff closest to the process, to implement the plan, and then to reevaluate the situation by recollecting and analyzing objective data. This process repeats itself until variation is reduced and improvement is demonstrated as depicted in the Plan-Do-Check-Act (PDCA) cycle (Figs. 2–5 and 2–6).

QA was defined, coordinated, and communicated by a few people in the organization, most often in a "top-down" manner. In CQI, however, obtaining input and involvement from all staff, especially those closest to the issue, is the responsibility of everyone in the organization. The use of CQI does not eliminate QA altogether because organizations cannot deny that problems do occur and that steps must be taken to fix them; rather, CQI builds upon QA to weed out the problems before they occur.

As in other industries, quality in health care means doing the *right* things *right,* melding traditional QA approaches of correcting problems, to make continuous improvements in the processes and system to achieve the optimal clinical outcomes: satisfaction of customers and meeting of financial and operational goals. For nursing, "doing the right things right" depends on leadership and staff first determining what the mission is—whether it is on a patient care unit or in a college of nursing—and then defining how to carry out the mission. The next step is to develop methods to monitor how well the job is being done. This

CONTINUOUS QUALITY IMPROVEMENT PROCESS (CQI)

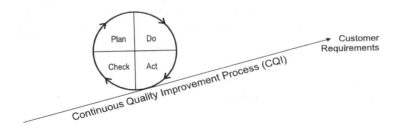

Figure 2–5
Graphic depiction of the continuous quality improvement process.

TOTAL QUALITY MANAGEMENT (TQM)

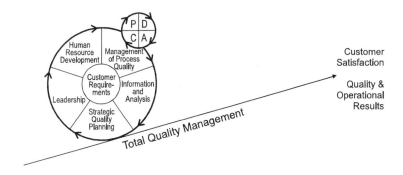

Figure 2–6
Graphic depiction of the total quality management process.

includes satisfying the customer (in this case patients, students, or colleagues as first priorities), and then developing and implementing plans to improve even further upon these processes and outcomes that have been identified.

Included in evaluating processes is cost analysis. This principle is applicable to evaluating products used in patient care. Because nurses are the end users of many health care products, it is vital that they be involved in evaluating the product in order to choose the best, not necessarily the least expensive, products used for patient care. Components of a thorough product evaluation include a cost analysis, responsiveness and flexibility of supplier to meet changing needs, availability of the product, quality of the product itself, ease of use for the nurse (customer), and effect of the product on achieving patient (customer) outcomes. Education of staff about the product is a vital part of the service delivery process. Once this process is completed, it is necessary to follow a CQI cycle of piloting the product, reevaluating the outcomes, implementing on a broader scale, and reevaluating again to ensure that desired outcomes are met across patient populations for which the product is used.

Total Quality Management

TQM embraces both QA and CQI and takes the quality approach one step farther. In TQM, a management philosophy that permeates the entire organizational structure, operations policies, and practices is used (Gaucher & Coffey, 1993). It emphasizes empowerment of employees in the organization

to practice QA and CQI to make TQM happen by providing high-quality, cost-effective care.

TQM philosophy implies that benchmarking partners are identified. These can include organizations or industries that are recognized for excellence or best practice in a particular process. Competitive health care partners with similar missions, processes, and product usage that are recognized for quality as well as internal best practices within one's own organization can be included in benchmarking. Customer and financial outcomes should be identified and benchmarked with other organizations locally, regionally, and nationally. The TQM philosophy requires effort across the institution for the quality program, without which lasting effects of efforts to improve quality and organizational performance are not realized. It involves leaders setting the stage with vision, mission, values, information analysis, strategic quality planning, human resources development for education of all employees in the CQI/TQM philosophy, and quality process management, and results in internal and external customer satisfaction and improved care outcomes and operational results.

ELEMENTS OF SUCCESSFUL QUALITY PROGRAMS

Malcolm Baldrige Award Criteria

One basis that is used for determining successful quality programs are those embodied in the seven categories of the Malcolm Baldrige Award criteria (Barber, 1996). Introduction to these criteria and training for all managers and staff are critical to the success of the quality program.

1. *Leadership.* Leaders are committed to CQI as a part of the organization's overall vision and to establishing an ongoing system for assessing and improving performance at the work unit level and throughout the organization.
2. *Information and analysis.* Key quality characteristics are carefully selected, prioritized, and performance data collected. Benchmarking partners are identified.
3. *Strategic quality planning.* Quality planning is an essential part of the strategic planning process. Plans that address both short-term and long-term goals for improvement are developed and deployed.
4. *Human resource development and management.* Human resource planning must address training for senior leaders, management, physicians, and all staff in recruitment, work design, compensation, and recognition programs and how these contribute to a high performance.
5. *Management of process quality.* Key quality characteristics for process performance must be monitored, trended, and analyzed using a systematic model to guide the improvement process. These include patient care functions, support functions, and administrative and financial operations, as well as suppliers' performance.
6. *Quality and operational results.* Attaining systematic improvement requires revising policy, procedure, and practices based on outcomes of management of process quality and comparing the organization's performance to that of competitors and benchmarking partners. Results are shared and communicated to all stakeholders of the process.
7. *Customer focus and satisfaction.* Needs of internal and external key stakeholders, such as patients, families, providers, payers, and members of the community at large, are monitored in ways such as surveys, focus groups, complaint management systems, and service follow-up systems. Systemwide trends are identified, and a plan for improvement is developed

and disseminated throughout the organization.

Management of Process Quality Using FOCUS-PDCA

Although there are a variety of processes and approaches that can be used to implement and guide quality activities, it is important to integrate an ongoing system into everyday practice for pursuing improvement opportunities and tackling problems. An approach that is used widely in health care is the 1991 FOCUS-PDCA model from the Columbia HCA Healthcare Corporation, Quality Resource Group, Nashville, TN, 1991:

F	Find a process to improve.
O	Organize a team that knows the process.
C	Clarify current knowledge of the process.
U	Understand causes of process variation.
S	Select the process improvement.
P	Plan the improvement and continue data collection.
D	Do the improvement, data collection, and analysis.
C	Check and study the results.
A	Act to hold the gain and to continue to improve the process.

Continuous Quality Improvement Tools

DATA COLLECTION/MEASUREMENT TOOLS

From the beginning of the CQI process, statistical methods are used to analyze data and to summarize results of benchmarking efforts. In addition, indicators are used to monitor and evaluate the quality of important patient care processes and outcomes, support services activities, and management functions that affect patient outcomes (Fig. 2–7). There are three types of indicators: outcome, process, and structure.

1. *Outcome indicator*—measures what happens or does not happen as a result of a process; measures the products of one or more processes. Examples are short-term results of specific treatments or procedures, longer-term

results of treatments or procedures, complications, adverse events, and health status and functioning.

2. *Process indicator*—measures an activity that is carried out either directly or indirectly to care for patients or for operational functions; measures activities provided that are believed to affect patient outcomes and system outcomes. Examples of clinical processes are assessment, planning, patient education, technical applications, and performing procedures and treatment; examples of system processes are care delivery models, admission systems, procurement of equipment and supplies, and the case management model.

3. *Structure indicator*—measures elements that determine ability to deliver care and whether these elements were appropriately used or applied; examples are staff assignments, equipment availability and functionality, bed availability, completion of forms, and signatures for documentation.

Indicators can be rate-based or triggered by a sentinel event. When indicators are rate-based, events that are expected to occur at some reasonable frequency are measured. The numerator is the number of occurrences and the denominator is the population measured. Thresholds may be set as a goal, but they are more effectively used as a signal to trigger action in the continuous improvement cycle. Indicators triggered by sentinel events are immediate, specific, in-depth case review and analysis for a serious, often avoidable event or wrong procedure, possibly involving the loss of a limb, function, or life.

Before the indicators are used on the entire population, it is important to test validity and reliability of the indicator. Applying the indicator to a small subset of the population and evaluating whether the instrument measured the intent for which it was designed can test validity. Reliability is the consistency of measurement over time, whether it provides the same results on repeated trials. Reliability can be tested by applying the instrument repeatedly to the same population or to different populations under similar circumstances. Because of changes in care practices and technology, reliability may be more difficult to evaluate

over time than validity if an indicator is used for long periods of time. Refer to Chapter 21 for more discussion on validity and reliability.

TOOLS FOR PROBLEM IDENTIFICATION, ANALYSIS, AND SUMMARY OF PROCESS

Several tools can be used for problem identification, analysis, and summary. Problem identification tools include nominal group technique and brainstorming. Data analysis tools that can be used are prioritization ratings, histograms, scatter diagrams, and control charts. Cause and effect (fishbone) diagrams, affinity charts, force field analyses, pareto charts, trend/run charts, and flowcharts may be used for problem identification and analysis. Processes may be summarized by using storyboards.

Problem Identification

Nominal Group Technique. The nominal group technique is used for generating and prioritizing ideas. Although it is similar to brainstorming, this process is more controlled because it balances participation. The group offers ideas one at a time, everyone takes a turn, then the group clarifies and ranks the ideas. Brainstorming may also follow after this technique.

Brainstorming. There are three phases in brainstorming: generation, clarification, and evaluation. During the generation phase, the group quickly generates thoughts or ideas in a very short time. As ideas are generated and listed using the speaker's own words, these are not judged or discussed because the focus is on the quantity of ideas rather than quality or clarification. Each idea is clarified in the clarification phase. In the evaluation phase, ideas are categorized, grouped, analyzed, and evaluated for their effect on an outcome. The cause and effect (fishbone) diagram or the affinity diagram may be used in evaluating the effect of an idea on outcome.

Data Analysis

Prioritization Rating. This is a technique that can be used to evaluate and compare a list of possible solutions against a set of guidelines. It is advisable to use this technique when there is uncertainty regarding

QUALITY MANAGEMENT   UNIVERSITY HOSPITAL

PATIENT RIGHTS INDICATOR
2nd Qtr. FY 1997–1998

KEY PROCESS: Patient rights: Advance directives

POLICY: Advance Directives/Personal Medical Care Decisions

INDICATOR: As attached.

TYPE OF
INDICATOR: Structure and process.

DEFINITION OF
TERMS: Advance Directives: refers to Living Will, or Special Power of Attorney for Medical
                    Treatment Plan. An instruction given in advance that tells others what health care you want
                    if you can't communicate because of illness or injury.

RATIONALE: -Patient Self-Determination Act of 1990, effective Dec. 1991
                    -Utah Personal Choice and Living Will Act
                    -University Hospital is committed to providing the highest quality of health care with regard
                    to human values
                    -Previous measurements indicate room for improvement; improvement activities have been
                    implemented.

DESCRIPTION OF
INDICATOR
POPULATION: Numerator: Number of patient medical records in compliance with each individual item of
                                  the indicator.

                    Denominator: All patient medical records on the patient care unit during one shift during
                                  the month of December.

METHODOLOGY: 1) Survey of patient medical records of inpatients as described in population denominator
                       for presence and completion of advance directives form.
                    2) Survey of same patient medical records for documents as listed on the data collection
                       form.

STANDARD: 100%

THRESHOLD: 100%

POSSIBLE
VARIANCES: Previous surveys have shown improvement needed in various areas of documenting that
                    patients are informed of their right to formulate advance directives.
                    The policy and form have been revised with minor changes; an audit by Health Information
                    Office showed improvement needed.

Confidential: This material is prepared pursuant to Utah Code Annotated § 26-25-1, et seq., and 58-12-43 (7, 8 and 9) for the purpose of evaluating health care rendered by hospitals or physicians and is **not part** of the medical record. It is also classified as "protected" under the Government Records Access and Management Act, Utah Code Annotated § 63-2-101 et. seq.

Figure 2–7
Patient rights indicator for measuring compliance to advance directives documentation.

PATIENT RIGHTS DATA COLLECTION FORM
2nd Qtr. FY 1997–1998

Patient name:

MR #:

Admit date:

Admitting RN:

Admitting Area:

	Yes	No	N/A	% Compli- ance
1. Patient survey form is in the front of the patient medical record. If no, please indicate where it is found _____				
2. Please check the written information sections completed: 　　a. Living Will section				
b. If yes, copy is in the patient medical record *or* context of advance directive is documented in the comments section of the form *or* context of advance directive is documented in the patient medical record.				
c. SPA for MT section.				
d. If yes, copy is in patient medical record.				
e. Medical Treatment section.				
f. If yes, copy is in the patient medical record *or* context of medical treatment plan is documented in the comments section of the form *or* context of medical treatment plan is documented in the patient medical record.				
g. Written information provided, *or* process not completed, *or* family given information section checked.				
h. Reinitiation section if applicable.				
i. Reinitiation RN signatures if applicable.				
j. Reinitiation pt/fam section if applicable.				
3. Form is signed by caregiver. (Please indicate the **position title** of the caregiver who signed the form *if* it is signed by a caregiver other than the RN.)				
4a. Form is signed by the patient/family.				
4b. If not signed by patient/family, valid reason is documented on the form. 　　(If the answer is yes, #4a and #4b are N/A.)				

Evaluate each item and score yes, no, or N/A according to hospital policy for each medical record surveyed.

Confidential: This material is prepared pursuant to Utah Code Annotated § 26-25-1, et seq., and 58-12-43 (7, 8 and 9) for the purpose of evaluating health care rendered by hospitals or physicians and is **not part** of the medical record. It is also classified as "protected" under the Government Records Access and Management Act, Utah Code Annotated § 63-2-101 et. seq.

Figure 2–7 *Continued*

which solution is best, when the team is divided and needs factual information to reach agreement, and when there is need to demonstrate that the team weighed possible solutions against the right variables. The processes used in prioritization rating include the following:

1. Determine the guidelines that the solution must meet.
2. List three to five of the most important guidelines across the top of a chart (assign a rating scale to each guideline).
3. List alternative solutions down the left side of the chart.
4. Rate how well each alternative meets each guideline.
5. Add scores.
6. Evaluate and plan action.

EXAMPLE: "U-CHOOSE" QI TEAM

The purpose of the team was to provide patients and families more control by providing as many choices in the delivery of patient care as possible. As the team evaluated implementing the options available to patients, they evaluated some possible aspects of the program against cost, time, acceptability, and authorization; with a total rating for each aspect, it became clear which aspects of the program might be more successful with patients, staff, and management.

Other tools for analysis include the following:

Histogram. This is used to display distribution of data showing variance within a process.

Scatter Diagram. This is used for correlation.

Control Chart. This is used to show variances from upper and lower limits of a process over time.

Problem Identification and Data Analysis

Cause and Effect (Fishbone) Diagram. The fishbone diagram is used to identify and illustrate the relationships between an effect, an outcome, or a problem and the hunches about factors that contribute to it. It is important that everyone agrees on an outcome statement. Some causes may show

up on more than one branch, all branches do not have the same number of causes, there is no specified number of branches, and having secondary branches is acceptable. Figure 2–8 is an example of a fishbone diagram.

There are four steps in developing the diagram.

1. Summarize outcome/goal/problem.
2. Determine headers.
3. Determine elements of each branch header that contribute to the effect.
4. Evaluate and draw conclusions, then begin to plan actions.

Affinity Charts. Affinity charts are used to organize ideas on the brainstorming list into natural clusters of related items and to assign cluster headings (for example, objectives to be accomplished or values) to discuss and manage ideas more easily and to identify patterns. Affinity diagrams are helpful because they tap creativity, relieve confusion, and acquire group consensus in a short time.

Force Field Analysis. This type of analysis is used to identify the *helping/driving forces* that will assist in achieving a goal and the *hindering/restraining* forces that block reaching a goal. The steps in doing a force field analysis are as follows:

1. Define goal. A goal may be stated in behavioral terms.
2. Draw line across or down middle of chart (can be horizontal or vertical).
3. List the driving forces on separate sides of the line during the team discussion.
4. Determine which forces are more powerful (heavier arrows); these are the priorities.
5. Plan actions for *minimizing* the *opposing* forces and maximizing the supporting forces (Fig. 2–9).

Pareto Charts. Pareto charts (see Fig. 2–2) can be used to prioritize problems that need to be solved by determining the origin of the greatest contributing factors or to show changes in factors over time. A series of vertical bars (bar graphs) are used. Each bar represents a value that can be numerical, time, action, or group of individuals such as a discipline or department. Categories are compared (for example, ranked from highest to lowest or vice versa).

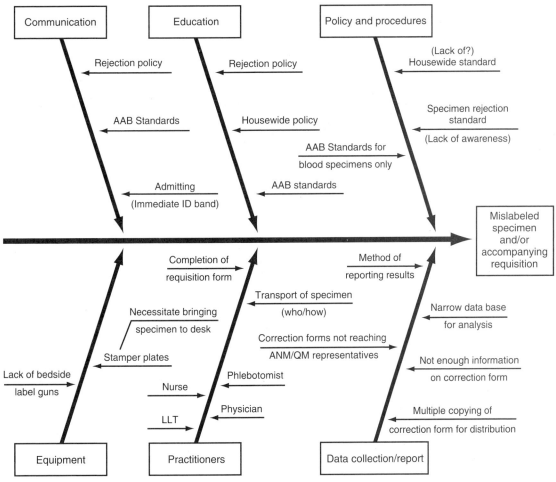

Figure 2–8
Specimen labeling cause and effect (fishbone) diagram.

Trend/Run Charts. Uses of the trend/run charts (Fig. 2–10) are for displaying, analyzing, and understanding the variation in data over time to evaluate impact of activities toward improvement in reaching goals. Each variable is plotted on the chart at progressing points in time.

Flowcharts. Flowcharts are used to identify the flow or sequence of events that leads to an outcome. Through this process, a team may gain greater understanding of the process and where action is needed. Steps in a process (for example, patient care, activities of a team, procedural steps) are listed and arranged in chronological order. A *symbol* is used around each step to depict the exact nature of that element in the process. It is vital to look at all "wait" symbols and ask why they are necessary and look at the decision points and clarify the criteria for making the right decisions. The following are benefits that may be accrued from using a flowchart:

1. Assists the team in making decisions about the scope or focus of their improvement
2. Assists the team in quickly determining the steps to modify
3. Engages people involved in creating the flowcharts in QI
4. Graphically depicts a simplification of the new process that can facilitate standardization of policy or procedure or help people better understand a new policy and procedure

Summary of Process

Storyboards. Visual summary of the process and outcomes can be displayed by using

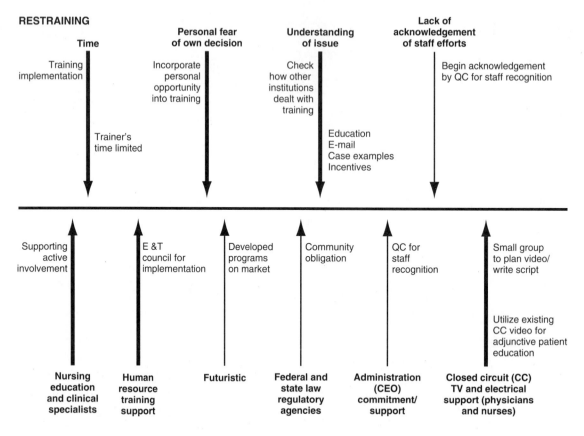

RESTRAINING

Time	Personal fear of own decision	Understanding of issue	Lack of acknowledgement of staff efforts

Training implementation

Incorporate personal opportunity into training

Check how other institutions dealt with training

Begin acknowledgement by QC for staff recognition

Trainer's time limited

Education
E-mail
Case examples
Incentives

Supporting active involvement

E & T council for implementation

Developed programs on market

Community obligation

QC for staff recognition

Small group to plan video/ write script

Utilize existing CC video for adjunctive patient education

Nursing education and clinical specialists

Human resource training support

Futuristic

Federal and state law regulatory agencies

Administration (CEO) commitment/ support

Closed circuit (CC) TV and electrical support (physicians and nurses)

SUPPORTING

Figure 2–9
Patient rights/advance directives force field analysis depicting the restraining and supporting forces for staff education issues.

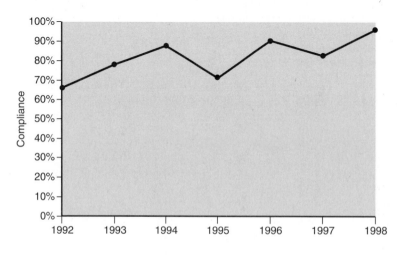

Figure 2–10
Advance directives documentation compliance trend/run chart.

storyboards. The FOCUS-PDCA may be used for format.

The reader is referred to *The Memory Jogger Plus+* (Brassard, 1989) for further information on CQI tools.

CONTINUOUS QUALITY IMPROVEMENT/ TOTAL QUALITY MANAGEMENT RELATIONSHIP TO RESEARCH AND PATIENT CARE DELIVERY

Health care institutions and providers are experiencing more pressure to verify the value and cost-effectiveness of services they deliver and the effects on patient recovery and health status outcomes. To accomplish this, the focus must be on gaining knowledge through QI and research about why work processes fail and not on assuming that the practitioners are incorrectly following the system (Neuhauser, McEachern, & Headrick, 1995). Physicians, nurses, administrators, and all disciplines need to acquire the following (Berwick, 1994a):

1. An understanding of the health care system as a whole
2. The ability to work effectively across disciplinary boundaries
3. The ability to collect, analyze, and interpret outcomes of care data
4. Participation in formal improvement teams
5. Trust in the motives and intelligence of people in different professional roles
6. A willingness to test new approaches to work
7. An interpretation of the underlying needs of patients and others who depend on the health care system

All human service professions are facing complex individual and family health problems that a single discipline cannot solve alone; therefore, it is necessary for disciplines and departments within an institution to work collaboratively to provide better quality care and reduce wasteful variation. Accrediting bodies also are focusing on the organization at the system level. There is need for a formal approach to understanding systems, gathering data, and enlisting those involved in the process and search for understanding.

The CQI and research processes can be used to provide outcomes data. After the focus of CQI projects is identified, a literature review is conducted. Identification or development of reliable and valid data collection tools follows. Sample selection procedures used in research can be applied to CQI projects. Problem identification, analysis tools, and statistical analysis methods used in research are similar to those that have moved into practice settings with the CQI movement. These replace the previous "clinician's impression" method of interpreting data. The common patient-focused goal of both CQI and research is to make improvements in patient care.

CQI and research data can be used to seek solutions to clinically related issues. As evidence-based protocols are developed and tested, the research process is useful in evaluating newly implemented action plans. A comparison of the CQI and research processes is in Table 2–1.

Research and CQI efforts can focus on establishing the balance between the cost of technology and its efficacy. This focus can take a variety of approaches, one of which is to look at cases that have traditionally generated high costs. Another approach is to focus on new procedures that are evolving from an experimental stage to more routine application, whereas another is to focus on well-established treatments that are high cost because of the complexity of the treatment or the seriousness of the patient's problem. In all cases, the aim of research and CQI should be to reduce costs while maintaining or improving patient outcomes (Nolan, 1994).

CQI and research differ as described in an editorial in the *Journal of the American Medical Association* (Berwick, 1996). Rules of science in the form of pure research and hiding variations in outcomes for competitive gain may have become too stringent and the costs too prohibitive for useful improvements to be made in care. When practitioners work collaboratively to understand differences in care and outcomes and to learn from each other, the results can produce better outcomes and reduced mortality rates in a timely manner. The CQI PDCA cycle reflects a general model of learning— to take action, guided by theory, and then to reflect on that action to gain knowledge—as opposed to the randomized clinical trial approach often used in research. The value of the PDCA cycle comes from involvement of practitioners who are closest to the issue

Table 2–1

Comparison of Continuous Quality Improvement/Total Quality Management and Research Process

CQI/TQM	USEFUL TOOLS	RESEARCH

Find a process to improve:
  Process prioritization
  Customer research
  Review strategic/operational
    plans
  Identify the key processes
    and outcomes
	Opportunity statement
	Pareto diagram
	Prioritization matrix
	Run chart
		Formulate and delimit the
		  research problem; clarify the
		  research question.

Organize to improve the
  process:
  Select a team/individual who
    has process knowledge
  Create a plan
	Process improvement plan
	Ground rules
		Identify principal
		  investigators, data collectors,
		  statisticians.

Clarify current knowledge of
  the process:
  Look at current process
  Identify quick and easy
    improvements
  Standardize best current
    method
	Flowchart
	Group decision making
	Tools
		Review related literature;
		  determine what is known
		  about the subject and what
		  gaps exist; develop a
		  theoretical conceptual
		  framework.

Understand the sources of
  process variation:
  Measure the key processes
    and outcomes
  Stabilize the process
  Identify process and outcome
    variables
  Measure possible variables
  Test whether there is a
    relationship between the
    process/outcome and
    potential variable
	Cause and effect diagram
	Data collection methods
	Flowchart
	Pareto diagram
	Run chart
	Scatter diagram
	Control charts
	Histogram
	Group decision-making tools
		Identify the variables;
		  formulate the hypothesis.

Select the process
  improvement:
  Evaluate improvement
    alternatives for their
    potential effectiveness and
    feasibility
  Select the improvement
	Flowchart
	Group decision-making tools
		Select a research design;
		  specify the population.

Plan the improvement:
  Plan the implementation of
    the improvement
  Plan continued data
    collection
	Data collection methods
	Group decision-making tools
		Operationalize; select the
		  sample.

Do the improvement to the
  process:
  Make the change
  Measure the impact of the
    change
	Flowchart
	Data collection methods
	Run charts
		Do a pilot study; measure
		  research variables; collect
		  the data.

Check the results:
  Examine data to determine
    whether change led to the
    expected improvement
	Pareto diagram
	Cause and effect diagram
	Run charts
	Control charts
	Histograms
		Analyze the data; interpret
		  results of the study.

Table 2–1 ....

Comparison of Continuous Quality Improvement/Total Quality Management and Research Process *Continued*

CQI/TQM	USEFUL TOOLS	RESEARCH
Act to hold the gain and continue to improve the process: Develop a strategy for maintaining the improvements Determine whether to continue working on the process	Flowchart Group decision-making tools	Communicate study findings to other researchers and clinicians; analyze implications for current practice; present ideas and recommendations for future studies (Mateo & Kirchhoff, 1991).

Adapted from IHI Process Improvement Models, 1995. Institute for Healthcare Improvement, Boston.

who see the processes at work and know so much about what happens. They are able to reflect step by step in real time, thereby possibly seeing causes and effects that a more distant investigator could only have discovered much more slowly with dissection of a randomized design. By implementing the PDCA cycle and using the strategic tools, careful inductive learning by experts who have knowledge of their own work produces powerful timely results, which are valid, creative, and potentially helpful to others.

Practitioners and organizations have an ethical obligation to inform others through presentations and publications of knowledge on reducing errors, easing pain, reducing delays, or decreasing waste. Medical journal editors have begun to provide space for clinical observations derived from studies less formal than randomized clinical trials. Reports on improvements achieved by careful clinicians using proper CQI methods represent real-time science and must be publicized so that patients reap the full benefits from all efforts at improvement.

This is not to say that research is not valid or needed. Some people would promote that the evolution of CQI is at a crossroads in that its value has not been proven in terms of actual breakthroughs in results, especially in total organizations and systems. They would also say that without formal research, CQI recommendations are matters of opinion (Berwick, 1994b).

SUMMARY

The processes of CQI and research are crucial to organizations in their quest for pro-

viding the best, most cost-effective care to patients. It is vital that organizations engage in institutionwide CQI efforts that meet the criteria for successful quality programs such as those defined by the Malcolm Baldrige Award criteria and integrate a system such as the FOCUS-PDCA for pursuing improvement opportunities and addressing problems. CQI is achieved when processes of care are examined from multidisciplinary perspectives as teams collaborate to define problems, seek solutions, and collect and analyze data.

Health care research offers a scientific basis for identifying promising improvement for clinical reform. It is essential to improve knowledge, and research has been useful in obtaining and applying knowledge for advances in health care throughout history. This is the way health care has traditionally been improved, including advances in organ transplantation, in vitro fertilization, and gene therapy. By interweaving the TQM approaches and research, in-depth validations of methods allow the development of a framework for continual improvement in health care. Members of the health care community have a choice: continue to engage in isolated efforts against the external forces or combine efforts of CQI and research and redesign the system to reduce costs while maintaining or improving outcomes.

REFERENCES

Barber, N. (1996). *Quality assessment for health care, a Baldrige-based handbook.* New York: Quality Resources, A Division of the Kraus Organization Limited.

Berwick, D. M. (1996). Editorial: Harvesting knowledge from improvement [Editorial]. *Journal of the American Medical Association, 275*, 877–878.

Berwick, D. M. (1994a). Eleven worthy aims for clinical leadership of health system reform. *Journal of the American Medical Association, 272*, 797–802.

Berwick, D. M. (1994b). QL perspective: Managing quality—the next five years. *Quality Letter for Healthcare Leaders, 6*(6), 1–7.

Brassard, M. (1989). *The Memory Jogger Plus +*. Methuen, MA: Goal/QPC.

Davis, E. R. (1993). There's more to quality improvement than a name change. *Journal for Healthcare Quality, 15*(6), 33–35.

Gaucher, E. J., & Coffey, R. J. (1993). *Total quality in health care*. San Francisco: Jossey-Bass, Inc.

Leebov, W., and Ersoz, C. J. (1991). *The health care manager's guide to continuous quality improvement*. Chicago: American Hospital Publishing, Inc.

Mateo, M. A., & Kirchhoff, K. (1991). *Conducting and using nursing research in clinical setting* (1st ed.). Baltimore: Williams & Wilkins.

Neuhauser, D., McEachern, J. E., & Headrick, L. (1995). *Clinical CQI*. Oakbrook Terrace, IL: Joint Commission on Accreditation of Healthcare Organizations.

Nolan, T. (1994). QL perspective: Integrating quality improvement and cost reduction. *Quality Letter for Healthcare Leaders, October,* 2–5.

Williams, T., & Howe, R. (1992). W. Edwards Deming and total quality management: An interpretation for nursing. *Journal for Healthcare Quality, 14*(1), 36–39.

SUGGESTED READINGS

Berwick, D. M. (1989). Sounding board: Continuous improvement as an ideal in health care. *New England Journal of Medicine, 320*, 53–56.

Berwick, D. M. (1996). We can cut costs and improve care at the same time. *Medical Economics, August,* 180–187.

Castaneda-Mendez, K., & Bernstein, L. (1997). *Journal for Health Care Improvement, 19*(2), 11–16.

Champagne, M. T., Tornquist, E. M., & Funk, S. G. (1997). Achieving research-based practice. *American Journal of Nursing, 97*, 16AAA–16DDD.

Gaucher, E., & Kratochwill, E. W. (1993). The leader's role in implementing total quality management. *Quality Management in Health Care, 1*(3), 10–18.

Harris, M. (1997). A breakthrough series—Update: Closing the gap between what we know and what we do. *Quality Letter for Healthcare Leaders, February,* 2–12.

Joint Commission on Accreditation of Healthcare Organizations. (1991). What is quality improvement? In *The transition from QA to CQI: An introduction to quality improvement in health care* (pp. 13–21). Oak Brook Terrace, IL: Author.

Kleeb, T. (1997). Collaboration: A framework for clinical quality improvement. *Journal for Healthcare Quality, 19*(4), 10–17.

Kleeb, T. (1997). Teaching total quality management: Developing and deploying education throughout a health care system. *Journal for Healthcare Quality, 19*(2), 17–26.

Miller, D., Smith, D. J., Brophy, M., Mollman, M., Owen, J., Smith, G., More, C. (1996). Total quality improvement: An example of an effective team. *Journal for Healthcare Quality, 18*(1), 20–23.

Ohm, B., & Brown, J. (1997). Quality improvement pitfalls and how to overcome them. *Journal for Healthcare Quality, 19*(3), 16–20.

Oleson, K. J., Jones-Schenk, J., & Tuohig, G. M. (1994). A quality improvement focus for patient rights: Advance directives. *Journal of Nursing Care Quality, 8*(3), 52–67.

Reinertsen, J. L. (1993). Outcomes management and continuous quality improvement: The compass and the rudder. *Quality Review Bulletin, January,* 5–7.

Tuohig, G. M., & Oleson, K. J. (1995). Enhancing clinical nursing research: A vital role for staff development educators. *The Journal of Continuing Education in Nursing, 26*, 147–149.

Wakefield, D. S., & Wakefield, B. J. (1993). Overcoming the barriers to implementation of TQM/CQI in hospitals: Myths and realities. *Quality Review Bulletin, March,* 83–88.

Youngberg, B. (1996). QRC advisor: Storyboards can showcase performance improvement efforts. *Quality, Risk, and Costs, 12*(9), 2–3.

Chapter 3

Exploring Innovative Ways of Giving Nursing Care

Mary G. Schira and Magdalena A. Mateo

Research-based practice, the ultimate goal of all research activities, can only be realized if practitioners in clinical settings apply research principles as well as findings in monitoring and evaluating care. Practitioners who read, critique, and evaluate research reports in terms of their applicability to patient care issues come to appreciate the value of research in practice and learn how to apply it to the clinical setting (Mateo & Schira, 1991).

Nurses have unique and challenging opportunities to involve themselves in the evaluation of nursing care and the discovery of answers to clinical problems. Using research findings in practice can improve patient outcomes, help contain health care costs, and create a professional practice environment (Bergstrom, 1991; Downs, 1991). Although the health care industry aspires to use the research process and research findings in clinical settings to discover new ways of improving patient care, this goal has not yet been accomplished. Despite the availability and significance of findings that can and should be used, nursing research findings are not being incorporated into practice (Bower, 1994).

How, then, does a nurse begin the process of using research to provide better patient care? As proposed in this chapter, sequential phases in delineating the problem stage and in exploring the solution stage can be used to solve clinical problems or address issues. These stages require a review of the literature in order to ensure that the nurse is up-to-date on the practice issue. Examples are given throughout the chapter to illustrate the phases in each stage.

This chapter also addresses criteria necessary for making changes in practice, such as determining applicability of the methods suggested in the literature, and compatibility of the research project with institutional policies, resources, support, and timing. Pragmatic factors to consider when introducing innovations in practice (for example, getting the cooperation of groups and conducting effective meetings) are also presented. Finally, suggestions for incorporating research findings into the development of standards of care, patient care protocols, or policies and procedures are addressed.

STAGES IN SOLVING CLINICAL PROBLEMS

Delineating the Problem

The four phases of delineating the problem include awareness, clarification, problem definition, and resolution. The activities suggested for each phase are illustrated in Figure 3–1.

AWARENESS

Recognition that a clinical problem exists is the first step to using research in practice. Initially, someone observes a discrepancy in practice or feels that something is not quite

right. In the awareness phase (Could there be a problem?), the applicability of a current intervention is challenged, or outcomes that were anticipated but not achieved are investigated. For example, a patient receiving intravenous patient-controlled analgesia (PCA) following surgery seems to be continually uncomfortable. The discomfort occurs despite the fact that, according to advocates of PCA, the patient should feel more comfortable because the individual determines when and how often to administer the medication. Proponents of this intervention also believe that patients on PCA require less nursing time. After observing discomfort in some patients, the nurse begins to think that something is not right. The nurse also notices that some patients on PCA require *more* nursing time than patients receiving intramuscular injections for pain management.

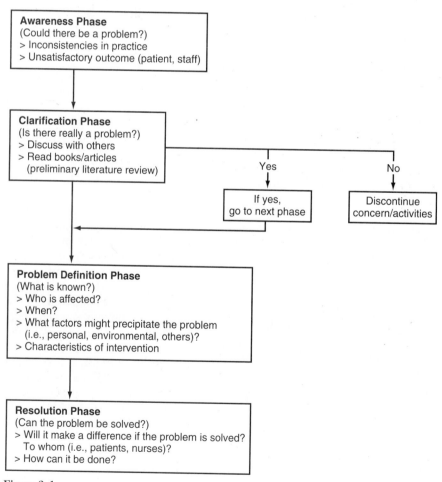

Figure 3–1
Delineating the problem.

CLARIFICATION

The answer to the basic question raised during the next step (Is there really a problem?) is sought by discussing observations with colleagues, by talking with patients, and by reviewing what has been written about the practice or phenomenon in question. With reference to the example on PCA, the nurse would (1) clarify whether other patients have shown signs of discomfort, (2) validate observations by questioning patients about pain relief and discomfort, (3) conduct a preliminary review of the literature on effects of PCA on postsurgical patients, and (4) review medical records for documentation.

PROBLEM IDENTIFICATION

In the question in this phase ("What is known?"), the nurse seeks answers by brainstorming with peers, reviewing information obtained in the literature, and identifying the following essential elements of a problem:

1. Individuals or groups who are affected
2. Time of day when incidents or situations are usually observed (for example, after activity, early in the morning)
3. Factors (personal or environmental) contributing to the existence of the problem
4. Characteristics of the intervention (treatment)

RESOLUTION

When details of the problem have been determined, the resolution phase ("Can the problem be solved?") begins. To answer this question, the following issues should be addressed:

1. Why is the problem important to patients and to nurses?
2. What difference will it make if answers are obtained?
3. What has to be done?

Exploring the Solution

Exploring the solution consists of five phases (Fig. 3–2), including discovery, using research findings, decision making, execution, and evaluation.

DISCOVERY

"How have others tried to solve the problem?" Finding solutions to clinical problems is challenging and often exciting, because, in the search, new and better methods for patient care can be discovered. Personal and organizational resources can be used during this first phase of the solution stage to expedite the search for solutions. The investigator determines the resources (personal and organizational) needed to solve the problem.

Personal resources include the nurse's critical thinking, problem-solving ability, creativity, and clinical knowledge. Organizational resources include human and material assets. Human resources within the organization can include other nurses, advanced practice nurses (clinical nurse specialists, nurse practitioners), nurse researchers, nursing administrators (clinical unit and organizational level), and other professionals (physicians and psychologists). Material assets include library and computer facilities.

USING RESEARCH FINDINGS

"What has been published?" Knowledge about published materials and what other people have tried is vital when exploring solutions to a problem. A computerized literature search (for example, using MEDLINE) is a good way to locate published references that are relevant to the clinical problem. A search generates a list of articles related to the clinical problem. Detailed information on conducting a literature search is discussed in Chapter 17.

Journal articles are generally better sources of information than books because they are more timely. Journal articles that summarize and analyze published research on a particular topic are especially helpful in adopting research findings into clinical practice. Review articles that list and discuss a number of related studies with similar findings provide the reader with more confidence in the findings than when only one report is cited. Meta-analysis is also an important tool. Meta-analysis is a statistical procedure that compares similar studies to determine readiness of the outcomes for implementation in clinical practice (Massey & Loomis, 1988). For example, Devine and Cook (1983) analyzed the results of 49 studies that examined the relationship between

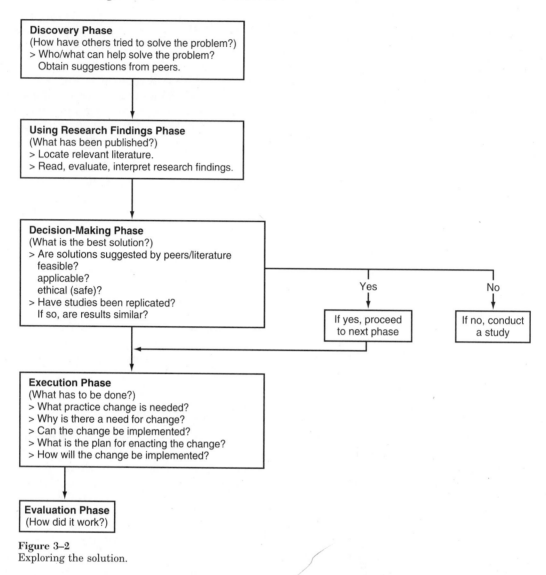

Figure 3–2
Exploring the solution.

brief psychoeducational interventions and length of postsurgical hospital stay of patients by using meta-analysis. Findings indicated that hospital stay was decreased up to 1.25 days. These findings supported the belief that psychoeducational interventions may be cost effective with various types of surgical patients because the hospital length of stay is reduced (Devine & Cook, 1983). Although not numerous in the nursing research literature, meta-analyses are very helpful in assisting nurses solve clinical problems using nursing research findings.

Although practicing nurses might initially find research articles challenging to read, this important skill can be acquired and improved with practice. Through read-

ing and evaluating research reports and interpreting findings, the nurse can determine the applicability of a study to the clinical problem and decide whether a change in practice is warranted (Rankin & Esteves, 1996). Nurses may find it helpful to read and discuss research articles as a group, thus helping each other learn how to critically evaluate the research literature (Kirchhoff & Beck, 1995).

Research findings can be used from either an instrumental or a conceptual perspective (Tanner, 1987). Instrumental utilization means that the nurse uses the study findings in specific ways. The findings may provide evidence for a solution to the problem, support the theory that guides practice, or provide measurement methods or tools to be used in practice. For example, Bergstrom, Braden, Laguzza, and Holman (1987) developed an assessment tool as part of their research that has come to be used in clinical practice to determine an individual's risk for development of skin breakdown (Braden, 1989). In conceptual utilization, the nurse uses clinical knowledge and experience to synthesize salient points and ideas from the literature and, out of that, arrives at an educated opinion of the clinical problem but with no specific approaches. For example, a study may identify that postoperative coronary bypass patients experience difficulty with concentration. The nurse may use this information to explain, at least in part, why these patients seem to exhibit poor retention of discharge medication instructions. Following the literature review, the nurse should consider whether a study has instrumental or conceptual applicability.

Research articles generally begin with an abstract and contain broad headings that include an introduction, literature review, methods, results, discussion, and references. Evaluating and interpreting results in an organized, stepwise fashion is helpful. Table 3–1 illustrates one such approach. For more information about the individual sections of a manuscript, refer to Chapters 17 and 27.

DECISION MAKING

In the decision-making phase ("What is the best solution?"), it is important to know whether a study has been replicated and whether the same results were obtained. Issues related to feasibility, applicability, and risk also should be considered (Haller, Reynolds, & Horsley, 1979).

Research findings should not be integrated into practice based on a single study. Replication is necessary because studies that have been repeated in different settings or with different populations ensure that the results are generalizable (that is, findings do not result from a particular setting or sample). Replicated studies yielding similar results provide the necessary support for using those findings in practice (Connelly, 1986).

After the nurse is convinced that research findings are supported by more than one study, the feasibility of using the findings in the practice setting must be addressed. To implement the findings, perhaps

a major change must be made in some aspect of nursing care or new equipment must be purchased. It is important to ensure that personnel and material resources are available before finalizing plans for changes. Other factors that should be assessed include the following:

1. Compatibility with institutional policies
2. Adequacy of resources (staff, equipment, funds)
3. Administrative support
4. Timing (too many recent changes on the unit)

The nurse must consider the similarities with or differences between the setting in which the studies were conducted and the current institution when assessing the applicability of research findings to the clinical problem. Similarities and differences in patients, staffing levels and mix, and organizational structure must be addressed. Whether or not differences exist, it is prudent to consider such possibilities before adapting research-based solutions to clinical problems. At this point in the process, the nurse must gain administrative support for the proposed solution (if not already done). Unit and organization level support is key to the success of the process.

After determining that the alternative approach supported by the research is likely to make a difference in practice or patient care outcomes, the nurse should consider the potential risk to the patient, staff, and organization. The risk of trying a new approach should be balanced against the risk of maintaining the status quo. Implementation of changes should be designed so that risk is minimized and benefit is maximized.

When all of the aforementioned factors have been considered and the nurse believes that the proposed solution to the problem is still desirable, the next step is to proceed with the execution phase. If, however, the solution is not feasible or questions concerning applicability persist, a study may need to be conducted. See Unit III for information on the essential activities to be undertaken in conducting research.

EXECUTION

After the plan for solving the clinical problem has been carefully thought out, put into writing, and reviewed, the most excit-

Table 3–1

Determining a Study's Applicability to a Clinical Problem

HEADING	CONTENT	APPLICABLE TO PRACTICE SETTING?	COMMENTS
Title	Study design	Was the study done to describe, compare, or test an intervention? Was it done to replicate another study?	_____
	Participants or phenomena	Who or what was studied?	_____
	Variables	What variables were examined?	_____
Abstract (overview)	Purpose of the study	Could the study assist in solving the clinical problem?	_____
Introduction	Literature review	How does this study fit with current knowledge?	_____
	Study purpose	What was studied? Is it clinically important?	_____
	Problem statement	Is the problem succinctly defined?	_____
Methods	Sample number of participants, criteria for inclusion (characteristics)	Are the participants and events similar to the clinical problem being studied? What are the similarities or differences? Characteristics of subjects, (sex, age)?	_____ _____
	Selection of subjects (random or convenience)	Method for subject selection?	_____
	Setting Study location (hospital, outpatient, home)	Is the study setting similar? If not, can the methods be adapted?	_____
	Design Method for answering the research question (experimental, nonexperimental)	Can the same method be used or adapted?	_____ _____
	Treatment or procedure used	Can the treatment or procedures be done?	
	Data collection Tools and instruments	Are the data collection methods feasible?	_____
	Type of information collected and frequency	Can the same data be obtained?	_____
Results	Answers to questions (findings)	Was each question addressed?	_____
	Data analysis	Were the results statistically significant? Clinically significant?	_____ _____
	Tables and figures	If frequencies were used, do the numbers add to the actual total?	_____ _____
Discussion	Review of results in relation to study purpose(s)	Do the findings make sense? How can the findings be used?	_____
	Explanation of results Implications and limitations for practice	Are there limitations in applying findings (to setting, patients, staff, organization, cost)?	_____ _____
References	List of publications used in preparing the report	Does the list include recent clinically relevant publications? Are there citations that might be useful?	_____ _____

ing phase begins. In the execution phase ("What has to be done?"), the nurse finally gets the chance to apply the solution that researchers have suggested to be the best approach to the problem. This is an exciting yet challenging time, because what was formerly proposed in the thinking stage is applicable in the reality stage. In addition, the solution entails changing something in the practice environment. Facilitating change requires careful planning and implementation.

The nurse who has been working toward implementing the long-awaited solution (innovation) may be tempted to go forward with the solution immediately. It is prudent, however, to first conduct and evaluate the solution in a small-scale trial of the plan (pilot test). Through a pilot test, the nurse has the opportunity to "work out the bugs"—for example, try the solution in one unit of the hospital instead of all units—and determine whether anticipated outcomes to the problem were achieved. The primary goal of a pilot test is to obtain feedback from the participants who will eventually help make the change in clinical practice, so that necessary revisions can be made. The pilot test also serves to preview what might become standard practice.

When presenting the plan, the nurse should remember that even in a pilot test, a change in existing practice is being proposed. Changing practice requires using a process of planned change (Goode & Bulechek, 1992). Individuals approach change differently and will therefore view the plan in different ways. Resistance to the plan may surface because individuals are poorly informed of the research base, fear interference with established practice patterns, or perceive a threat to professional autonomy (Titler et al., 1994). Therefore, the nurse should communicate openly and frequently with all individuals involved in all phases of exploring the solution.

The nurse should also consider the characteristics of the target group and the environment before presenting the plan. Techniques used to encourage the organization to accept the plan ("buy in") include presentations, conducting research, publications, and incentives, such as cost savings and staff job satisfaction (Brett, 1989). It is also important to identify the best way to communicate the plan to whomever will be involved. For example, if the audience consists

of management staff, the presentation should include the cost-effectiveness, efficiency, and increased productivity of the new method. If the audience consists of unit nurses, however, the ease of using the new method as opposed to the difficulties of the old method and the impact on quality of care should be highlighted. Environmental factors (staff turnover, workload, morale, and organizational priorities and characteristics) could also affect the acceptance of the plan and should be addressed when the plan is presented.

It is important to give details to the persons involved in the pilot test. This information should include the "who, what, when, and why" of the study, the name of the contact person, and progress reports. Information can be disseminated to the staff through written communication or a meeting.

If the decision is to use written communication, a short summary (1 to 2 pages) of the plan can be developed and distributed. This summary should be attractive so that it is not considered just another "handout" or piece of paper. Make announcements and handouts attractive by using brightly colored card stock or create heading in bold and capital letters, giving brief descriptions under each heading. A flowchart or diagram may be used as a visual way of presenting the important aspects of the plan.

The meeting notice example provided (see box) stresses the following points: (1) The word "Our" was used to underline the ownership nature of the project, (2) inclusive dates for incorporating the new method were given to indicate that staff feedback would be used in adopting the new approach to care, (3) methods of evaluation were listed, and (4) all possible ways of addressing staff questions or concerns were included.

Although presenting the plan at a meeting can be time-consuming, such personal communication permits the clarification of issues or concerns. Preparations for this meeting are important because it is at this time that staff support can be gained, increasing the possibility of a successful project and adoption of a change in practice (see box). During a meeting, administrative and organizational support for the plan can also be explained. Visible support can be shown by ensuring that a member of the organization's administrative group (for example, pi-

➤ Example of an Announcement to Implement a New Approach to Patient Care

ATTENTION NURSES!! PHYSICIANS!!

WHO: Our patients with central lines and whose hospital identification ends in an odd number.

WHAT: New central line dressing method that will be changed once a week. (Current policy/procedure is dressing change every 3 days.)

WHEN: September 1 – December 31

WHY: Studies indicate that changing the dressing once a week can decrease infection, inflammation, and patient care cost.

CONTACT: Jane Smith for patients that qualify for the study, or for more information, questions, ideas, concerns, etc. Phone 555-4536 (can leave a message) or Pager 555-1127.

PROGRESS: A monthly update will be posted concerning our progress. We will keep you informed if our average infection rate and patient care cost decreases as compared with our current method.

lot test site unit manager) is present at the meetings to indicate support and answer additional questions about the organization's role in the proposed plan.

Starting and ending dates for implementing the project give the staff a sense of direction. It is also recommended that one person be responsible for answering questions and clarifying issues during the implementation phase. The nurse responsible for the project needs to be on the unit and readily accessible to staff during the first few days of the project if possible. This way, questions can be answered immediately and the nurse is available to help with any additional work that starting up the project might entail. Staff members may feel less overwhelmed by the change and any additional work if they have assistance.

Staff cooperation for trying new methods and maintaining enthusiasm are crucial to any project. If staff members experience difficulty implementing or following the new method, the nurse must talk with the staff to determine the source of the difficulty. In many cases, problems can be corrected with additional information or encouragement. There are several ways of keeping staff members energized during the implementation phase. Strategies include the following:

1. Present progress reports at formal and informal meetings (see box) and during casual conversations. Change of shift report may be an excellent time to update staff on the status of a project (especially for those unable to attend a formal meeting).
2. Communicate appreciation by sending or posting thank you notes.
3. Provide small incentives (donuts, snacks, coffee) occasionally.
4. Keep the time for the pilot as short as possible in order to maintain commitment and staff interest.

➤ Guidelines for Holding Successful Meetings

1. When sending the meeting announcement, attach a brief overview of the plan listing the salient points (clinical problem, proposed solution, protocol, outcome measurements).
2. Establish the meeting time and stay within the schedule.
3. Keep the group focused on topics relevant to the plan.
4. Identify persons who are the formal and informal leaders and seek their support before the meeting. Formal leaders are those in leadership positions. Informal leaders are those not in leadership positions but with influence, either positive or negative.
5. At the end of the meeting, summarize salient points (when the plan is to be initiated, whom to call for questions or other concerns, and what methods will be used to monitor progress) and thank the group for their help.

(Lancaster, 1981; Jay, 1982)

➤ **Meeting Announcement Example**

> !!!!!COME ONE—COME ALL!!!!!
>
> Please join us for a progress report on the successful implementation of the pilot test of "The Central Line Dressing Change Method."
>   Coffee and donuts will be served
>   Mark your calendars for:
> **Wednesday, October 12**
>   10:00–10:30 AM, 2nd floor Conference Room
>   **YOUR HELP IS TRULY APPRECIATED!!**

After the pilot test has been run, the nurse reviews staff comments and responses based on the evaluative or outcome criteria identified earlier. To a large extent, the decision to proceed with large-scale implementation of the project is based on revisions that reflect the comments and responses gleaned from the staff. If the protocol is realistic and met the outcomes identified in the pilot test, the nurse should develop a plan for selling or marketing the innovation to the larger organization. The previously mentioned strategies can be used to prepare the full project implementation.

EVALUATION

Although continuous monitoring during the adoption phase provides some kind of evaluation, it is during the actual evaluation phase ("How did it work?") that the nurse reviews the innovation totally and questions whether outcomes were met and what benefits were achieved. The outcomes can be analyzed after a specified time or after a specified number of trials have been carried out. Usually, three main areas are analyzed during the evaluation phase: patient care outcome, nurse and staff satisfaction, and organizational considerations. In the example of a new approach to patient care for central line dressing changes, patient outcomes related to infection and inflammation, staff satisfaction outcomes regarding ease of the method, and organizational outcomes specific to dressing change material and staff time costs could be evaluated. Results of the project should be shared with all participants through a short meeting or written summary. A short written summary of the project submitted to the nursing administrator often serves to conclude the project for the nurse and participants. In addition, the nurse may wish to publish the pilot test process and results in the organization's internal newsletter. A newsletter article also gives the nurse an opportunity to publicly recognize and thank all participants in the pilot test.

INCORPORATING RESEARCH FINDINGS INTO POLICIES AND PROCEDURES

A research-based practice (the desired result for the conduct of clinically relevant research) emerges from standards of care or policies and procedures based on study findings. As discussed earlier in this chapter, before research results can be applied to practice, nurses must consider replication, feasibility, and risk (Haller, Reynolds, & Horsley, 1979). Other considerations include leadership, involvement of staff, and the mechanisms for updating information.

Leadership

An effective leader for a project is often a person in the setting with clinical and management experience. Clinical experience is helpful in establishing realistic standards of care and policies and procedures. Management experience is helpful in identifying and delegating responsibilities to others. An effective leader also has a thorough understanding of the change process and how to facilitate change in an organization.

Staff Involvement

Staff involvement is crucial to the development and implementation of research-based standards of care, protocols, or policies and procedures. Although some staff might be enthusiastic about trying new ways of providing care, there are others who prefer the old practices. Both types of staff need to be involved in planning for and implementing new ways of providing care. It is essential to minimize resistance from persons who are comfortable with the status quo and maximize the enthusiasm of those who welcome the change.

Staff involvement can be fostered by working with established committees in the organization, such as policy and procedure committees. Committees usually comprise different levels of staff representing various clinical and support departments within the nursing organization. If various levels of nursing staff and departments participate in the project, the procedures that result and the documentation that supports the procedure are not only realistic but also timely. Furthermore, there is a greater possibility of employing the procedures in practice because the staff have a sense of ownership.

Adopting a consistent and acceptable research-based format for the whole organization is vital. One way of organizing research-based policies and procedures is to devise a prospectus with three columns: column 1, procedure steps; column 2, rationale—a single sentence summarizing study findings (numbers can be placed after the rationale that indicate the source of the information in a reference list at the end of the procedure); column 3, special considerations (patient- or unit-specific information).

Updating Information

Once it has been decided that research-based standards of care and policies and procedures are essential, the next step is to determine how the standards and policies will be updated. The Joint Commission on Accreditation of Healthcare Organizations requires periodic revision of such documents; therefore, most organizations already have a method in place. An additional method has to be established for updating research findings as new information is discovered. This can be done in two ways: (1) by reviewing journal publications as they are released and (2) by reading publications such as *The Online Journal of Knowledge Synthesis for Nursing* (an online journal of Sigma Theta Tau, the International Honor Society of Nursing). The index of relevant journals can also be photocopied and circulated to the appropriate groups, making it easier to scan the research-based journals for new practice developments.

SUMMARY

Innovation through research-based nursing care can be beneficial to the patient (because the best care is provided) and to the nurse (because a professional practice environment that contributes to the expansion of nursing science exists). The organization also gains because improved patient care is provided in an efficient, cost-effective manner, resulting in patient and staff satisfaction.

Nurses in practice settings have the unique opportunity to make a difference in patient care by using research to delineate problems and explore solutions. "Delineating the problem" includes an awareness of the problem, along with clarification, definition, and resolution. "Exploring the solution" requires discovery of prior studies, use of research findings, execution of the protocol, and evaluation of the outcomes. It is crucial to address all issues pertaining to the replication and feasibility of the study, as well as potential risks and benefits to patients, caregivers, and the organization.

It is also crucial to determine and gain support from staff before planning new approaches in practice. Support from the administration and those affected by the change contributes to successful implementation of new interventions. Establishment of a research-based practice is fostered by adopting standards of care, protocols, and policies and procedures that incorporate tested interventions. It is equally important, however, that documentation be continually updated to be meaningful. A method for updating information that is both efficient and easy will facilitate the process.

REFERENCES

Bergstrom, N. (1991). Scientific base for nursing practice is goal of ANA. *Council of Nurse Researchers, 18* (2), 1, 7.

Bergstrom, N., Braden, B., Laguzza, A., & Holman, V. (1987). The Braden scale for predicting pressure sore risk. *Nursing Research, 36,* 205–210.

Bower, F. (1994). Research utilization: Attitude and value. *Reflections, 4*(2), 4–5.

Braden, B. (1989). Clinical utility of the Braden scale for predicting pressure sore risk. *Decubitus, 2,* 44–46.

Brett, J. (1989). Organizational integrative mechanisms and adoption of innovations by nurses. *Nursing Research, 38,* 105–110.

Connelly, C. (1986). Replication in research in nursing. *International Journal of Nursing Studies, 23,* 71–77.

Devine, E., & Cook, T. (1983). A meta-analytic analysis of effects of psychoeducational interventions on length of postsurgical hospital stay. *Nursing Research, 32*, 267–274.

Downs, F. (1991). How to make a difference. *Nursing Research, 41*, 323.

Goode, C., & Bulechek, G. (1992). Research utilization: An organizational process. *Journal of Nursing Care Quarterly* (Special Report), 27–35.

Haller, K., Reynolds, M., & Horsley, J. (1979). Developing research-based innovation protocols: Process, criteria, and issues. *Research in Nursing and Health, 2*, 45–51.

Jay, A. (1982). How to run a meeting. *Journal of Nursing Administration, 12*(1), 22–27.

Kirchhoff, K. T., & Beck, S. (1995). Using the journal club as a component of the research utilization process. *Heart & Lung: The Journal of Critical Care, 24*, 246–250.

Lancaster, J. (1981). Making the most of meetings. *Journal of Nursing Administration, 11*(10), 15–19.

Massey, J., & Loomis, M. (1988). When should nurses use research findings? *Applied Nursing Research, 1*, 32–40.

Mateo, M., & Schira, M. (1991). Exploring innovative ways in giving nursing care. In K. Kirchhoff & M. Mateo (Eds.), *Conducting and using nursing research in the clinical setting* (pp. 81–92). Baltimore: Williams & Wilkins.

Rankin, M., & Esteves, M. (1996). How to assess a research study. *American Journal of Nursing, 96* (12), 32–37.

Tanner, C. (1987). Evaluating research for use in practice: Guidelines for the clinician. *Heart & Lung, 16*, 424–431.

Titler, M., Kleiber, C., Steelman, V., Goode, C., Rakel, B., Walker, J., Small, S., & Buckwalter, K. (1994). Infusing research into practice to promote quality care. *Nursing Research, 43*, 307–313.

Chapter 4

Integrating Research and Practice

Ada M. Lindsey

Research is essential to professional nursing practice. Many nurses are just getting started with research; however, there is an imperative to engage in research to build the science base for nursing practice, ultimately to improve the health outcomes for all people. To increase this science base for practice, nurses need to expand their research efforts. The clinical relevancy of some nursing research has been questioned, and the majority of nursing efforts in this arena have been fairly modest in scope. Particularly at this time of change in health care delivery, there is increased urgency to move beyond these beginnings, to move to evidence-based practice. The process of integrating research and practice can be a major catalyst in building the science base and in moving nursing practice toward increased research-based practice.

It is the professional responsibility of nurses to determine the best practice, under what conditions, and in which set of circumstances. To enhance the integration of research and practice, nurses must have an organizational environment in which inquiry and critical thinking are valued. In the current era of resource constraints experienced in most health care environments, it may be difficult to find the requisite infrastructure support, but fostering the development of research-based practice, determining the most effective practices, is best for the long-term success of the organization,

their patients, and the health care system. The American Nurses' Association, in partnership with the American Association of Critical Care Nurses, has launched an initiative, the Best Practice Network, which includes a Web site (www.best4health.org) and a directory for innovative ideas and best practices. The Web site facilitates communication about creative solutions and best practices. This illustrates the increasing value placed on research-based practice and the opportunity and necessity for comparing practices and outcomes.

Many of the clinically focused activities that have gained some prominence during the relatively recent changes in health care systems also provide favorable conditions and opportunities for enhancing the integration of nursing research and practice. Examples of these activities include quality improvement efforts, practice guidelines development, implementation of managed care and case management models, development and use of critical paths, implementation of computerized patient records, clinical practice improvement efforts, measuring, monitoring, and comparing patient and health system outcomes, and, in some places, employment of nurse researchers.

In this chapter, several of these activities are used to illustrate the potential for facilitating the integration of nursing research and practice. Summaries of nursing studies are included as examples of the integration of research and practice.

ENVIRONMENT FOR HEALTH CARE DELIVERY

In addition to the focus on cost of health care, there has been a tremendous movement on the part of the public, employers, insurers, and government to demand data about practices and health care outcomes, a demand for increased accountability. This focus has resulted in the development of clinical practice guidelines and critical paths (for example, clinical progressions, care maps). The clinical practice guidelines and critical paths have helped to define the expected standard of care for achieving the best patient care outcome. From the resulting accumulation of data, it has been possible to determine variations in practice and variations in patient outcomes. Both of these types of variations have become critically important to the public, to health care providers, and to health care systems as part of this demand for increased accountability. Comparative analyses (benchmarking) of practices and outcomes across providers, settings, and geographical regions are used in determining best practices. There clearly has been an increased interest in evidence-based best practices and the resulting health care outcomes (for the individual and health care systems).

These changes in the health care environment have influenced nurses and nursing practice. They also make a clear case for the need to integrate nursing research and practice. Clinical practice improvement is a professional responsibility. Nurses must continue to examine the effectiveness of their current practices—which requires research. Nurses must demonstrate accountability in improving practice—which requires research. Practice related patient outcomes must be examined—which requires research.

It is essential for nurse researchers and nurse clinicians to work together to investigate and study a question or problem that is significant for improving practice, that will result in better health, better outcome, and better quality of life, and that will be more cost-effective. In this way, the work of nurses will be evidence-based and have a visible impact on the health of people and on health care delivery.

Practice Guidelines

One goal in developing practice guidelines is to improve practice that ultimately will improve health outcomes of individuals in specific settings and across settings. Practice guidelines have been developed under the Agency for Health Care Policy and Research (AHCPR), and some professional specialty organizations also have produced practice guidelines. Development and incorporation of practice guidelines provide an opportunity for the integration of research and practice. The clinical practice guidelines Cardiac Rehabilitation and Cardiac Rehabilitation as Secondary Prevention developed under the auspices of the AHCPR are used here to illustrate this integration opportunity (Wenger et al., 1995a, 1995b). To develop these practice guidelines, multidisciplinary panels examined research pertinent to the specific practice to determine whether there was sufficient evidence upon which to base recommendations for practice guidelines. The scientific evidence was summarized in brief detail (patient/sample characteristics, intervention, follow-up period, outcomes) for each study cited and the strength of the evidence was rated (well designed and controlled trials, trials with less consistent results, observational studies, supported by expert opinion). Conclusions derived from the composite review of scientific evidence were used in the practice guideline development. Tables 4–1 and 4–2 are illustrative of the evidence cited for cardiac rehabilitation outcomes from studies examining the effects of exercise training and/or the effects of education, counseling, and behavioral interventions (Wenger et al., 1995b).

In this example, the practice guideline panel concluded that the most substantial benefits of multifactorial cardiac rehabilitation included improvement in exercise tolerance, symptoms, blood lipid levels, and psychosocial well-being and reduction of stress, cigarette smoking, and mortality (Wenger et al., 1995a). In their report, need for additional research was identified; several of the recommendations of interest to nurses include (1) identification of factors that enhance adherence to cardiac rehabilitation, (2) development of optimal education and counseling strategies for cost-effective coronary risk reduction, and (3) development and assessment of valid psychosocial measures to quantify improvement in psychological functioning and quality of life in patients following participation in multifactorial rehabilitation. These and other recommendations for research have implica-

Table 4-1

Summary of Evidence for Cardiac Rehabilitation Outcomes: Effects of Exercise Training

OUTCOME	Total Number of Studies	EVIDENCE BASE*			STRENGTH OF EVIDENCE†
		Randomized Studies	Nonrandomized Studies	Observational Studies	
Exercise tolerance	114	46	25	43	A
Exercise tolerance (strength training)	7	4	3	0	B
Exercise habits	15	10	2	3	B
Symptoms	26	12	7	7	B
Smoking	24	12	8	4	B
Lipids	37	18	6	13	B
Body weight	34	11	7	16	C
Blood pressure	18	9	6	3	B
Psychological well-being	20	9	8	3	B
Social adjustment and functioning	6	2	2	2	B
Return to work	28	10	9	9	A
Morbidity	42 (+2 survey reports)	15	14	13	A
Mortality	31 (+2 survey reports)	17	8	6	B
Pathophysiological measures:					
Changes in atherosclerosis	9	5	1	3	A/B
Changes in hemodynamic measurements	5	0	0	5	B
Changes in myocardial perfusion/myocardial ischemia	11	6	2	3	B
Changes in myocardial contractility, ventricular wall motion abnormalities, and/or ventricular ejection fraction	22	9	5	8	B
Changes in cardiac arrhythmias	5	4	0	1	B
Heart failure patients	12	5	3	4	A
Cardiac transplantation patients	5	0	1	4	B
Elderly patients	7	0	1	6	B

* Number of studies from scientific literature by type of study design.
† Rating for strength of evidence:

A = Scientific evidence from well-designed and well-conducted controlled trials (randomized and nonrandomized) provides statistically significant results that consistently support the guideline statement.

B = Scientific evidence is provided by observational studies or by controlled trials with less consistent results.

C = Guideline statement supported by expert opinion; the available scientific evidence did not present consistent results or controlled trials were lacking.

From Wenger, N. K., Froelicher, E. S., Smith, L. K., et al. (1995). Cardiac rehabilitation as secondary prevention. Clinical practice guideline. Quick reference guide for clinicians, No. 17. (AHCPR Pub. No. 96-0673). Rockville, MD: U.S. Department of Health and Human Services, Public Health Service, Agency for Health Care Policy and Research and National Heart, Lung, and Blood Institute.

44

Table 4–2

Summary of Evidence for Cardiac Rehabilitation Outcomes: Effects of Education, Counseling, and Behavioral Interventions*

OUTCOME	TOTAL NUMBER OF STUDIES	RANDOMIZED STUDIES	NONRANDOMIZED STUDIES	OBSERVATIONAL STUDIES	STRENGTH OF EVIDENCE†
Smoking	7	5	1	1	B
Lipids	18	12	3	3	B
Weight	5	3	1	1	B
Blood pressure	2	0	2	0	B
Exercise tolerance	3	1	1	1	C
Symptoms	4	2	1	1	B
Return to work	3	2	0	1	C
Stress/ psychological well-being	14	7	5	2	A
Morbidity	3	3	0	0	B
Mortality	8	8	0	0	B

* Number of studies from scientific literature by type of study design.

† Rating for strength of evidence:

  A = Scientific evidence from well-designed and well-conducted controlled trials (randomized and nonrandomized) provides statistically significant results that consistently support the guideline statement.

  B = Scientific evidence is provided by observational studies or by controlled trials with less consistent results.

  C = Guideline statement supported by expert opinion; the available scientific evidence did not present consistent results or controlled trials were lacking.

From Wenger, N. K., Froelicher, E. S., Smith, L. K., et al. (1995). Cardiac rehabilitation as secondary prevention. Clinical practice guideline. Quick reference guide for clinicians, No. 17. (AHCPR Pub. No. 96-0673). Rockville, MD: U.S. Department of Health and Human Services, Public Health Service, Agency for Health Care Policy and Research and National Heart, Lung and Blood Institute.

tions not only for researchers but also for directing practice. Researchers and clinicians can work together in implementing the practice changes and in determining the effectiveness of the changes on the most pertinent outcomes of interest. The identified questions for additional research can serve as a basis to design and conduct a study. This practice guideline development illustrates the need and a way for integration of research and practice to occur. The ultimate goal of improving practice is to improve health outcomes.

The process used in developing practice guidelines is similar to those processes previously used in nursing research utilization projects with the goal of determining whether there is sufficient scientific evidence to provide the basis for a change in practice. Quality improvement efforts also have included the development and implementation of practice guidelines and use of other evidence-based tools to improve care.

It is important for the team of nurses or others involved in these processes to include people with clinical skills and those with research skills. Use of these processes to develop and implement practice guidelines and to evaluate the effect of the guideline implementation will facilitate development of evidence-based practices in the clinical setting and across settings. For nurses, the imperative is to continue to create the clinical nursing research base, because the research is essential for these processes to yield credible recommendations/directions for practice changes.

Comparative Analyses

To be able to compare practices and outcomes across providers, units, settings, and patients, it is necessary to have similar data elements available for comparative analyses. One critical area where nursing practice and research must become more integrated is in deriving agreement on the patient care data elements that need to be "captured." Agreement on the patient care data elements to be recorded will facilitate the documentation of important aspects of nursing practice and the related patient care outcomes; these data elements (care processes and outcomes) will then be available and retrievable for research. This is important not only for one unit or one practice setting but also for making certain that it is possible to conduct comparison studies of the effectiveness of nursing practices in an integrated delivery system or across multiple sites and systems. Nationally, as a result of recognition for the need of a uniform minimum health data set and of the work of the National Committee on Vital and Health Statistics, three large health care data sets were developed. These are the Uniform Hospital Discharge Data Set, the Long-Term Health Care Minimum Data Set, and the Uniform Ambulatory Medical Care Minimum Data Set. However, none of these national data sets include essential data elements relevant to nursing practices. An example of work that has been done to encourage the "capture" of common data elements for nursing practice is the development of the Nursing Minimum Data Set (NMDS) (Werley, 1986; Werley, Lang, & Westlake, 1986; Werley, Devine, & Zorn, 1988a, 1988b; Werley & Lang, 1988; Werley, Devine, & Zorn, 1990; Ryan & Delaney, 1995). The NMDS was constructed to include data in three categories: nursing care elements, patient demographic elements, and service elements (Ryan & Delaney, 1995). The nursing care elements to be documented are nursing diagnosis, nursing intervention, nursing outcome, and intensity of care. The service elements include unique agency, patient, and provider identification numbers; admission/encounter and discharge dates; disposition of the patient; and expected payer. This data set does not include medical diagnosis or treatment; it is projected to be a standardized approach to collecting minimum common, essential data for describing nursing practice. Studies that have examined aspects of the use of NMDS have been reviewed (Ryan & Delaney, 1995).

Even though this work on the NMDS has been progressing for more than a decade, in most clinical settings, and even in those settings with computerized information systems, it is difficult to retrieve information that links identified patient problems, specific nursing practices, and related patient outcomes. It is this linkage, in addition to documentation, that is critical for nursing practice and research. Another major consideration is having one computerized patient record for the health care continuum across ambulatory as well as acute care or long-term care or other community settings where health care is accessed. In this era of accountability and managed care scenarios, there is an increasing demand for demonstrating cost-effectiveness of health care in general, and professional nursing practice cannot ignore the usefulness of evidence-based practices in documenting the cost-effectiveness of clinical work. This effort can be facilitated greatly if persons in practice and those who have research skills can work together, if the essential data elements related to nursing practices and patient outcomes have been documented (captured), and if those that are captured relate or link nursing practices to patient outcomes to allow the study of practice or outcome comparisons across sites. Major considerations for this minimum nursing data set effort are the differences in how nurses within and across settings document their nursing practices, interventions, and outcomes; how and if they are linked in the documentation; and how intensity of nursing care is determined, rated, and documented. There is a potentially more problematic issue: With the move toward standardized care maps and computerized patient records, there is also a move toward charting and documenting by exception. If documenting by exception becomes the norm, it will be difficult to determine what constitutes nursing practices and the effect these practices have on health outcomes for individual patients or for the system. It is through systematic comparisons from large data sets and samples that variations in practices and their effectiveness in achieving the desired outcomes will yield knowledge about which are "best practices" under various conditions and circumstances.

Holzemer (1997) makes a case for addressing and understanding the difference in the variations in nursing practice that occur from the intentional individualizing of patient care and those variations that occur that are unintentional. Unintended variation can result in unsatisfactory patient outcomes. To identify variations in practice with use of nasogastric tubes (NGTs) in adult patients, an investigator-developed survey was mailed to 350 randomly selected staff nurses in 11 acute care hospitals in Rhode Island (Schmieding & Waldman, 1997). The investigators reported the survey findings from 153 staff nurses (43% return rate) pertinent to use of NGTs for gastric decompression. There was a broad range of years of work experience in this sample, with 63% of respondents having worked 5 or more years and 16% having worked 2 years or less. The researchers examined the reported suction pressures used, the irrigation frequency, methods for maintaining patency when a vented NGT was used, assessment of secretions, and use of NGTs for medication administration. A majority (68%) of nurses reported using low suction pressure (90 mmHg or less); however, 20% reported using high pressure (120 mmHg or greater). Even though low suction pressure is recommended, the investigators noted a paucity of research about the suction pressure that is necessary to promote gastric drainage. Almost half the nurses reported irrigating NGTs every 4 hours or more. The investigators questioned whether this frequency is necessary to maintain patency or whether it is a result of physician orders. Even though the vents on the NGT are designed to facilitate the drainage action of the tube, reflux of gastric contents through the vent can occur; 15% of the nurses reported clamping the vent. Other solutions to the problem of reflux are more appropriate. About half of the nurses reported testing gastric secretions routinely for blood and pH. Seventy percent of nurses reported using Hemoccult; however, Gastroccult is recommended for testing for blood because Hemoccult can yield false-negative results in presence of low pH (less than 4). These findings provide evidence of variation in practice of staff nurses in 11 different acute care hospitals. However, these findings do not yield information about the "best practice," which is yet to be determined. The investigators concluded that the reported practices were not reflective of the available limited research. There is minimal research to direct specific practice changes. If NGTs continue to be used for gastric decompression following some types of abdominal surgery, then the cost-effectiveness of these practice variations warrant further study

to yield evidence-based rationale to inform practice. For example, does the routine, every-4-hour NGT irrigation improve NGT patency? That is, is it cost-effective, or is some other practice more cost-effective in ensuring patency?

Comparative analyses help to determine variations in practice and to identify best (most effective) practices. This is another example in which nurse researchers and clinicians can work together to conduct research that has impact for practice improvement and better patient outcomes.

Outcomes

With the attention to cost and accountability, there is intense interest and debate about outcomes and about which outcomes need to be measured. The debate is fueled, in part, because outcomes are viewed from several different perspectives. For example, there are clinical outcomes such as improved functional mobility and decreased asthmatic episodes in children with asthma; there are system-based outcomes such as decreased number of hospitalizations, decreased number of procedures, and decreased costs of care; there are population-based clinical outcomes such as improved breast cancer screening rates in women at increased risk for breast cancer; there are provider-based clinical outcomes such as improved health promotion behaviors in patients cared for by nurse practitioners; and there are patient-based outcomes such as degree of participation in care decisions, satisfaction with care provided, and satisfaction with adequacy of information provided. There are patient outcomes such as mortality, morbidity, infection, quality of life, functional status, pain, weight changes, and satisfaction with care; there are health care system outcomes such as length of stay, time in intensive care, time on ventilator, and number of procedures and readmissions; and there are family and community outcomes such as role changes, time off from work, and caregiver responsibilities, especially with early discharge and with increased chronic illness. With emphasis on managed care it is critical to incorporate the whole health continuum and not focus just on one acute episode of illness. This shift in creating an integration of health care into a system of care is still not fully accomplished; however, the emphasis on managing outcomes and cost will facilitate this system integration. These changes have had and will continue to have an impact on the development of research-based nursing practices. Nursing practices must become more data driven; nurses can use the data to determine the best practices—comparing practices and outcomes across settings. Technological advances and development of the computerized patient record help to make these data and outcome comparisons possible, to track the outcomes and health over time from the inpatient and ambulatory care settings, from home visits, and from work and school sites.

At a 1996 conference, Cronenwett (1996) challenged nurses to choose to be knowledge workers, that is, to be in a position to make decisions about their practices. This position requires the integration of research and practice. The current emphasis in health care on examining practices and measuring outcomes creates a push, a tension, that can be facilitative in the development of research-based practice.

A study to test effectiveness of a systematic oral hygiene teaching program and two mouthwashes in preventing oral mucositis in cancer patients receiving chemotherapy is an example of research that has potential for impact on nursing practice, on improving patient outcomes, and on cost savings for the patient, the health care system, and third party payers (Dodd et al., 1996). The clinical significance of this study was the potential of the intervention to prevent, delay onset, or minimize development of oral mucositis. Ulcerations, pain, oral infections, and decreased intake that are associated with oral mucositis occur in an already compromised patient population. The investigators note there was no "best practice" identified for treating chemotherapy-induced mucositis, especially in outpatient settings. This is an example of a study in which there is real clinical significance for determining a best practice.

The study design was a randomized clinical trial conducted in 23 outpatient settings with a sample of 222 cancer patients who were beginning mucositis-inducing chemotherapy (89 were lost to follow-up, yielding a total of 133 subjects). All the subjects received the teaching program but were randomized to one of the two mouthwashes (0.12% chlorhexidine or sterile water),

which were used over three cycles of chemotherapy. Using the Oral Assessment Guide, patients' oral cavities were assessed monthly in conjunction with the chemotherapy cycles and when any oral changes were reported between cycles. The investigators found no significant difference in incidence, days to onset, or severity of mucositis between the two types of mouthwash. Thus, use of sterile water as a mouth rinse saves the cost of using chlorhexidine ($20/pint); an apparent decrease of 44% in predicted incidence of mucositis to less than an observed incidence of 26% was associated with the use of the systematic teaching program. The investigators concluded that introduction of a systematic oral hygiene teaching program using sterile water as the mouth rinse may be effective in preventing chemotherapy-induced mucositis and is cost-efficient.

This is a study that can be replicated by clinicians and researchers working together. If findings are congruent, they can serve as a basis to change practice and that practice will be evidence-based, improving a patient outcome, that is, preventing or decreasing incidence of oral mucositis, and decreasing cost of oral care over time.

Development and testing of the Oral Assessment Guide (that was used in the cited study) was completed previously by another group of investigators (Eilers, Berger, & Peterson, 1988). It was designed for use by nurse clinicians to rate oral mucosal changes in eight parameters and is not specific for mucositis. Thus, it may be necessary to adapt this instrument to achieve specificity for mucositis. However, the study testing the effectiveness of two mouthwashes on mucositis has significant clinical relevance and reflects well the integration potential of research and practice.

Symptom management is of considerable importance to nurse clinicians and researchers. In addition to the management of mucositis and pain, fatigue is another commonly experienced symptom for which little research has been conducted to determine which strategies are most effective for symptom management. Examining the effectiveness of various strategies in symptom control in specific patient populations represents the type of studies that have tremendous potential for the integration of research and practice in influencing patient outcomes.

Two examples of outcomes research conducted in different settings (hospital and long-term care facility) illustrate the potential that this kind of study has on practice and health care delivery. (They are illustrative of the research potential and of one direction that nurses need to move.) The hospital study examined the outcomes of hospital-based managed care intervention on cost, quality of care, and physical recovery of women who underwent cesarean section (Blegen, Reiter, Goode, & Murphy, 1995). This example has both a patient and a system outcomes focus. Two groups of women were used: one group (N = 100) before implementing the managed care intervention and one group (N = 107) following the intervention implementation. Data were collected at discharge and 1 month after discharge. The managed care intervention included three components: (1) a care map that had a set of expected patient outcomes and a critical path for cesarean section delivery, (2) a nurse case manager who implemented the care map and coordinated the care, (3) and a lay-language care map that was given to the intervention group women 8 hours after surgery and that was explained to them by the nurse case manager. The critical path had been developed by a multidisciplinary team and included multidisciplinary care activities. The outcomes examined were length of stay, cost of care after cesarean section delivery, patient ratings of the quality of care, and physical recovery as rated by the patient at discharge and 1 month after discharge. The three measurement instruments used were Patient Perception of Quality of Care, Perceived Quality of Maternity Care, and Physical Recovery, and system data on cost and length of stay were obtained. In comparing the two groups (before and after the managed care intervention), the researchers found that the intervention group had decreased length of stay, decreased cost after cesarean section delivery, increased perceived quality of care, and no difference in physical recovery at discharge. However, at 1 month after discharge, the intervention group rated their physical recovery lower than the nonintervention group, which suggests a question for further study. This study illustrates the use of a system intervention (that is, managed care) in one setting, with one nurse case manager and in one type of patient. The potential is to test

this intervention in more settings, moving to a multisite study, with more than one nurse case manager (to help determine whether it is the individual or the intervention that makes a difference), and ultimately testing the effectiveness of the intervention model in other types of specific patient populations.

The second example of outcomes research was conducted in long-term care facilities with an elderly population as a demonstration of the cost-effectiveness of the use of a gerontological nurse practitioner (GNP) and physician (MD) team (Burl, Bonner, & Rao, 1994). The purpose of the study was to compare cost and utilization of health care services in nursing home patients cared for either by the GNP-MD team or by an MD alone. The researchers used three GNPs, each of whom had a caseload of 100 patients and each of whom worked with an MD. The sample included 87 elderly patients with health plans who resided in seven nursing homes. Those in the subacute and intermediate care units were included. The researchers examined the patient demographics, costs of medications, use of emergency room, hospital admissions and length of stay, and visits by attending MD and by specialty MD. This was mostly a systems outcome focused study; that is, it examined the use of resources as affected by provider group (GNP-MD team or MD alone). For elderly patients cared for by the GNP-MD provider teams, the study found significantly lower rates of emergency department transfers from the long-term care facility, lower rates of hospital admissions, decreased length of stay for those hospitalized, and fewer visits by MD specialists. The researchers concluded that use of the GNP-MD teams resulted in overall lower costs and fewer specialty referrals, and that effective episodic care was provided by the team and use of the team provided a more comprehensive approach. The potential for this kind of study is to incorporate the examination of patient outcomes as well, for example, to include level of pain, functional status, and quality of life. Both of these outcomes research examples demonstrate the integration of research and practice as well as the influence that this type of research can have on practice and health care delivery.

There is another shift that is occurring, changing the focus from one of examining practice variations and patient outcomes to a focus on outcome management. This latter focus is more inclusive of cost (bottom line), quality (competence), and service (care and satisfaction). These are the components that frame clinical effectiveness and outcomes management, measurement, and resource allocation. Research is essential to clinical effectiveness and outcomes management. In addition to the benefit that can be derived from the integration of nursing research and practice, these efforts will be most effective with the involvement of multidisciplinary teams.

Clinical guidelines, critical paths, clinical paths, clinical progressions, and clinical processes also are used as tools in outcomes management (Spath, 1994). However, reporting variances from the paths has been a barrier to use for a variety of reasons. One is the time and effort involved in tracking the variances; this may impede effective clinical path implementation. Information technology support is essential to track the variances.

The book *Nursing Practice and Outcomes Measurement* (Joint Commission, 1997) provides case examples, demonstrates accomplishments, and suggests work that needs to be done. The important goal is to move beyond measuring outcomes, to managing outcomes, and to use the data to work at improving the outcomes. Changing clinician practices will continue to be a challenge in achieving this goal. However, there still is much discussion about what outcomes are important to measure, what measures should be used, and what are the computer software and hardware requirements for the aggregation and comparative analyses of data. Nurses at some institutions have taken the lead or have been critical to the development of outcomes measurement and in the move to manage outcomes (Spath, 1994). Outcomes management has been viewed as a way to improve quality of care while controlling costs, and the use of guidelines is the basis for such practice. Measurement is systematic—data are pooled, findings are disseminated, and feedback is given to providers for improvement.

Clinical Performance

The Joint Commission on Accreditation of Healthcare Organizations (JCAHO) began an initiative, ORYX, in 1997, to integrate performance measures into the accreditation process. Hospitals were required to select a performance measurement system by the end of 1997 and to begin to collect data by January, 1998, on two clinical performance indicators that are related to at least 20% of their patient population (inpatient and outpatient). Each year for 4 years the number of clinical performance indicators to be tracked will be increased by two, and the percentage of patient population to be covered also will be increased. The hospitals can select a performance measurement system from an approved list, they can develop their own system and submit it for approval, or they can use the Joint Commission's Indicator Measurement System (IM-System). Examples of measures that are more likely to include 20% of the patient population served are a general surgical or obstetrical measure, a cardiovascular measure, possibly an infection control measure. The Joint Commission plans to monitor the clinical performance indicators for trends, significant variances, and for comparison across institutions. The interest is in determining how the institutions use the data to improve and the results of the improvement. This initiative has considerable potential for the integration of nursing practice and research. Clinicians and nurse researchers must become engaged in this process at their institutions, which include not only hospitals but also ambulatory care and long-term care settings. One clinical performance measure that has long been of interest to nurses is functional status. This is an area where nurse clinicians and nurse researchers could make a substantial contribution in assisting their respective institution to meet JCAHO requirements and ultimately to monitor and work at improving the functional status of a patient population. Nurses can also work on interdisciplinary teams to contribute to the measurement of other selected clinical performance indicators.

Even before this new initiative was implemented, many institutions already had a performance measurement process in place and were tracking more than two indicators, but the point is that this represents another substantial opportunity for the integration of nursing practice and research, and the research activity has a meaningful practical application.

NURSING PRACTICE AND RESEARCH UTILIZATION

The Individual and Research

In the early 1990s, more than 1200 nurses employed at nine health care agencies were surveyed to determine their research attitudes, work environment, and research involvement. Although the respondents acknowledged valuing research, only 24.6% (<25%) reported using research findings as a basis to change practice (Rizzuto, Bostrum, Suter, & Chenitz, 1994). Even though changes in the health care delivery environment have occurred since that study and more nurses have had research preparation, there is still a great need for more clinically relevant research and a need for more effort directed to integrating nursing research and practice.

An example of a study from which it is reasonable to consider application of the findings to the practice setting is the examination of the effectiveness of adding wheat fiber to the diet in preventing constipation in postsurgical orthopedic patients (Ouellet, Turner, Pond, McLaughlin, & Knorr, 1996). The intervention was shown to promote spontaneous bowel movements and to decrease the number of elimination interventions needed (for example, laxatives, suppositories, and enemas). The investigators reported that bowel function for the group receiving supplemental wheat bran was five times better than in the control group. Using a log linear model for analysis of the bowel efficiency data and controlling for possible influences of age, gender, type of orthopedic surgery, and adherence to the dietary wheat bran supplement, the investigators suggest the magnitude of this effectiveness of the intervention has practical (clinical) significance. The investigators attributed part of the successful outcome to the mean intake of 7.5 glasses of water each day.

In considering the clinical and research applications of the study, the investigators noted a high attrition rate ($\sim 30\%$), primarily because of postoperative complications, withdrawal of subjects, and inability to begin the supplement according to study protocol. In this study, two groups were used: one (N = 41) was a control group that received 20 g of a crushed cereal, and the other group (N = 40) received 20 g of wheat bran. Subjects in both groups were encouraged to drink at least six glasses of water each day. Assessments were done for a period of up to 8 days; a panel of expert judges reviewed the records and assigned a value from 1 = good (spontaneous bowel movement) to 5 = poor (many elimination interventions used). The median of the assigned values was the bowel efficiency. The investigators also commented that inclusion criteria for the study stringently controlled who could participate as subjects, eliminating those with certain types of orthopedic surgery, those who were unable or unwilling to consume six glasses of water each day, and those with bowel dysfunction. In comparing their findings to those of other similar studies, the wheat bran intervention did not eliminate constipation for all subjects; 55% of the study group needed some elimination intervention. They noted that the assessments and ensuring the availability of sufficient water were labor intensive. Cost or cost-effectiveness or patient satisfaction with the intervention and outcome was not addressed in this study. Thus, some questions remain relative to the adoption of these findings to practice, but it is a beginning to create an evidence-based practice protocol.

Findings from a qualitative study of parents' experiences in becoming effective in managing their children's asthma provide background information for designing interventions to assist parents in being successful in incorporating asthma management in their lives (Jerrett & Costello, 1996). This is an example for application of findings in a community setting. The 39 subjects who were interviewed in their homes included 30 families (30 mothers and 9 fathers) who had at least one child aged 2 to 13 years with asthma.

The investigators characterized the process as one of gaining control and suggested the parents experienced three phases. One was being out of control, running around and seeking help; a second phase was being involved, trying out new ways, making changes; and a third phase was being in control, able to take charge, and becoming competent relative to the child's illness. Using these findings and other similar information, the next most critical step is to develop and test the effectiveness of interventions to assist parents whose child has asthma to gain control quickly and to become competent in the management of the child's asthma, for the benefit of the child, the parent, and the health care system. Because asthma is a chronic childhood illness that can result in increased visits to the emergency department and hospitalizations and may affect the daily lives and activities of children and their families, determining which strategies are most effective in improving the management of asthma is of great clinical importance. Particularly in the current state of evolution of health care delivery and attention to cost-effectiveness, nurses can no longer delay in determining which of their interventions, practices, or strategies is the most effective in which specific context. This is indeed a new era in which evidence-based practice and accountability for outcomes are inherent to professional nursing practice; thus, nurses must be engaged in integrating research into their professional practice.

Integrating research and practice often has been characterized as research utilization, and certainly research utilization is one process that requires the use of research findings in determining evidence-based practice changes (Goode, Lovett, Hayes, & Butcher, 1987; Nolan, Larson, McGuire, Hill, & Haller, 1994; McGuire, Walczak, & Krumm, 1994; Crane, 1995; Cronenwett, 1995). Research utilization is another example in which there is a natural interface between nurse researchers and nurses in practice.

The Organization and Research

In writing about the future of research utilization, Crane (1995) acknowledged that it is both an individual professional responsibility and an organizational process. In the organization, the research utilization process can result in planned change. In preparing nurses to participate in this organizational process, Crane (1995) suggested there is a need in graduate education programs (master's) to shift the focus from the conduct of research to a focus on evaluation of practice and patient outcomes using research methods to evaluate and document outcomes of care, and to the pilot testing of research-based interventions. This shift in focus would facilitate collaborative research and practice efforts and would speed the incorporation of research utilization in prac-

tice settings and the adoption of evidence-based practice changes. In addition, research utilization would benefit greatly from having more publications in which there is a synthesis of findings from studies examining practice problems. Creating the synthesis of findings from multiple studies and publishing the critical reviews centered on practice problems can be undertaken jointly by nurses primarily engaged in practice and those engaged in research. However, there are practice problems in which there are no studies or only single studies reported. Cronenwett (1995) acknowledged that integrating research literature into a practice innovation can be difficult; however, she also recognized the accountability that each professional nurse has to use new knowledge in practice. Within a professional practice model (data-based decision making), a decision-driven model occurs when there is an integration of research with practice.

There is some urgency to generate the clinically relevant science base for incorporation into nursing practice. Generation of the science base includes conducting research and testing the outcomes of evidence-based practice changes.

A brief summary of major tasks involved in using research findings to change practice is given in Table 4–3. From this brief overview it is apparent that collaboration between nurse researchers and those primarily engaged in practice is likely to yield a better result.

Titler and colleagues (1994) described a

Table 4–3

Summary of Tasks for Incorporating Research into Practice

Identify practice problem, document pertinent current patient outcomes

Do integrated research review—create synthesis of findings focused on specific practice problem/questions

Translate synthesis of findings into research-based practice protocols or guidelines

Plan for and implement practice change (considering resources: for example, personnel needed, training for implementation, materials)

Measure effectiveness of practice change on the pertinent patient outcomes and on resource use process used to infuse research into practice to promote quality patient care and identify factors to consider in making the changes; for example, competency of staff to carry out change, impact of change on iatrogenic injury, and whether the change requires a multidisciplinary team. Several practice change examples are given; for example, one resulted in decreased urinary tract infections and dysuria after Foley catheter removal and one resulted in improved pain management. The authors recognized the necessity of helping nurses view research as an important part of their practice that promotes quality care. Nurse researchers can contribute to this view by including nurses engaged in practice in the entire research endeavor and by studying questions that are viewed as being important to direct practice that has the potential to improve patient care outcomes. It is through this process that research increasingly will form the basis for professional nursing practice.

Fitch and Thompson (1996) describe strategies used to foster research-based oncology nursing practice in their setting. This is one example of how a nurse researcher employed in the clinical setting can facilitate development of research-based practice. In addition to working on research projects with individual nurses, the nurse researcher worked closely with staff nurses serving on quality assurance, professional nursing development, nursing standards, and strategic planning committees. Through these efforts, it is possible to show how research approaches and findings can be used in daily practice. The authors characterized this strategy as influencing "research-mindedness" with a goal of encouraging the nurses to ask questions such as "how do we know that?" Integrating research and practice also is facilitated when research expectations are clearly articulated and used in performance evaluations. This, however, implies that there is organizational commitment to and infrastructure support for staff nurses to engage in research activities.

In contrast to the organizational support for research evident in the foregoing examples, Anderson and colleagues (Anderson, Foreman, Theis, & Helms, 1997) briefly described some of the difficulties they experienced in conducting a study to examine the continuity of care in the discharge transitions of 30 elderly patients who had an epi-

sode of acute confusion while hospitalized. They conveyed well the influence that the chaotic nature of health care systems has on the conduct of clinical research and the collaborative efforts of the research team with the nursing staff. For example, the nursing staff were perceived to have limited assistance in caring for a significant number of very ill patients, nurses were not assigned to care for the same patients each day, there were float nurses who did not know the units or the patients, work schedules varied, and units were not consistently staffed. The researchers reported observing little coordination in patient care. They also reported that the elderly patients were not moved through an integrated network of health care settings, making follow-up difficult. Involving very busy clinicians who are working in this kind of clinical environment in research team activities is and will continue to be a challenge. The authors stress the importance of developing strategies to involve nursing staff in research, to have them be real collaborators, and to help create an organizational climate receptive to research.

Engagement in clinical research activities takes time, for both the clinicians and the researchers, but research must be valued and useful to practice for it to be a visible, viable attribute of the organizational culture. Determination of the focus of the clinical studies to be conducted is of critical importance to achieving an integration of practice and research.

McSkimming (1996) reported her experience of being employed as a nurse researcher in a practice setting to facilitate clinical nursing research and research utilization. She briefly described the change in the practice culture that occurred over 7 years, a change into a culture in which the use of research in practice was valued. She began with the traditional strategies of providing research classes and seminars, research-related staff development, and continuing education activities, and establishing journal clubs and a nursing research committee. As an outcome of this beginning work, a statement was developed to guide a change in thinking: "the vision was that nurses would practice with a spirit of inquiry" (McSkimming, 1996; p. 607). Additional strategies for the continued development of the culture change included providing administrative support for making research-based practice changes, for example, secretarial time, consultation time, data management, and analysis assistance. Schools with graduate nursing programs were invited to have their graduate students conduct their research in the clinical setting, and students periodically presented the results of their work to the staff. McSkimming noted that a key strategy in moving the culture change was to align clinical advancement and reward and recognition with the expectation of the conduct of research and research utilization. There was acknowledgment that research is "essential to achieving excellent patient care." She reports that approximately six clinical studies or research utilization projects are conducted each year and that these efforts have led to practice changes. McSkimming recognizes the need for continued development such as having a specific budget for nursing clinical research, granting time for clinicians to be engaged in research, and contracting with researchers to develop and conduct research relevant to the priorities of the institution.

SUMMARY

Although there are many uncertainties in current health care systems, it is especially critical at this time to facilitate a research culture in nursing practice arenas; it is essential to expand evidence-based nursing practices and to contribute to the improvement in patient care outcomes. To achieve these goals, clinicians and researchers must work together in integrating research and practice.

REFERENCES

Anderson, M. A., Foreman, M. D., Theis, S. L., & Helms, L. B. (1997). Unanticipated results of continuity of care research with the elderly, Part 2—Health system issues. *Western Journal of Nursing Research, 19*(4), 531–535.

Blegen, M. A., Reiter, R. C., Goode, C. J., & Murphy, R. R. (1995). Outcomes of hospital-based managed care: A multivariate analysis of cost and quality. *Obstetrics and Gynecology, 86*, 809–814.

Burl, J. B., Bonner, A., & Rao, M. (1994). Demonstrating the cost-effectiveness of a nurse practitioner/physician team in long term care facilities. *HMO Practice, 8*(4), 157–161.

Crane, J. (1995). The future research utilization. *Nursing Clinics of North America, 30*(3), 565–577.

Cronenwett, L. R. (1995). Effective methods for disseminating research findings to nurses in practice. *Nursing Clinics of North America, 30*(3), 429–438.

Cronenwett, L. R. (1996). Keynote address. State of the Art Conference. University of Nebraska Medical Center, Nursing, Omaha, NE.

Dodd, M. J., Larson, P. J., Dibble, S. L., Miaskowski, C., Greenspan, D., MacPhail, L., Hauck, W. W., Paul, S. M., Ignoffo, R., & Shiba, G. (1996). Randomized clinical trial of chlorhexidine versus placebo for prevention of oral mucositis in patients receiving chemotherapy. *Oncology Nursing Forum, 23*(6), 921–927.

Eilers, J., Berger, A. M., & Peterson, M. C. (1988). Development, testing and application of the oral assessment guide. *Oncology Nursing Forum, 15*, 325–330.

Fitch, M. I., & Thompson, L. (1996). Fostering the growth of research-based oncology nursing practice. *Oncology Nursing Forum, 23*(4), 631–637.

Goode, C. J., Lovett, M. K., Hayes, J. E., & Butcher, L. A. (1987). Use of research-based knowledge in clinical practice. *Journal of Nursing Administration, 17*(12), 11–18.

Holzemer, W. L. (1997). Variation in nursing practice: Asset or liability? *The Science of Caring.* School of Nursing and Nursing Alumni Association, University of California San Francisco, *9*(2), 34–40.

Jerrett, M. D., & Costello, E. A. (1996). Gaining control, parents' experiences of accommodating children's asthma. *Clinical Nursing Research, 5*(3), 294–308.

Joint Commission. (1997). *Nursing practice and outcomes measurement.* Oakbrook Terrace, IL: Joint Commission on Accreditation of Healthcare Organizations.

McGuire, D. B., Walczak, J. R., & Krumm, S. L. (1994). Development of a nursing research utilization program in a clinical oncology setting: Organization, implementation, and evaluation. *Oncology Nursing Forum, 21*(4), 704–710.

McSkimming, S. A. (1996). Creating a cultural norm for research and research utilization in a clinical agency. *Western Journal of Nursing Research, 18*(5), 606–610.

Nolan, M. T., Larson, E., McGuire, D., Hill, M. N., & Haller, K. (1994). A review of approaches to integrating research and practice. *Applied Nursing Research, 7*, 199–207.

Ouellet, L. L., Turner, T. R., Pond, S., McLaughlin, H., & Knorr, S. (1996). Dietary fiber and laxation in post-op orthopedic patients. *Clinical Nursing Research, 5*(4), 428–440.

Rizzuto, C., Bostrum, J., Suter, W. N., & Chenitz, W. C. (1994). Predictors of nurses' involvement in research activities. *Western Journal of Nursing Research, 16*, 193–204.

Ryan, P., & Delaney, C. (1995). Nursing minimum data set. *Annual Review of Nursing Research, 13*, 169–194.

Schmieding, N. J., & Waldman, R. C. (1997). Gastric decompression in adult patients. *Clinical Nursing Research, 6*(2), 142–155.

Spath, P. L. (1994). *Clinical paths tools for outcomes management.* Chicago: American Hospital Publishing, Inc.

Titler, M. G., Kleiber, C., Steelman, V., Goode, C., Rakel, B., Barry-Walker, J., Small, S., & Buckwalter, K. (1994). Infusing research into practice to promote quality care. *Nursing Research, 43*(5), 307–313.

Wenger, N. K., Froelicher, E. S., Smith, L. K., Ades,

P. A., Berra, K., Blumenthal, J. A., Certo, C. M., Dattilo, A. M., Davis, D., DeBusk, R. F., et al. (1995a). *Cardiac rehabilitation as secondary prevention. Clinical practice guideline. Quick reference guide for clinicians, No. 17.* (AHCPR Pub. No. 96–0672). Rockville, MD: U.S. Department of Health and Human Services, Public Health Service, Agency for Health Care Policy and Research and National Heart, Lung, and Blood Institute.

Wenger, N. K., Froelicher, E. S., Smith, L. K., et al. (1995b). *Cardiac rehabilitation as secondary prevention. Clinical practice guideline. Quick reference guide for clinicians, No. 17.* (AHCPR Pub. No. 96–0673). Rockville, MD: U.S. Department of Health and Human Services, Public Health Service, Agency for Health Care Policy and Research and National Heart, Lung, and Blood Institute.

Werley, H. H. (1986). National invitational work conference to develop a nursing minimum data set. *Research Alert, 7,* 4, 8.

Werley, H. H., Devine, E. C., & Zorn, C. R. (1988a). The nursing minimum data set: Effort to standardize collection of essential nursing data. In M. J. Ball, K. J. Hannah, U. G. Jelger, & H. Peterson (Eds.), *Nursing informatics* (pp. 160–167). New York: Springer-Verlag.

Werley, H. H., Devine, E. C., & Zorn, C. R. (1988b). Nursing needs its own minimum data set. *American Journal of Nursing, 88,* 1651–1653.

Werley, H. H., Devine, E. C., & Zorn, C. R. (1990). The nursing minimum data set: Issues for the profession. In J. C. McCloskey & H. K. Grace (Eds.), *Current issues in nursing* (3rd ed., pp. 64–70). St. Louis: Mosby.

Werley, H. H., & Lang, N. M. (Eds.) (1988). *Identification of the nursing minimum data set.* New York: Springer Publishing.

Werley, H. H., Lang, N. M., & Westlake, S. K. (1986). The Nursing Minimum Data Set Conference: Executive summary. *Journal of Professional Nursing, 2,* 217–224.

Chapter 5

Strategies in Research Utilization, One Form of Evidence-Based Practice

Karin T. Kirchhoff

There is a need to keep up to date with changes in nursing, technology, medical care, and health care. All of these impact the practice of nursing. There are many ways to keep up with these changes, and research utilization is only one. In addition, research results are not the only data that should be used to make changes. The term *evidence-based practice* is a way of accounting for the many types of information used to make changes in practice. Forms of evidence, other than research, are addressed later in this chapter.

Although numerous publications address the need for the use of research in practice, the efforts required to do this work, the steps in the process, or strategies used are infrequently documented. Research utilization cannot be undertaken without active plans to disseminate research findings and to make the needed changes. Funk, Tornquist, and Champagne (1995) documented the "barriers to research utilization." These barriers were divided into four scales or categories: the characteristics of the adopter (nurse's research values and skills), the organization (limitations of the setting), the innovation (qualities of the research), and the communication (presentation and accessibility of the research).

White, Leske, and Pearcy (1995) compared several models of how research utilization can occur. In the first model, the Conduct and Utilization of Research in Nursing project, the investigators focused on reviewing research on selected clinical problems. The investigators used a knowledge-based approach and tried to match their findings to clinical sites needing that information.

The Stetler Model has six phases: preparation (purpose of the review), validation (the critique process with a decision about the results), comparative evaluation (fit with the setting), decision making (to use, to consider use, to delay use, or not to use), translation and application, and evaluation.

The Iowa model showed that triggers for change could be either problem or knowledge focused. Following the identification of a trigger, the research literature is evaluated. If sufficient, the change process included identifying outcomes to measure, beginning with the change on a pilot unit and evaluating effectiveness.

It is possible that research utilization ac-

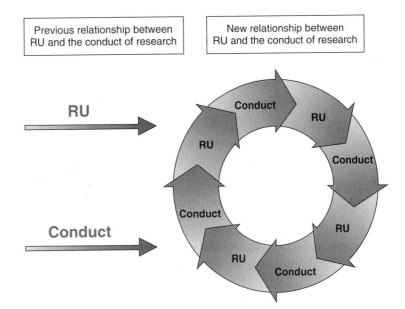

Figure 5–1
Relationships between research utilization (RU) and conduct of research.

tivities will be more tightly linked to the conduct of research in the future; these have been viewed as separate activities in the past. With utilization of many types of findings leading to studies to improve patient outcomes and with the use of those data, a circle or, better yet, an upward spiral may result in which the two activities are more integrated (Fig. 5–1).

This chapter suggests several strategies to promote the use of research findings and other forms of evidence. Access to research is only the first step in the process, but it is a necessary beginning before the subsequent steps can occur (see box).

ACCESS TO RESEARCH FINDINGS

Sharing Articles

Personal subscriptions to publications provide the easiest and most rapid way to have access to research findings; obviously, cost

➤ **Access to Research Findings**

- Sharing articles
- Journal clubs
- Literature reviews
- Computer searches
- Conferences

is an issue and the nurse's specialty and interests would dictate the choice of journals. A less costly source of journals is the hospital or a nearby university library, but the needed journals may or may not be available. Some hospital libraries have only medical journals. If so, personal subscriptions are the best option.

Publications of the nursing department or nursing unit could be a place to include a summary of articles that provide a solution to a clinical problem. This avenue has potential for wide distribution.

Distribution of articles could be one of the tasks of a research committee (Cronenwett, 1995). Some screening could occur in the committee to assess whether the author's recommendations are warranted. A portion of the staff bulletin board on the nursing unit could be used for posting articles of interest, or a bulletin board could be dedicated for such postings. The librarian can be asked to do a search on a topic of current interest and to post the search strategy and the relevant articles. The staff could then take the articles as they have time to read them.

Journals have many approaches to dissemination of research. Some publications (for example, *Nursing Research*) have as their primary purpose the dissemination of original research results for the profession. Some clinical journals (for example, *Heart & Lung*) publish research articles in the specialty area as well as clinical articles. Some newsletters publish a compilation of published abstracts across journals but on a specific topic. Some journals provide research summaries on a topic. Examples are *Applied Nursing Research* and *Knowledge Synthesis in Nursing* (an online journal of Sigma Theta Tau International). The more that has been done to summarize the research on a topic across several studies, the easier it is for nurses at the bedside to use the results. With subscriptions to these varied offerings, a member of a research committee could quickly review the abstracts of research or research summaries, check for relevance to various nursing units, and either distribute the abstracts or obtain the full report for dissemination to the staff who care for that type of patient.

Journal Clubs

The use of journal clubs (see box) is an established tradition among physicians who meet in their specialty groups. They usually select one or two articles on a topic, read them before the meeting, and share their opinion of the articles. Because these physicians govern their own practice, they may decide, for example, to add an additional preoperative blood test based on what was read at their meeting.

➤ Organizing Journal Clubs

- Someone needs to take responsibility for organizing the group.
- The topic is selected ahead of time by the attendees.
- A computer search of research articles should be done.
- The topic selected has to be appealing to all of the group members.
- During the journal club meeting, each member briefly reviews an assigned study.
- A decision should be made about what is the desirable practice.
- Someone should follow through with the needed change strategies.
- Efforts then need to turn to maintaining the change over time.

Journal clubs have not been used with the same frequency in nursing. Nurses, especially those paid by the hour, have difficulty in getting away while on duty, and they may be unwilling to do the preparatory reading and the journal club on their own time. In addition, they might be reluctant to read the selected research articles. Even nurses who have taken a research course may not have learned how to critique research articles, or, more important, how to do research utilization.

Many times only quantitative research reports are seen as ready to be critiqued and utilized. Sandelowski (1997) argued that qualitative studies change the way the world is viewed and that, in effect, changes the world. In the same vein, Stetler, Bautista, Vernale-Hannon, and Foster (1995) argue for different types of application—instrumental, conceptual, and symbolic.

To have a successful journal club, someone must be responsible for making room arrangements, distributing correspondence, and undertaking other organizational tasks. Responsibility can be shared or delegated, but placing responsibility with one individual facilitates the process. Kirchhoff and Beck (1995) described their process used at a university hospital. The topic for discussion was preselected by the attendees who were clinical specialists, educators, quality assurance, and research personnel—individuals who are better able to schedule their own time. A member of the group in conjunction with one of the researchers completed the computer search of research articles relevant to the topic. Article selection was based on accessibility of the journal, relevance to the topic, and number of articles found. If there were few articles, they might all be considered; if there were many, the most relevant or the better studies were selected, the exact number based on the number of nurses attending the next scheduled meeting. If studies were generally consistent in their findings and there were fewer attendees, then only representative articles were selected.

The topic selected and the content of the selected articles must be appealing to all of the group members; otherwise, attendance diminishes. With large department-wide groups, choices of topics can be general (for example, "pain") to keep members interested. Then articles can be assigned by specialty such as pediatric pain, cancer pain, and postoperative pain to engage the entire group. Having separate journal clubs for specific clinical nursing units or cluster groups is preferable to having a journal club for all of the clinical specialists because the topics can be narrowed. The trade-off may be in the reduction of available members.

During the journal club meeting, each member briefly reviews an assigned study. Articles can be presented in the order in which they were published or by some other method that is more meaningful. Following review of most of the related literature, it is recommended that a decision be made about what is the desirable practice. Sometimes not enough is known or the results of published studies are inconsistent. When research results are consistent or the inconsistencies can be explained, a comparison between the research base and the present practice will yield information about whether change needs to occur. When practice is in line with the research base, no change needs to be pursued. When there are discrepancies between practice and what the research seems to dictate, some action should be decided upon as a consequence. Before action is taken, a final check of the literature is needed. If research reports exist with different results than those reviewed, an incorrect decision could result.

Changing Practice as a Result of Journal Club Findings

The change process is frequently enacted through committee work. Pharmacy and therapeutics committees, administrative groups, and policy and procedure committees are examples of common places where these ideas can be brought. Although it is time-consuming to work through these groups, there is a higher likelihood of institutionalizing the change, once it is enacted. It is more important to make the change endure than to rapidly implement a change that will not be maintained when the stimulus for change disappears.

The usual strategies used in Lewin's change theory apply here. The unfreezing of "how we always do things" needs to occur. People affected by the change need to be involved in the process; they could read the articles or be given a summary of the studies. Their time and the amount of involvement needed will dictate the best approach. Informal leaders facilitate the process

through their own channels if their support can be garnered. The use of pressure in making the change is seldom helpful. Even if some movement in the right direction occurs, the likelihood of return to past practices is high.

Once the change is in place, efforts then need to turn to maintaining the change over time. Turnover in personnel and lack of attention will reduce the impact of the change unless efforts are made to ensure that the new practice continues.

Haller, Reynolds, and Horsley (1979) recommended a three-step process for research utilization. The first step is evaluation and integration of studies, which involves assessment of whether replication has occurred, evaluation of the scientific merit of the studies, and a determination of the risk to the patient. If risk is high, there must be strong replication and scientific merit. If risk is low, the stringency with which the criteria are applied can be relaxed somewhat. The second step is assessing the finding for practice relevance. Is it feasible? Does nursing have the resources to do it? Is the cost-benefit analysis positive? The third step is clinical evaluation following implementation of the change. It is possible that the literature directs practice one way but, in a specific clinical setting, the predicted results do not occur.

Using Literature Reviews

Frequently, literature reviews done by graduate students and faculty as part of theses or grant proposals are not read or even accessible to staff who commonly perform the intervention or care for the patient group under study. Faculty and student reviewers should share their research literature at a unit meeting or other gathering of nursing staff. In this way, the nursing staff have access to the research findings as well as analysis of the results, with a smaller investment of their time.

Avenues for sharing literature reviews need to be developed. A head nurse or clinical specialist could take time in a monthly unit meeting, in clinical conferences, or in patient care conferences to share pertinent literature. In so doing, the staff comes to expect to hear literature shared and cited.

Computer Searches

Some hospitals have the capacity to do literature searches. At times, there is no charge if the search is related to a patient problem. Knowing how to take advantage of this benefit is one way to increase access to research findings.

Conferences

A few research conferences are targeted toward summarizing research in an area; however, most are geared toward the reporting of single studies that are less useful for clinicians. Even the report of single studies may include a summary of research on that topic. Attendance at these meetings can be stimulating for nursing staff who sometimes garner answers for practice problems. The chance to have a discussion with the investigator is an added benefit. Regional research meetings may be a good place to start, with smaller travel expenses being an added incentive.

LEARNING RESEARCH UTILIZATION

Development of the nursing staff in research utilization is needed before research articles are critiqued for changes in practice. Research utilization is facilitated by being familiar with content on research utilization models, the critique process, Haller and colleagues' steps to take before making a change, and Lewin's change theory. Content on research utilization is usually omitted or minimally presented in research courses. The focus of many research courses is on the conduct of research rather than on the use of research. Sometimes, content on how to critique research is presented, but that is only an initial step in using research.

Many nurses have not taken any research courses because such courses are usually offered at the bachelor's level and the majority of nurses have diploma degrees (Kirchhoff, 1983). Research articles can be difficult to understand, even with a bachelor's level research course as a background. However, the American Nurses' Association (1989) expects that the nurse with a baccalaureate degree can read research critically and determine the readiness of research for utilization in clinical practice.

Another obstacle in using research is that the educational process for most nurses consisted of reading textbooks. Seldom are research articles assigned as sources of information. By habit and by education, then, most nurses look to textbooks for answers to clinical problems. Some textbooks include research articles in their references, but many textbooks do not include research-based clinical practice. Guidelines on critiquing research articles are presented in Chapter 17.

Research utilization may need to be taught in the clinical setting in order to promote an environment in which research is used as a base for practice. Persons responsible for staff education (for example, staff developmental educators, clinical specialists, or master's-prepared head nurses) should have been so educated, or they should be given opportunities to obtain such content. Workshops for nursing staff using packets of research articles on a selected topic are one method of providing such content.

Consultation may be needed for the educational process to continue or for clinical decisions to be made based on research findings. For example, faculty or students might join such an endeavor as a journal club or at workshops staged at a local college of nursing.

Other Evidence for Practice

When the literature yields insufficient information to guide practice, sometimes using a search engine to query the World Wide Web by topic yields information. Web sites for nurses to explore have been suggested by Lybecker (1997).

Suggestions for how to interpret or critique these findings are as follows:

1. Look for multiple sources of information—similar to the idea of replication in research utilization.
2. Use information from national foundations over local information.
3. Check the credentials of the source of information.
4. Determine the funding source of the information.

A fruitful source of evidence is to find national guidelines, organizational stands on practices, or other opinions that might be considered expert (see box). The American Association for Critical-Care Nurses has developed protocols for practice that assist clinicians in understanding and integrating the latest findings into practice. The topics completed thus far are (1) noninvasive monitoring, (2) care of the mechanically ventilated patient, (3) hemodynamic monitoring, and (4) creating a healing environment.

In the hierarchy of information, expert opinion has credibility, although not as much as research-supported practice. With the development and dissemination of national guidelines, an expectation may arise that such guidelines should be followed blindly. However, the guidelines are only recommendations and need to be evaluated for applicability with individual patients. Murphy (1997) cautioned about the dangers of not following the guidelines. Clear documentation should be provided when deviations are chosen because of individual circumstances.

In the midst of uncertainty or lack of information, expert opinion provides some guidance. This information should be evaluated as to which group had the opinion. Was it the Centers for Disease Control and Prevention providing the latest accident statistics, or was it a local chapter of Mothers Against Drunk Driving? What is the basis for the opinion? Are recommendations research based, expert opinion, or just a statement of recommendation by a group or individual with experience?

How strongly the organization holds that opinion is another issue. The Agency for Health Care Policy and Research (AHCPR) lists the strength of their recommendations in each guideline. However, the strength rating is not consistent across guidelines. The range of support is A to C in some guidelines and A to D in others. Some of the recommendations are research based but

> Other Evidence for Practice

- National guidelines
- Consensus statements of professional organizations
- Expert opinion
- Internal data
- Continuous improvement
- Benchmarking information

several are just the best judgment of the assembled panel of experts. AHCPR is a cosponsor of an Internet-based clearinghouse for guidelines to provide access to major guidelines as well as to provide comparisons of different guidelines on the same topic (Agency for Health Care Policy and Research, 1997). This site will provide a common place to find all of the information, even that which is in conflict.

Other evidence that should be considered is the internal data from the clinical setting. Some is obtained from quality improvement activities, which provide opportunities for improvement. Teams frequently collect data at a single time point or over time. The impact of those data to improve patient care should be assessed.

Janken, Rudisill, and Benfield (1992) suggested that product evaluation can be a research utilization strategy. They added two elements to the usual procedure for product evaluation. A clinical conference summarizing the research on the procedure was used to initiate the process, and the evaluation tool was augmented to include patient outcomes data.

Other similar data are the outcomes of patients following clinical paths. These paths should be developed through research utilization of achievable outcomes and the interventions required to achieve them. Over time data should be collected to assess whether the path was structured appropriately for that population. Results of outcomes studies on these patients can be fed back into further refinement of the path and the needed interventions.

Internal data can be strengthened by comparisons with like institutions and is called *benchmarking*. These comparisons show when patients' outcomes, costs, and length of stay data are out of line with the usual. At times, information is needed about just how similar are the comparison units. When they are similar and the comparison unit has better outcomes, information should be shared to facilitate change.

Resources Required for Research Utilization

Nurse administrators need to support efforts in research utilization. Allowing time for someone to review and disseminate research literature is critical. Providing support for such activity in the organizational structure takes some of the burden from staff nurses who are frequently seen as the ones responsible for using research. The nurse researcher, if available, would be a powerful resource for obtaining such literature and assisting the staff in decision making.

Administrators can give powerful messages in response to suggestions about changing practice, in that they need to have a basis for change. Thus the staff person who suggests the change would be required to provide corroborating literature.

There is a financial element involved in acquiring research resources. Online searches through the National Library of Medicine and Sigma Theta Tau have a cost, and subscriptions to selected journals may be needed. Attendance at research meetings and clinical meetings where research is presented are fruitful for the nursing staff, for which allowances for travel and educational leave must be budgeted. Staff who attend these meetings become more critical of continuing outdated practices and may obtain skills or ideas to improve care. At the annual Research Utilization Conference at the University of Iowa, ways to change practice are showcased and attendees are taught how to implement the changes.

Policy and procedure development should involve the use of research findings. The committee responsible needs to use the resources already mentioned, such as searches, educational opportunities, and meetings. Even if no studies can be found on a specific procedure, guidelines or consensus statements may be found if a search is made.

The expectation of research utilization needs to be set in job descriptions and performance appraisals. At beginning levels, the expectations may be to raise issues for research utilization or to assist in the implementation of change. Higher levels would involve critique, accessing the literature, and leading the change process.

Problems identified in quality assurance circles become good mechanisms for initiating a literature search and forcing decisions about needed change. If the problem is commonly found and of a serious nature, the likelihood of others having studied it increases. Conversely, it is also possible that only an anecdotal report of what happened in a single setting will be found.

ENVIRONMENT

An environment that is supportive of questioning and change is one in which research utilization is possible. Some administrators do not wish to be questioned and, in that stance, do not provide an atmosphere for change. Expecting research to be used in that environment is unrealistic. Discussion about the basis of practice and about the questionable need for continuing traditions occurs in healthy environments.

Lack of time and lack of nursing support were identified as the two top discouragers of research utilization in a regional survey (Pettengill, Gillies, & Clark, 1994). These are obstacles that can be minimized by administrators.

SUMMARY

Research utilization is an active process for which many nurses have not been prepared. If practice is to change to be in accord with the latest research findings, then faculty, students, and nurse administrators need to work with and support those at the bedside to promote research utilization.

REFERENCES

Agency for Health Care Policy and Research. (1997). AHCPR to focus on strengthening the evidence base about proven clinical practices. *Research Activities, 206,* 10.

American Nurses' Association. (1989). *Education for participation in nursing research.* Kansas City, MO: Author.

Cronenwett, L. R. (1995). Effective methods for disseminating research findings to nurses in practice. In M. G. Titler & C. J. Goode (Eds.), *The Nursing Clinics of North America, Research Utilization, 30*(3), 429–438.

Funk, S. G., Tornquist, E. M., & Champagne, M. T. (1995). Barriers and facilitators of research utilization: An integrative review. In M. G. Titler & C. J. Goode (Eds.). *The Nursing Clinics of North America, Research Utilization, 30*(3), 395–407.

Haller, K., Reynolds, M., & Horsley, J. (1979). Developing research-based innovation protocols: Process, criteria, and issues. *Research in Nursing and Health, 2,* 45–51.

Janken, J. K., Rudisill, P., & Benfield, L. (1992). Product evaluation as a research utilization strategy. *Applied Nursing Research, 5,* 188–201.

Kirchhoff, K. T., & Beck, S. (1995). Using the journal club as a component of the research utilization process. *Heart & Lung: The Journal of Critical Care, 24*:246–250.

Kirchhoff, K. T. (1983). Should staff nurses be expected

to use research? *Western Journal of Nursing Research, 5,* 245–247.

Lybecker, C. J. (1997). A nurse explores the Internet. *American Journal of Nursing, 97,* 42–51.

Murphy, R. N. (1997). Legal and practical impact of clinical practice guidelines on nursing and medical practice. *The Nurse Practitioner, 22,* 138, 147–148.

Pettengill, M. M., Gillies, D. A., & Clark, C. C. (1994). Factors encouraging and discouraging the use of nursing research findings. *Image: Journal of Nursing Scholarship, 26,* 143–147.

Sandelowski, M. (1997). "To be of use": Enhancing the utility of qualitative research. *Nursing Outlook, 45,* 125–132.

Stetler, C. B., Bautista, C., Vernale-Hannon, C., & Foster, J. (1995). Enhancing research utilization by clinical nurse specialists. *The Nursing Clinics of North America, 30*(3), 457–473.

White, J. M., Leske, J. S., & Pearcy, J. M. (1995). Models and processes of research utilization. *The Nursing Clinics of North America, 30*(3), 409–420.

Chapter 6

Research Skill Development

Magdalena A. Mateo, Karin T. Kirchhoff, and Mary G. Schira

Nurses in clinical practice settings have responsibilities to enact research roles. The American Nurses' Association (1981) listed the responsibilities of nurses according to their educational preparation. They are as follows:

1. Graduates of *associate degree* programs in nursing assist in the identification of problems and collection of data.
2. Nurses with *bachelor of science degrees* in nursing read and critique research for its applicability to practice, identify problems for investigation, and share research findings with colleagues.
3. Nurses with *master's degrees* in nursing assume an active role in facilitating research and research-related activities. This role includes (1)

redefining nursing practice problems so that solutions based on scientific knowledge and methods are used, (2) monitoring the quality of nursing practice in a clinical setting by using a systematic method of inquiry, and (3) promoting collaborative research endeavors.

4. Nurses with *doctoral degrees* in nursing or a related field provide leadership for integrating research with practice through (1) development of methods to evaluate and monitor nursing procedures in the clinical setting, (2) conduct of research that contributes to the advancement of nursing practice through the development of theoretical explanations of phenomena, or (3) discovery of ways to apply existing scientific knowledge.

This chapter discusses the development and refinement of research skills and the importance of attending educational programs, becoming a research assistant, pursuing graduate education, and gaining research skills through other opportunities. Learning how to assume a leadership role when facilitating research is vital to the development of these skills.

Productive researchers are active in publication. Chapters 27 and 28 offer guidelines for developing skills in publication. A mentor can facilitate the development of writing and publishing skills. Other benefits gained through mentoring are familiarization with organizational politics and acquisition of the skills necessary to becoming an independent researcher—proposal writing, conducting research, funding, presenting, and publishing research.

PARTICIPATING IN RESEARCH AND RESEARCH-RELATED ACTIVITIES

Nurses in practice settings can acquire skills in using and conducting research by participating in research and research-related activities. Examples of such activities include solving clinical problems, presenting research findings at patient care conferences and nursing grand rounds, and participating in continuous improvement (CI) projects, patient classification systems, organizational initiatives related to performance measures, and product evaluation. Other examples are facilitating others' research and serving as members of research committees.

Solving Clinical Problems

The nurse is often faced with conflicting views from peers or other members of the health care team regarding procedures or certain interventions. These conflicts can be resolved by calculating the consensus of peers and by reviewing the literature to learn how others have dealt with the same issues. A meeting directed at discussing ways of resolving issues can be held. Research articles addressing this issue can be distributed for review before the meeting date. Nurses gain familiarity with the research process as well as with the focus

of studies relevant to practice by reading research articles. Journal articles about possible solutions to a clinical problem can confirm or deny a good "hunch." It is important when reading research articles to use guidelines to determine whether a study has merit and is applicable to the setting and the clinical problem. (Refer to Chapters 3 and 4.)

Patient-Focused Conferences

Patient care conferences and nursing grand rounds, which are often used in practice settings as forums for discussing clinical issues, serve as avenues for presenting applicable research findings. Research literature can be used to support an intervention by providing background information. For example, studies comparing clean versus sterile dressings for patients with tracheostomies report no differences in the incidence of infection. These findings can support the practice of applying clean dressings on patients with tracheostomies.

When research publications are used to support practice, the nurse becomes more aware of terminology and learns how to identify pertinent studies. In addition, reading and critiquing skills are further developed. Chapter 17 explains how to find research articles.

Once an article has been retrieved, the nurse should review its content to ascertain its applicability to the clinical issue (patient population, setting, diagnosis). If there is a similarity between the article and the clinical issue, the nurse can then present highlights of the study at a patient care conference. Before any change can be made in practice, a literature review on the topic must be performed to look for support or contradictions in findings across similar studies. When results are similar and a sufficient number of studies are found, results can be implemented in practice after evaluating the risk to patients in making such a change.

Continuous Improvement

By using the CI process, nurses examine issues and concerns relevant to practice in an organized manner. This examination includes the following:

1. Identification of the problem, target population, and setting
2. Review of the literature and current practice
3. Standardized collection of data
4. Analysis and interpretation of results
5. Recommendations for practice changes

For example, if there is an increase in infections around central lines in a given unit, the nurse could collect information to examine this trend. Data collection might include patient information (age, medical diagnosis, medication, and orientation—confused, disoriented, oriented to time, place, and person), time of day, location of infection, insertion site, type of dressing, frequency of dressing change, and who inserted the line. Based on analysis and interpretation of results, recommendations are made for practice changes, such as cleansing the site or different care of the dressing. A researchable problem emerges when the literature does not contain clear recommendations.

Patient Classification System

Nurse workload based on patient needs for nursing care is measured by a classification system. A patient classification system allows for categorization of patients according to predetermined characteristics. Participation in patient classification system activities gives the nurse an appreciation for a vital aspect of research—the utility of numbers to describe characteristics and the use of reliability and validity estimates in measurement.

The quantification of patient care requirements is an excellent method for learning the relationship between two variables, namely, types of patients and staff requirements (number and skill mix). Participation in patient classification provides the nurse with the following experiences:

1. Classifying patients according to required levels of care, which are reported in numerical form
2. Using predetermined, standardized criteria (definition of terms and a specified classification time each day) when categorizing patient care needs
3. Ensuring that data collected are reliable (by establishing reliability among raters) and valid (by participating in time and motion studies)

Organizational Initiatives Related to Performance Measures

The emphasis on clinical and financial outcome measurements within organizations offers numerous opportunities for nurses to develop research skills. Initiatives to integrate performance measures into the accreditation process, such as the ORYX by the Joint Commission on Accreditation of Healthcare Organizations, highlight the vital aspect of measuring outcomes of care. In addition, more organizations are conducting benchmarking efforts to determine their status when comparing their performance to that of similar organizations. Further information regarding outcome measurement is in Chapters 4 and 7.

Evaluation of Products

Almost daily, new products are introduced for use in the care of patients. Deciding on the adoption of a new product requires the use of an evaluation process. This process includes establishing and monitoring adherence to a protocol, ensuring approval from the Food and Drug Administration, and establishing criteria by which a product will be evaluated (Mateo, 1993). Criteria often considered in product evaluation are quality, cost, safety, serviceability, and standardization (Larson & Maciorowski, 1986).

Facilitating Others' Research

Nurses are intimately involved in patient care. For this reason, they are often asked to participate in research, either as subjects (to complete questionnaires) or as collaborators (to collect data, serve as liaisons for research projects, identify subjects, or assist in developing protocols). Participation in research done by others provides an opportunity to become familiar with the research process and to gain needed skills. Successful participation in research, as well as acknowledgment of that participation, is important in the continued pursuit of knowledge.

Nurses develop research skills and learn ways to examine problems by assisting in problem identification and data collection, evaluating research for its relevance to practice, and sharing research findings with colleagues. Firsthand research experience involves developing data collection protocols, helping identify subjects, and collecting data. This experience helps the nurse to understand the many aspects of conducting research. Some examples are the criteria for the inclusion of subjects in a study, how those subjects are selected, the use of instruments, ensuring the integrity of the intervention, and analysis procedures. Nurses begin to perceive the rudiments of scientific inquiry and collaborative work through facilitation of others' research.

Research Committee Membership

Research committees may be departmental or unit based. Most departmental-based research committees are charged with the review of research proposals or promotion of research activities through educational offerings within the nursing department. The committee often is composed of nurses with varied educational backgrounds and job titles. Consequently, the nurse who is beginning to develop research skills might profit from the knowledge and experience of other more experienced committee members.

Unit-based committees may have a focus on conducting or using research, or both. The conduct of research may emerge when clinical issues arise from CI efforts, thereby giving rise to the need to identify trends that may be influencing the occurrence of incidents. The action plan may be in the form of patient care guidelines, which are developed through research use, implemented, and followed by an evaluation of changes in practice and their effect on outcomes. Research utilization is promoted when staff nurses are knowledgeable about the relevance of research findings to their practice (Logan & Davies, 1995).

REFINING RESEARCH SKILLS

After having participated in research activities, the nurse might decide to refine the research skills already developed. Ways of accomplishing this include (1) attending

continuing education programs in research or courses offered by graduate programs of nursing, (2) assuming a research assistant role, (3) pursuing graduate education, or (4) gaining experience through other opportunities. Graduate education (master's degree and doctoral degree) is a formal way of developing independent research skills. Nurses acquire vital skills for assuming leadership roles in research endeavors by taking research courses, completing a thesis or dissertation, and working with faculty who are actively involved in research. The nurse who enters graduate school with clinical research experience is often more motivated to meet research requirements than the nurse without such experience.

Educational Programs

Skills required for conducting research and integrating research into practice can be acquired by attending classes in graduate schools or in research seminars. With the increasing emphasis on research in practice, there are numerous professional organizations and institutions that offer programs designed to augment the nurse's understanding of how to conduct research or how to use it. Programs are offered over a period of time (for example, 4 weeks) so that participants are able to apply learned concepts. Although various approaches are used in continuing education programs, each syllabus must be reviewed carefully to determine whether the program meets specific learning needs.

Research Assistantship

Research assistants perform many tasks, including reviewing the literature, writing study abstracts, developing questionnaires, managing funds, collecting and coding data, analyzing data, and reporting findings (Werley, Murphy, & Newcomb, 1981). Basically a research assistant has the opportunity to "learn by doing" and, perhaps, gain an appreciation for the number of research applications made to the nursing profession. Usually an investigator pays the research assistant an hourly wage. The nurse's contribution to the study might be acknowledged in publications, but this is not likely and, because of the monetary compensation, is not required. Some investigators promise research assistants authorship to ensure their commitment. The research assistantship might be combined with graduate study as a method of funding education and enhancing research skills.

Other Research Positions

Research skills could also be attained by assuming roles such as a staff nurse in a clinical research center or as a coordinator for funded projects in which principal investigators are from other departments. These studies might be in health services, survey research, drug studies, or clinical trials by physicians. The nurse learns protocol development, implementation, and troubleshooting of issues in data collection. When working with persons in other disciplines, the nurse develops research skills; however, it is necessary to be cognizant of differences in research methods among disciplines.

Graduate Education

MASTER'S DEGREE

Graduate education gives a nurse the opportunity, particularly while developing the thesis, to conduct research with experienced faculty. Many graduate programs in nursing give students the option of either completing a project (developing a proposal for an educational program) or conducting a study. Although there are many different reasons for choosing each of these options, a project not requiring actual data collection is often selected by students who want to graduate soon, or who have limited interest in conducting research. However, if a nurse intends to refine research skills, conducting a study provides hands-on experience under the supervision of an expert advisor or committee. A study rather than a project provides the opportunity to apply knowledge gained in the classroom to the experience of implementing research. A research practicum provides opportunity for graduate students to experience the frustrations and excitement intrinsic to the research process (Howard, Beauchesne, Shea, & Meservey, 1996).

Once a nurse decides to conduct a study, the first step is to select the research topic.

Students are often encouraged to conduct replication studies or to take part in the advisor's research, if the topic is of interest. Replicating a published study helps the student learn the research process and, at the same time, validates or invalidates results that have already been reported. A study that is of personal interest to the student can serve as an excellent start for launching a research career. A study related to the advisor's area of research, however, offers a unique opportunity to gain experience from someone with extensive knowledge in the area and experience with research methods. This experience could also be the beginning of a collaborative relationship that might continue beyond graduate school.

The accrual of in-depth, research-based knowledge in a specialty area while acquiring a master's degree is beneficial. Expertise in a clinical area gives the nurse the confidence to suggest changes in practice. When the nurse is familiar with organizational characteristics, this increases the likelihood of a successful plan for making changes in practice.

Nurses with master's degrees play a key role in facilitating research by promoting conduct and use of research among staff nurses and nurses in management (assistant nurse managers, nurse managers, directors of nursing). This is particularly important because nursing job descriptions and evaluations stress increasing levels of research activity for higher levels in the organization.

DOCTORAL DEGREE

Prospective students should inquire about the research activities and interest areas of faculty at each school before deciding on a doctoral program. For example, if the nurse's interest is in oncology research, it is appropriate to inquire about faculty who are conducting research in this clinical area. In the pursuit of a doctorate, it is vital to participate in research-related activities (attendance at research-reporting sessions) and to continue membership in organizations and regional research societies. This establishes the groundwork for collaborative relationships and keeps the nurse-student abreast of advances in nursing research.

Although research skills are refined in doctoral programs, further sharpening is re-

➤ The Successful Researcher

---

1. Has in-depth knowledge, mastery of basic methodological skills, and advanced skills relevant to the researcher's area of investigation
2. Possesses an understanding of the values, expectations, and sanctions of a research career
3. Acquires and maintains scholarly habits (publishes, produces research, works simultaneously on numerous projects, and schedules time to work on research)
4. Is autonomous (self-directed, highly motivated, creative)
5. Has skill in interpersonal relationships

---

quired to become an accomplished researcher. Successful researchers possess distinct characteristics (see box) (Bland & Schmitz, 1986).

The characteristics of a productive researcher are enhanced, facilitated, and nurtured through the following:

1. Continued assistance from advisors and mentors, particularly in the early stages of career development (Bland & Schmitz, 1986)
2. Professional contacts with peers and colleagues from other institutions through collaboration and networking activities (Hunt et al., 1983)
3. Employment in a supportive and stimulating environment in which research is valued and rewarded

ENACTING THE RESEARCH ROLE: A KEY TO SKILL DEVELOPMENT

Research skills can be attained first by assuming the role of facilitator followed by a leadership role. Activities that facilitate the conduct and use of research (serving as a collaborator or assisting staff to acquire clinically relevant research literature) help develop these skills. Once the nurse has successfully acted as a facilitator and feels ready to expand the role, the next logical step is leadership (conducting research and then integrating the findings into practice).

Facilitative Role

Research can be facilitated through the following:

1. Using research methods to seek answers to clinical questions and to evaluate clinical nursing practices
2. Assuming a collaborator role for the research of others
3. Attending research conferences
4. Joining research organizations and encouraging others to join

USE OF RESEARCH METHODS

The conduct and use of research is fostered by citing and evaluating relevant research literature when (1) suggesting changes in practice, (2) examining problems encountered in a defined patient population, (3) explaining phenomena in nursing grand rounds presentations, (4) consulting with staff about challenging patients, and (5) investigating CI issues.

COLLABORATION

The nurse can assume the role of coinvestigator (member of the research team) or consultant (clinical expert) to facilitate research. Conducting research as a team member is particularly helpful when it is the nurse's first research experience. When clinical expertise is needed for tool development or testing a protocol, the nurse can act as a consultant. The role of collaborator affords an excellent opportunity to gain firsthand experience in conducting research, writing a proposal, and presenting and publishing results. Experienced researchers help the novice acquire needed skills gradually without assuming ultimate responsibility. Refer to Chapter 15 for information on working with other researchers.

RESEARCH CONFERENCES

Research conferences generate research ideas, keep researchers abreast of advances in research, and offer strategies for poster and paper presentations. The conference activities of experienced researchers give nurses the opportunity to appreciate the personal characteristics of productive researchers.

RESEARCH ORGANIZATIONS

Membership in research organizations teaches the nurse how to identify potential research collaborators or mentors. Professional organizations exist at the regional, state, and national levels. The Midwest Nursing Research Society (MNRS), for instance, has interest groups in many areas, two being "administration" and "pain management." The group members pursue research in a specific area only. Nurses who align themselves with such special interest groups not only acquire firsthand knowledge about current target research topics but also establish professional relationships with experts in these areas. Membership application forms usually include information about special interest groups inside professional organizations.

Leadership Role

After the nurse has succeeded as a facilitator, the next step in refining research skills is to gain experience in leadership. Although the nurse has acquired beginning skills in integrating research with practice, credibility still needs to be established. The nurse must be perceived as someone whose research abilities have been sanctioned by other researchers or by research organizations. This credibility is gained by continually pursuing research activities, such as the following:

1. Developing research-based protocols from policies and procedures
2. Participating actively in research organizations
3. Making presentations at research conferences
4. Conducting research alone or in collaboration
5. Organizing special research interest groups
6. Serving as primary investigator for a study
7. Assisting other nurses in identifying research ideas—proceeding on to a proposal or critiquing studies for applicability to practice
8. Directing the implementation of studies
9. Assuming a mentor role

PARTICIPATING IN MENTORING ACTIVITIES

Mentoring is an active process in which an experienced person (mentor) assists a novice to advance within a given organizational or professional structure (Alleman, Cochran, Doverspike & Newman, 1984; Campbell-Heider, 1986; Bidwell & Brassler, 1989). The mentor relationship is directed toward the stepwise integration of talented nurses into influential positions (Kelly, 1978).

Depending on the stage of research skill development, a nurse might serve as a mentor to another nurse yet be a novice when working with a more experienced person. For instance, a clinical nurse specialist might be a mentor for a staff nurse, whereas a director of nursing research at the doctoral level might be a mentor for a nurse manager with a master's degree, a clinical nurse specialist, or a staff nurse. As the mentor-novice relationship develops, a mutual exchange based on the performance of both persons can result in invaluable rewards: career and professional advancement for the novice and affirmation of skills for the mentor.

Mentors foster the novice development by assuming various roles, including the following: inspirer, investor, and supporter (Darling, 1984); coach, counselor, and teacher (Kapustiak, Capello, & Hofmeister, 1985); guide, tutor, and confidant (Bohannon, 1985); adviser and sponsor, yet peer (Levinson, Darrow, Klein, Levinson, & McKee, 1978). Mentors can assist the novice in orienting to institutional and professional protocols, including appropriate dress at functions, when to speak at meetings and what to say, and whom to contradict and with whom to agree (Hunt & Michael, 1983). In addition, the mentor can foster the novice's socialization to the researcher role by encouraging and sponsoring membership in professional organizations and attendance at scientific conferences. The mentor can provide experiences to the novice by working as a collaborator on a research project, by serving as a consultant in preparing research proposals, by assisting with manuscript preparation, or by helping present findings at conferences (Werley & Newcomb, 1983).

Mentoring relationships occur over a period of time and consist of four phases: (1) initiation, (2) cultivation, (3) separation, and (4) redefinition (Kram, 1983).

Initiation

Activities during the initiation phase range from mentor/mentee selection to establishing a relationship. Considering that mentors are individuals who have attained recognition in research, it is not surprising to find that they may have limited time to assist those who are pursuing research skill development. In addition, there is also a limited number of doctorally prepared experienced researchers, both in academic and practice settings, who can or are willing to serve as mentors (Werley & Newcomb, 1983). It is therefore important that young professionals actively seek a mentor who may be able to meet their needs and who has a reputation for developing novice researchers.

Having a good fit for the mentor/mentee relationship is crucial to its success. Various factors should be considered when launching a mentoring relationship (see box) (Hunt & Michael, 1983; Darling, 1985b; Bohannon, 1985; Lough, 1986).

Defining goals early in the mentoring relationship is important so activities can be

 ## Mentor/Mentee Relationships: Considerations

Mentee Characteristics

1. Experience with authority figures, modes of learning, and stage of professional development
2. Performance, character, energy, ambition, social affiliation with the mentor, and high visibility

Mentor Characteristics

1. Research interest, time availability, willingness to assist in the mentee's project without taking it over
2. Interpersonal skills such as setting objectives, delegating, supervising, and coordinating

directed toward the desired outcomes. Once mentoring has started and the relationship begins to have meaning for both individuals, the cultivation phase follows.

Cultivation

The cultivation phase usually ranges from 2 to 5 years, and this phase could be a turning point in the relationship. Both individuals may gain maximum benefits, or they may decide that the situation is not working. During this stage, interaction between the mentor and mentee increases through modeling, acceptance and confirmation, counseling, and friendship, eventually resulting in a deeper bond.

Assessing outcomes for both the mentee and the mentor are important in order to determine whether continuing the relationship will be meaningful to both. Indices that could be used to assess outcomes of the relationship include evaluation of the mentee's knowledge and skill development, such as the ability to complete projects or acquire traits reflecting refinement of research skills. Equally important to determining whether the relationship is productive is assessment of the mentor's enactment of the role. The mentor should be conscious of his or her mentoring style and stage of professional development, as well as have an understanding of the mentee's needs. An awareness of undesirable characteristics or behaviors of mentors may be helpful (Darling, 1986):

1. "Avoiders," those who are neither available nor accessible
2. "Dumpers," those who put mentees into a new role and let them either sink or swim
3. "Blockers," those who continually refuse requests, withhold information, take over the mentee's project, or supervise too closely
4. "Destroyers/criticizers," those who focus on inadequacies

Separation

The separation stage is often reached following a significant change in the mentee/mentor role or an emotional experience in the relationship. Several factors are associated with a conclusion to mentoring relationships (Blotnick, 1984; Darling, 1985a):

1. The mentee wants to be autonomous.
2. The mentor no longer has the time to assist.
3. There are not enough rewards for both mentor and mentee.
4. The mentee is leaning excessively on the mentor.
5. A change in position or location no longer permits interaction.
6. There is a mismatch between mentee/mentor in professional or personal goals.
7. The relationship is used by the mentee primarily to advance professionally without regard for the mentor.

Depending on the reason for ending the mentoring relationship, the redefinition stage may follow.

Redefinition

This phase is characterized by the emergence of a peerlike relationship between the mentor and mentee over an indefinite period of time following the separation phase. If the separation occurred in an amicable manner, the mentoring relationship is replaced by one that is friendly and collegial.

DEVELOPING A RESEARCH FOCUS

Working toward a research focus entails progressive activities that are aimed at undertaking continuing and cumulative research, thereby increasing the substantive and research expertise of the individual. For example, an individual might choose to focus on the topic of pain. One study might focus on identifying factors associated with the decision to administer pain medications based on the patient's need. Another study might examine factors that contribute to differences in doses of pain medications required by patients (for example, based on family background, use of other drugs and alcohol). Yet another study might investigate the effect of selected nursing interventions, such as the use of relaxation techniques, on the patient's experience with pain.

The nurse's experience and interest need to be considered when deciding on a research focus. Having a research focus may result in the nurse's being recognized as an expert in a designated field, thereby resulting in requests from other researchers to collaborate as a coinvestigator, serve as a consultant, or be a speaker at conferences. A focus also facilitates accruing materials, because friends and colleagues might send articles and information pertaining to the topic. While having a study focus is beneficial, there are some disadvantages. The individual may feel (1) understimulated, (2) lacking in knowledge of other areas of research, or (3) pressured to have students or staff work only in the designated research focus. However, at the master's and doctoral levels, researchers are frequently evaluated for their ability to achieve such a focus. In academic settings, one criterion for faculty to receive promotion and tenure is to have a research focus. In clinical settings, a research focus permits the development of expertise needed for additional research in an area or for utilizing recent findings in practice.

SUMMARY

Numerous avenues can be used to acquire research skills. By engaging in the clinical problem-solving process, an individual gains experience in seeking solutions from literature review, discussions with colleagues, and subjective and objective evaluations of outcomes. Identifying ways of assigning values to aspects of patient care (for example, classifying patients according to required hours of care) is a beginning step in learning how to collect and analyze data—a critical aspect of research.

Colleagues and other researchers are invaluable resources as one begins to acquire skills. By working with collaborative groups, the nurse learns practical aspects of conducting and using research. When possible, participation in mentoring activities should be sought because both the mentor and the mentee benefit during the phases of initiation, cultivation, separation, and redefinition.

Refinement of research skills is a continuing and building process that requires purposeful activities directed at mastery of tasks at specific stages of the nurse's career. Participation in research and research-related ac-

tivities enables the nurse to develop skills in a stepwise manner to attain the eventual goal of being an independent researcher.

REFERENCES

American Nurses Association. (1981). Guidelines for the investigative function of nurses. Kansas City: Author.

Alleman, E., Cochran, J., Doverspike, J., & Newman, I. (1984). Enriching mentoring relationships. *The Personnel and Guidance Journal, 62*, 329–332.

Bidwell, A. S., & Brassler, M. L. (1989). Role modeling versus mentoring in nursing education. *Image: Journal of Nursing Scholarship, 21*, 23–25.

Bland, C. J., & Schmitz, C. C. (1986, January). Characteristics of the successful researcher and implications for faculty development. *Journal of Medical Education, 61*, 22–31.

Blotnick, S. (1984). *The corporate steeplechase: Predictable crises in a business career.* New York: Facts on File.

Bohannon, R. W. (1985). Mentorship: A relationship important to professional development. *Physical Therapy, 65*(6), 920–923.

Campbell-Heider, N. (1986). Do nurses need mentors? *Image: Journal of Nursing Scholarship, 18*, 110–113.

Darling, L. A. W. (1984). What do nurses want in a mentor? *Journal of Nursing Administration, 14*(10), 42–44.

Darling, L. A. W. (1985a). Endings in mentor relationships. *Journal of Nursing Administration, 15*(11), 40–41.

Darling, L. A. W. (1985b). Mentor matching. *Journal of Nursing Administration, 15*(1), 45–46.

Darling, L. A. W. (1986). What to do about toxic mentors. *Nurse Educator, 11*(2), 29–30.

Howard, E. P., Beauchesne, M. A., Shea, C. A., & Meservey, P. M. (1996). Research practicum: Linking education to practice. *Nurse Educator, 21*(6), 33–37.

Hunt, D. M., & Michael, C. (1983). Mentorship: A career training and development tool. *Academy of Management Review, 8*, 475–485.

Hunt, V., Stark, J. L., Fisher, F., Hegedus, K., Joy, L., & Woldum, K. (1983). Networking: A managerial strategy for research development in a service setting. *Journal of Nursing Administration, 13*(7&8), 27–42.

Kapustiak, M. M., Capello, S. M., & Hofmeister, L. R. (1985). The key to your professional success is you: Networking, mentor-mentee relationships, and negotiation. *Journal of the American Dietetic Association, 85*(7), 846–848.

Kelly, L. Y. (1978). Power guide—the mentor relationship. *Nursing Outlook, 26*, 339.

Kram, K. E. (1983). Phases of the mentor relationship. *Academy of Management Journal, 26*, 608–625.

Larson, E., & Maciorowski, L. (1986). Rational product evaluation. *Journal of Nursing Administration, 16*(7,8), 31–36.

Logan, J., & Davies, B. (1995). The staff nurse as research facilitator. *Canadian Journal of Nursing Administration, 8*(1), 92–110.

Levinson, D. J., Darrow, C. N., Klein, E. B., Levinson, M. H., McKee, B. (1978). *The seasons of a man's life.* New York: Knopf.

Lough, M. E. (1986). Networking and working with a mentor: Keys to eliciting support for clinical research as a staff nurse. *Heart & Lung, 15*, 525–527.

Mateo, M. (1993). Unit-based product evaluation. *Dimensions of Critical Care Nursing, 12*(2), 88–91.

Werley, H. H., Murphy, P. A., & Newcomb, B. J. (1981). Student research assistant: Tomorrow's nurse researcher. In S. D. Krampitz & N. Pavlovich (Eds.), *Readings for nursing research* (pp. 180–192). St. Louis: Mosby.

Werley, H. H., & Newcomb, B. J. (1983). The research mentor: A missing element in nursing? In N. L. Chaska (Ed.), *The nursing profession: A time to speak* (pp. 202–213). New York: McGraw-Hill.

SUGGESTED READINGS

Allen, D. S. (1986). Promoting professional career development: A case for mentors. *Educational Directions in Dental Hygiene, 11*(3), 25–31.

Arvidson, A. C. (1986). Mentoring experiences: Much can be gained if we are aware of their potential. *AORN Journal, 43*, 1197, 1200.

Bajnok, I. J., & Gitterman, G. (1988). Nurses as colleagues and mentors. *Canadian Nurse, 84*(2), 16–17.

Beaulieu, L. P. (1988). Preceptorship and mentorship: Bridging the gap between nursing education and nursing practice. *NSNA/Imprint, 35*(2), 111–115.

Bell, C. R. (1975). Career planning & development: A resource system. *Training and Development Journal, 29*(8), 32–35.

Bell, R. M. (1987, November). Presidential Address: Of mentors and academic responsibility. *The American Journal of Surgery, 154*, 465–469.

Bunjes, M., & Canter, D. D. (1988). Mentoring: Implications for career development. *Journal of American Dietetic Association, 88*(6), 705–707.

Conant, L. H. (1968). On becoming a nurse researcher. *Nursing Research, 17*, 68–71.

Kim, M. J., & Felton, G. (1986). Research mentoring. *Journal of Professional Nursing, 2*, 142.

Kleinknecht, M. K., & Hefferin, E. A. (1982). Assisting nurses toward professional growth: A career development model. *Journal of Nursing Administration, 12*(7, 8) 30–36.

Larson, B. A. (1986). Job satisfaction of nursing leaders with mentor relationships. *Nursing Administration Quarterly, 11*(1), 53–60.

Lenz, E. R. (1987). Developing a focused research effort. *Nursing Outlook, 35*, 60–64.

Lepping, G. (1985). Mentorship in occupational health nursing. *Occupational Health Nursing, 33*, 547–551.

Mayer, G. G. (1983). The clinical nurse-researcher: Role-taking and role making. In N. L. Chaska (Ed.), *The nursing profession: A time to speak*, (pp. 216–223). New York: McGraw-Hill.

Megel, M. E. (1985). New faculty in nursing: Socialization and the role of the mentor. *Journal of Nursing Education, 24*(7), 303–306.

Mercer, R. T. (1984). Student involvement in faculty research: A mentor's view. *Western Journal of Nursing Research, 6*(4), 433–437.

O'Connor, K. T. (1988). For want of a mentor: Does nursing nurture or obstruct its young practitioners? *Nursing Outlook, 36*(1), 38–39.

Pilette, P. C. (1980). Mentoring: An encounter of the leadership kind. *Nursing Leadership, 3*(2), 22–26.

Policinski, H., & Davidhizar, R. (1985). Mentoring the novice. *Nurse Educator, 10*(3), 34–37.

Puetz, B. E. (1985). Learn the ropes from a mentor. *Nursing Success Today, 2*(6), 11–13.

Rogers, J. C. (1986). Mentoring for career achievement and advancement. *American Journal of Occupational Therapy, 40*, 79–82.

Sirridge, M. S. (1985). The mentor system in medicine—How it works for women. *Journal of the American Medical Women's Association, 40*(2), 51–53.

Sovie, M. D. (1983). Fostering professional nursing careers in hospitals: The role of staff development, part 2. *Journal of Nursing Administration, 13*(1), 30–33.

Talarczyk, G., & Milbrandt, D. (1988). A collaborative effort to facilitate role transition from student to registered nurse practitioner. *Nursing Management, 19*(2), 30–32.

Webb, J. W. (1986). The art of growing professionally. *American Journal of Hospital Pharmacy, 43*(8), 1923–1926.

Using Research to Evaluate Practice

Chapter 7

Outcomes Evaluation

Karin T. Kirchhoff and Barbara A. Rakel

Today there is an increased demand for providers to show that interventions and systems of care result in improved patient lives and that the costs of care are considered in evaluating treatment outcomes (Burns & Grove, 1997). Health care providers strive to discover which interventions improve patient outcomes in multiple practice settings, by multiple health care providers. As part of routine practice, there has been a movement toward evaluation of these therapies under *usual* practice conditions rather than the *ideal* conditions of controlled clinical trials (Johnson & Maas, 1997). One of the reasons for this new focus is that measurement of intervention effectiveness with heterogeneous populations and in the hands of nonacademic practitioners has frequently had little or no correlation with efficacy data. This finding, combined with the documented variations in patterns of care across settings, the cost of health care, the focus on health care reform by state and federal governments, and the subsequent need to make resource allocation decisions, has stimulated an increased interest in outcome management. This chapter provides a description of outcomes evaluation, including

its history, reasons for importance, difference between outcomes research and management, measurement issues associated with both techniques, examples of outcome measures, and criteria for the selection of outcome instruments.

HISTORICAL FORCES IN OUTCOMES EVALUATION

Other authors have provided detailed synopses of the historical events leading to the current knowledge and emphasis on outcomes evaluation (Marek, 1989; Jacox, 1994; Griffiths, 1995; Burns & Grove, 1997). This discussion highlights some of the key aspects from these reviews.

The focus on outcomes is not new. The systematic use of patient outcomes to evaluate health care began with Florence Nightingale, who used mortality and morbidity statistics to illustrate the impact of environmental factors on these rates (Nightingale, 1858).

In the early 1900s, Ernest Codman, a Boston surgeon, proposed the use of outcome-based measures as indicators of medical care quality. His work is considered the precursor of modern outcomes research and his ideas formed the basis for the Joint Commission for the Accreditation of Healthcare Organizations (JCAHO) (Reverby, 1981).

In the late 1950s, Aydelotte (1962) attempted to investigate the relationship between nursing care and specific behavioral and physical patient characteristics, labeled "patient welfare." This study shed light on the complexity of this type of investigation by raising issues of tool reliability, validity, and sensitivity related to outcome evaluation.

Donabedian, in the mid-1960s, introduced a model for assessing the quality of medical practice (Donabedian, 1966). This model, which emphasized structure, process, and outcome, has gained wide use as the preferred method of evaluating health care services. However, the complexity of problems inherent in identifying and measuring patient outcomes resulted in measures of structure and process developing more rapidly than measures of patient outcomes. Mortality and morbidity statistics served as traditional outcome measures until emphasis was placed on effectiveness in the mid-1980s, which was fueled by political pressure and the availability of large data sets as a result of computerization (Johnson & Maas, 1997).

The political focus is apparent in the development of various agencies to study the effectiveness of health care services. In 1968, the National Institutes of Health initiated a Health Services Research Study Section, which eventually became the Agency for Health Services Research. Two projects from this initiative have had a large impact. They were the small area analyses conducted by Wennberg and others and the Medical Outcomes Study (MOS). Wennberg used claims data to find important differences in the outcomes of care between individual hospitals and physician practice patterns (Wennberg & Gittelsohn, 1982; Wennberg, Roos, Sola, Schori, & Jaffe, 1987). The MOS used four broad categories to measure the effect of physician structure and process on patient outcomes (Tarlov, Greenfield, Nelson, Perrin, Zubkoff, 1989). With this study came the birth of the "MOS Short Form—36 Questions" (SF-36) used to measure functional health status (Ware &

Sherbourne, 1992). This study has been criticized because it failed to control for the effects of nursing interventions, staffing patterns, and nursing practice delivery models on medical outcomes (Kelly, Huber, Johnson, McCloskey, & Maas, 1994).

In 1989, the Agency for Health Care Policy and Research (AHCPR) was created and replaced the Agency for Health Services Research. The primary mission of the AHCPR was to conduct medical effectiveness research, develop clinical practice guidelines, and disseminate information about effective treatments and interventions (U.S. Department of Health and Human Services [DHHS], 1992a). In 1991, they sponsored a conference, titled "Medical Effectiveness Research: Data Methods," to address strategies for dealing with large administrative databases and secondary data analyses (U.S. DHHS, 1991).

This agency also established the Medical Treatment Effectiveness Program (MEDTEP), which funded Patient Outcomes Research Teams (PORTs). PORTs were large-scale, multifaceted, multidisciplinary projects designed to examine the outcomes and costs of current practice patterns, identify the best treatment strategy, and test methods for reducing inappropriate variations in practice. Numerous patient conditions have been studied by PORT projects, including total knee replacements, pneumonia, back pain, biliary tract disease, stroke prevention, acute myocardial infarction, cataracts, and diabetes (Goldberg et al., 1994). One outcome of these projects was the development of clinical practice guidelines. These guidelines incorporate the available evidence on specific topics into sets of recommendations concerning appropriate management strategies for patients with the studied conditions. Of the 14 PORTs funded, none involved nurses as principal investigators, suggesting that the effects of nursing care will likely go unnoticed.

The American Nurses Association (ANA) has been an active proponent of outcomes evaluation over the years. In 1976, they emphasized outcomes as a measure of quality care. Their 1980 Social Policy Statement stated that one of the four defining characteristics of nursing is the evaluation of the effects of actions in relation to phenomena. Then, in 1986, the ANA board of directors approved policies related to the development of a classification system, inclusive of outcomes. Most recently, the ANA developed a Nursing Report Card for Acute Care Settings that lists indicators for patient-focused outcomes, structures of care, and care processes (American Nurses Association, 1995). These patient-focused outcome indicators are listed in Table 7–1.

In 1991, the National Center for Nursing Research (NCNR) sponsored a State of the Science conference, titled "Patient Outcomes Research: Examining the Effectiveness of Nursing Practice" (U.S. DHHS, 1992b). This conference outlined the existing body of knowledge concerning nursing interventions and patient outcomes, identified measurement issues pertinent to outcomes research, and made recommendations for future directions in this area (Hinshaw, 1992).

A strong recommendation has been the need to standardize nursing language so that activities that nurses perform can be included and evaluated as a component of outcomes evaluation. The Nursing Minimum Data Set was developed to establish uniform standards for the collection of minimum essential nursing data that may then be captured in large administrative data sets (Werley & Lang, 1988). Included in this data set are nursing care elements such as nursing diagnoses, interventions, and outcomes. Various groups have worked to provide standardized languages for these elements. To date, the classifications of the North American Nurses Diagnosis Association, the Nursing Interventions Classification, the Omaha System, and the Home Healthcare Classification have been recommended by the American Nurses Association Steering Committee on Databases to Support Clinical Practice for inclusion in national and international databases. There is also a classification of 190 nurse-sensitive patient outcomes, called the Nursing Outcomes Classification, which has been developed to facilitate the evaluation of nursing care (Johnson & Maas, 1997).

Despite the active agenda related to outcome research over the past decade, relatively little work that explicitly addressed the interactive effects of organizational factors in care delivery with client outcomes had been reported. Thus, in 1996 the American Academy of Nursing held an Invitational Conference on Outcome Measures and Care Delivery Systems. The conference brought together health services research-ers, nursing investigators, health care purchasers, and policy makers to identify and clarify outcome indicators shown to be sensitive to organizational factors (Mitchell, Heinrick, Moritz, & Hinshaw, 1997). The conference was organized around the outcome indicators of (1) achievement of appropriate self-care, (2) demonstration of health-promoting behaviors, (3) health-related quality of life, (4) patient perceptions of being well cared for, and (5) symptom management. Linkages of organizational factors with the more commonly used outcomes of mortality, morbidity, adverse events, and costs were also considered. The recommendations of the conference were presented to an invitational conference convened by the Agency for Health Care Policy and Research, with the National Institute for Nursing Research, and the Health Resources and Services Administration, Division of Nursing, to develop a research agenda regarding nursing staffing in hospitals.

WHY THE FOCUS ON OUTCOMES EVALUATION?

The outcomes movement of the 1990s is directly related to the crisis in the health care system caused by the dramatic increase in the expense of health care. The percent of the gross domestic product spent on health care went from 9.3% in 1980 to 14% in 1995 (U.S. Bureau of Census, 1997) and is projected to be as high as 16.4% in the year 2000 (Sonnefeld, Waldo, Lemieux, & McKusick, 1991).

Escalating health care costs have stimulated efforts to control expenses with prospective payment, capitation, and managed care. Business executives and other payers, in choosing where to purchase health care for their employees and customers, have demanded information about the results of care to help make these decisions. Because of this demand, various initiatives have developed. For example, HEDIS (the Health Plan Employer Data and Information Set), developed by the National Committee for Quality Assurance (NCQA), provides information on effectiveness of care, access or availability of care, satisfaction with care, health plan stability, use of services, cost

Table 7–1
ANA Nursing Report Card Patient-Focused Outcome Indicators

INDICATOR	DEFINITION
Mortality rate	A measure of the number of patients who die following admission to a hospital for care (can be examined over a number of different time periods)
Length of stay	Duration of the inpatient hospital component of a defined episode of illness
Adverse incident rate (total)	Measures the rate at which patients admitted to a hospital for care experience adverse incidents during the course of their stay that are not directly related to the reason for their admission
Medication error rate	Rate at which errors in the administration of medications occur within a given institution
Patient injury rate	Rate at which patients fall or incur physical injuries (unrelated to a surgical or diagnostic procedure) during the course of their hospital stay
Total complication rate	Rate at which additional diseases or conditions that are related to the patient's original diagnosis are developed in patients receiving care at a hospital
Decubitus ulcer rate	Rate at which patients receiving care at a hospital experience skin breakdown
Nosocomial infection rate (total)	Rate at which patients experience infections (all sites) originating in the hospital
Nosocomial urinary tract infection rate	Rate at which catheterized patients experience urinary tract infection originating in the hospital
Nosocomial pneumonia rate	Rate at which inflammation of the lungs with exudation and consolidation develop in patients during the course of their hospitalization
Nosocomial surgical wound infection rate	Rate at which patients experience surgical wound infections
Patient or family satisfaction with nursing care	A patient's or family's opinion of care received from nursing staff
Patient/family willingness to recommend hospital to others or to use hospital again	Rate at which patients or family would recommend the hospital providing their care to others or agree to return to the hospital for care in the future
Patient adherence to discharge plan	Rate at which patients fully and correctly execute the therapeutic regimen established for the period immediately following discharge
Readmission rate	Rate at which patients return to the hospital within a defined period of time following a hospital stay for unplanned or emergent care related to the same diagnosis addressed during the prior admission
Postdischarge emergency room visits	Number of patient visits to the emergency room, for preventable complaints related to a previous hospital stay, during a defined time period following discharge
Postdischarge unscheduled physician visits	Number of unplanned physician visits, for preventable complications related to a previous hospital stay, during a defined time period following discharge
Patient knowledge	The extent to which patients possess the knowledge and skills necessary to care for themselves following discharge, or if the patient is unable to do so, an appropriate member of the patient's social support network is able to provide that care

Definitions taken from American Nurses Association. (1995). Nursing report card for acute care settings. *Washington, DC: Author.*

of care, informed health care choices, and health plan descriptive information on approximately half of the health maintenance organizations in the United States. NCQA accreditation requires health plans to report 75 standardized measures, including the Short Form-36 Health Status Survey (Anonymous, 1996; Jones, Jennings, Moritz, & Moss, 1997).

These rapidly changing economic conditions are dramatically altering health care systems (Mark, 1995). Hospitals throughout the country are restructuring to cut costs and work more efficiently. In many hospitals, this translates to nursing departments being forced to cut budgets. Administrators everywhere are asking for data to help them make these difficult decisions.

Another factor behind this movement is the availability of large computerized data sets and the subsequent realization that dramatic geographical variations exist in the use of various medical treatments for the same diagnosis (Titler & Reiter, 1994). Wennberg and colleagues found that hysterectomy rates, for example, were four times higher in one city compared to another only 20 miles away (Wennberg & Gittelsohn, 1982).

Health care reform has also emerged as a top priority of state and federal governments. This issue has led to a variety of legislative rulings that have changed the landscape of health care over recent years. Examples of these include the Health Care Financing Administration's Medical Effectiveness Initiative launched to improve the quality of medical information available for practice (Roper, Winkenweder, Hackbarth, & Krakauer, 1988) and the creation of the AHCPR with responsibility for the Medical Effectiveness Treatment Program (Wood, 1990).

In addition to the costs and variation of health care is the realization that much of current health care remains untested. Even though efficacy research has provided insights into the impact of certain interventions on uncomplicated, compliant patients, to date, many acute and chronic diseases are more difficult to treat definitively when taken out of the controlled research environment (Greene, Maklan, & Bondy, 1994).

Schalock (1995) took a more inclusive view in identifying six major trends that have led to the importance of outcome-based evaluation:

1. The quality revolution that focuses on quality of life, quality management techniques, and so on
2. Consumer empowerment
3. Increased demands for accountability
4. The "supports paradigm," a change in the way people with special needs are viewed and served
5. The emphasis on enhanced functioning
6. The "emerging pragmatic evaluation paradigm," or the shift from the experimental approach to a more practical, problem-solving orientation to program evaluation

DEFINITION OF TERMS

The importance of outcome evaluation has led to conflicting terminology and definitions among authors. Commonly used terms—outcomes, risk adjustment, outcomes research, and outcomes management—are defined to provide clarity regarding their meaning and appropriate use.

Outcomes

Donabedian (1985) defined outcomes as "those changes, either favorable or adverse, in the actual or potential health status of persons, groups, or communities, that can be attributed to prior or concurrent care" (p. 256). More simply put, outcomes are the end results of treatments or interventions (Titler & Reiter, 1994; Jennings, 1995). These end results are influenced by several factors: risk factors such as baseline status, clinical status, and demographic/psychosocial characteristics; and treatment factors, such as setting and treatment interventions.

Risk Adjustment

The goal of outcome evaluation is to isolate the relationship between the outcomes of interest and the treatment provided by controlling for the effects of other relevant factors (Kane, 1997). This analysis is referred to as risk adjustment. The purpose of risk adjustment is to "level the playing field" in comparing outcomes across providers and sites. Although this concept is straightforward, performing clinically credible risk adjustment is difficult, especially given the widespread data constraints (Iezzoni, 1994). For example, a medical center may have a larger percentage of older patients receiving a procedure. When outcomes of the procedures are compared with centers having younger patients, statistical adjustments would be made.

Outcomes Research and Outcomes Management

The evaluation of outcomes can take different forms, depending on the purposes of the analysis. Two commonly used terms associated with outcomes evaluation are *outcomes research* and *outcomes management*. Outcomes research is the study of the effects of a specific intervention. Methods are designed to answer specific research questions regarding the intervention under study. This type of research activity is directed toward discovering and disseminating new knowledge, and it involves standardized methods for design, measurement, data collection, and data analysis (Joint Commission for Accreditation of Healthcare Organizations [JCAHO], 1994). The ability to generalize to specific populations beyond the boundaries of clinical settings or provider practices is a goal of this type of evaluation.

Outcomes research methods can take the form of *efficacy* studies, by providing stringent controls over the phenomena under study to achieve pure (or ideal) testing of an intervention. Outcomes research can also take the form of *effectiveness* research, which is conducted without stringent controls and sets out to answer the question of how an intervention, or set of interventions, impacts specific outcomes given the multiple intervening or confounding variables inherent in a clinical setting. The latter type is the more common form of outcomes research and considered by some to be conceptually similar to the study of outcomes (Guadagnoli & McNeil, 1994). Most investigators use either observational techniques, in which patient cohorts are evaluated prospectively or retrospectively to assess exposure to certain factors and compare outcomes of interest, or clinical and administrative database analyses to describe

individuals with particular diagnoses or those undergoing specific procedures (Wennberg, Roos, Sola, Schori, & Jaffe, 1987; Tarlov et al., 1989; Champion et al., 1990; Greene, Maklan, & Bondy, 1994; Greenfield et al., 1994).

In contrast, outcomes management incorporates aspects of both research and operations. Research provides the methodological foundation, whereas operations call for continuous monitoring of routinely delivered care; exploratory, descriptive, and predictive data-analytic techniques; and a shift toward an empirical basis for routine clinical decision making (JCAHO, 1994). Outcomes management focuses on specific outcomes in an attempt to identify areas of variation or inefficiencies so that appropriate changes in practice can be made. The focus is on individuals within a specific setting or under the care of specific providers.

Outcomes management collects and analyzes data over time in contrast to the evaluation of end results at prespecified time periods (although this approach is also used). Quality control techniques, such as run charts and statistical control limits, are frequently used to identify common and special causes of variation over time. These techniques flush out the processes that are stable and can be systematically improved from those that are affected by special causes of variation, such as equipment failure or changes in staffing levels, for which efforts are needed to control the process before improvements can be made (JCAHO, 1997). Even though both outcomes research and management may result in changes in practice, outcomes management is more directly concerned with closing the loop between assessment and improvement. Getting "buy-in" of providers to change practice and use of strategies such as internal or external benchmarking to identify areas of needed improvement are important considerations in outcomes management.

MEASUREMENT ISSUES

Measurement is fundamental to conducting outcomes evaluation and is linked to all steps of the scientific process. Kane (1997) stated, "One's measures are only as good as one's conceptualization of the concept, one's data are only as good as one's measures, and one's results are only as good as one's data" (p. 213). One must consider what needs to be measured, why it is important to measure it, and how the information will be used. All measurement is imperfect for two reasons: (1) anything investigators measure is an abstraction from reality and (2) anything measured is measured with error (Kane, 1997).

Several issues must be considered when measuring outcomes. These include the following:

• Timing of the measurement
• Attribution
• Database
• Level of analysis
• Episode of care
• Care continuum

Timing of Measurement

An important consideration is the timing of the measurement. One must specify the period of time in which certain outcomes should be measured or achieved (Hegyvary, 1991). Outcomes can be short-term or long-term. For example, one might assess the effectiveness of a smoking cessation program by determining whether the client remained abstinent 2 weeks after his or her quit date. But the assessment might also be made in terms of the patient's status 6 months or 1 year after quitting, which some might argue is a better indicator of success. However, such an approach must take into account the additional variables that may contribute to those results. It is generally acknowledged that long-term outcomes are less specific to the treatment or process of care because of the probability of numerous intervening variables that makes attribution of cause and effect difficult to ascertain (Lohr, 1988; Hegyvary, 1991; Crane, 1992).

According to Strickland (1997), measurement time points should be matched carefully to when an intervention most likely will have a measurable effect. Because outcomes can vary over the course of a hospital stay or over the trajectory of an illness, short-term, intermediate, and long-term intervals for measurement of outcomes may all be appropriate.

Attribution

Attribution of cause and effect is a complex issue that is also influenced by other things,

such as the type of outcomes being studied. For example, length of stay, mortality, and quality of life can all be influenced by multiple factors beyond a specific intervention. Demographic and social characteristics of patients can influence their quality of life apart from interventions performed to improve this outcome. Likewise, length of stay is influenced by cultural, geographical, and resource variables beyond the effectiveness of a specific intervention. Hegyvary (1991) stated that health is interrelated with every part of human existence and cannot be simplistically achieved through the application of isolated interventions. Approaches to the assessment of health care outcomes must recognize this complexity by conducting comprehensive analyses, such as multivariate analytical approaches, to determine the relative importance of each variable, and their interactive effects.

Another approach might be the development of more precise measurements. Crane (1992) suggested a need for precise measurements of the differences among and changes in health-related quality of life measures with respect to the sociodemographic characteristics of patients, the cultural and ethnic characteristics of patients, and the severity of illness.

Database

A related issue is which data to collect and include in a database. Hegyvary (1991) stated that the complexity of issues related to outcomes and results of treatments necessitates an extensive database for assessing outcomes. Various factors should be taken into account, such as demographic, structural, process, and provider-specific data. Constructing such a database requires the compatibility of measures and usually depends on access to other data sets. Such a requirement lends itself to issues of security and confidentiality that need to be honored and taken seriously.

In addition, when other data sets are used, it is also important to know how the data were collected and understand the definitions and categorizations behind the database. For example, if diagnostic related groups are used to identify patients, one needs to understand that group assignment is driven to maximize reimbursement and that these categorizations change each year toward groupings of similar resource utilization. If this identifier is being used, it is important to know what adjustments are needed so the data will reflect the clinical populations of interest.

Level of Analysis

The level of analysis is another issue to consider when evaluating outcomes. Different levels require different types of indicators and methodological approaches (Hegyvary, 1991). If interested in how individual patients are influenced by a specific treatment or intervention, analyses may include a baseline assessment so that comparisons can be performed after an intervention. For example, measurement of health status at an individual level may involve a baseline assessment before surgery and another health status assessment 6 months after surgery so that comparisons can be made to determine the impact of the interventions. If interested in groups of patients receiving specific interventions, the level of analysis would be at a group or aggregate level. In this case, only one measurement of health status may be used to determine the function of specific patient populations because of treatments. These results might be compared across institutions to benchmark practice and identify improvement opportunities.

The level of analysis may also have implications for the type of measure that is chosen. Stewart and Archbold (1992) cautioned that measures designed to assess individual differences might be inadequate for evaluating outcomes of intervention studies. The established psychometric properties no longer apply or indicate the degree to which the measure will be sensitive to the treatment condition under study.

Another issue related to level of analysis is how the data will be categorized and presented. For example, will it be around patient population or provider of care? The priorities of the audience are often a strong force in dictating this approach, particularly with outcomes management. If current structures for decision making are clinical departments, the data are best addressed if they reflect categorizations of patients served by staff in those departments. On the other hand, if product or service line structures exist, data can be categorized around appropriate patient population groups consistent with these structures.

Episode of Care

The definition of episode of care during which the outcomes are to be measured is a vital issue. There is often considerable uncertainty over when an "illness" or "condition" starts and ends, or at what specific period of an illness or condition outcome measurements should be made (Crane, 1992). The ANA wrestled with this issue during discussions of the ANA Report Card. Is the episode of care defined as equivalent to an encounter with a patient? For example, if a patient is seen in a clinic or home, or is admitted to a hospital for a period of time, is that encounter considered an episode of care, and, therefore, is evaluation related to those interventions appropriate? Or, should an episode of care be defined as synonymous with an illness or condition and start at the time of diagnosis and end at the time of cure or death? If this is the approach, outcome evaluation might be periodic throughout the episode of care unrelated to specific clinic encounters, home visits, or hospitalizations.

Care Continuum

Measurement of outcomes across the care continuum present other pressing issues, according to Lamb (1997). These include (1) the identification of severity and risk adjustment measures to ensure comparability of study groups, (2) access to usable data across multiple settings, (3) determination of and allocation of the contribution of selected components of a multifaceted intervention to quality and cost outcomes, and (4) decisions about the most effective integration of disease-specific, population-specific, and general outcome measures. Lamb stated that new methods of longitudinal research design are needed to bring together systems, quality, and cost perspectives to capture the impact of multifaceted interventions across time and settings.

TYPES OF OUTCOME MEASURES

Outcomes can include familiar clinical measures, such as signs and symptoms or death.

They can be expressed as complications, such as infections, or they can be used in a larger context, relying on patient-centered information obtained by means of questionnaires, such as patient satisfaction and functional health status (Kane, 1997). Many authors have identified outcomes for both broad and specific patient groups (Haussmann & Hegyvary, 1976; Horn & Swain, 1978; Hover & Zimmer, 1978; Lohr, 1988; Marek, 1989; Lang & Marek, 1990). Lang and Marek (1990) provide one of the more comprehensive listings. They reviewed nursing quality assurance and research studies to identify which outcome indicators were used by investigators. They found various outcomes and classified them into 15 categories: physiological outcomes, psychological measures, functional status, behavior outcomes, knowledge, symptom control, home maintenance, well-being (quality of life), goal attainment, patient satisfaction, safety, frequency of service, cost, rehospitalization, and resolution of nursing diagnoses or nursing problems.

A recent approach for measuring value, called the "Clinical Value Compass," describes a conceptual framework for identification of outcome measurements to facilitate changes for improving outcomes and lowering costs of patient care. This compass includes four major parts: (1) functional status, risk status, and well-being, (2) costs, (3) satisfaction with health care and perceived benefit, and (4) clinical outcomes, such as mortality and clinical symptoms (for example, relief of angina) (Nelson, Mohr, Batalden, & Plume, 1996).

Titler and Reiter (1994) suggested that any generic core of outcome data should include some measure of functional status and patient satisfaction. These measures, they stated, "provide a common denominator with which to make comparisons across diverse populations, thus making their application useful for evaluating the effectiveness of treatments in clinical practice, health care management, and health policy analysis." Examples of these measures are provided in the following section.

PATIENT SATISFACTION MEASURES

Patient satisfaction is an important indicator of care as perceived by the patient. The importance of this measure has been recognized by accrediting agencies such as the National Committee on Quality Assurance and by payers such as Medicare and Medicaid, who have mandated evaluation of patient satisfaction (National Committee for Quality Assurance, 1996). In addition, patient satisfaction ratings correlate positively with compliance with medical regimens, return for follow-up care, and continued enrollment in health plans (Ware & Hayes, 1988; Rubin et al., 1993; Williams, 1994; Zapka et al., 1995). Patient satisfaction data may also provide insight into opportunities to improve care by changing delivery systems, facilitating patient and staff communication, and improving overall efficiency. For these reasons, this outcome is of high interest and is evaluated by most providers of health care services.

Although many patient satisfaction measures exist, the two most utilized patient satisfaction surveys, either in full or in part, are the Group Health Association of America (GHAA) Consumer Satisfaction Survey (Davies & Ware, 1991) and the Picker/Commonwealth survey (University HealthSystem Consortium and the Picker Institute, 1998). The GHAA survey was developed primarily for employers who offer their employees one or more health benefit options and who want to obtain valid and comparable information on employee satisfaction. It contains two major sections: a three-part satisfaction battery, including 47 items, and a core set of additional items. The content is broken down into the following subscales:

Multi-Item Scales:	Access, finances, technical quality, communication, choice and continuity, interpersonal care, services covered, information, paperwork, costs of care, and general satisfaction
Single-Item Scales:	Overall care, time spent, outcomes, overall quality, overall plan, and plan satisfaction

Internal consistency reliability was estimated for the 11 multi-item scales using Cronbach's Alpha and fell in the range of .80 to .97. Evidence of three kinds of validity is also available on this survey (Davies & Ware, 1991). The strengths of this survey include the breadth of topics addressed and its usability by hospitals, providers, employers, and insurers. It also uses an excellent to poor Likert-type response set, which Ware and Hayes (1988) revealed as superior to strongly agree—strongly disagree metrics. The largest weakness is the lack of specific measures about outpatient services, although the questions can be revised for outpatient settings (Kane, 1997).

The Picker/Commonwealth hospital satisfaction survey was developed as part of a larger initiative to emphasize patient-centered care in partnership with the University HealthSystem Consortium (UHC). A series of 52 questions were developed to explore specific action taken by hospital staff. Most of the response options are dichotomous. However, follow-up questions are sometimes used to elicit more information about the problems reported (Kane, 1997). General headings include communication, financial information, patients' needs and preferences, emotional support, physical comfort, pain management, education, family participation, and discharge preparation/continuity of care. Benefits of this tool are primarily the benchmarking capabilities provided to UHC members who receive reports comparing the satisfaction of their institution to that of their peers and other nonacademic hospitals in the Picker database. Other benefits include the assistance that UHC provides in identifying and sharing best practices and the ability to link patient satisfaction with other UHC databases (University HealthSystem Consortium Web site, 1997).

FUNCTIONAL HEALTH STATUS MEASURES

When evaluating health status, it is important to first develop a conceptual model and define what aspects of health and range of dysfunction are to be measured. Measures of health status can include everything from mortality to health-related quality of life. In addition, there are unidimensional versus multidimensional tools as well as generic versus condition-specific measures from which to select. The domains that tend to be included in health status evaluation are the following: physical functioning, emotional or mental functioning, cognitive functioning, social functioning, pain, vitality, and overall well-being (Kane, 1997).

Unidimensional health status measures assess only one aspect and can be either a single indicator based on one question or a single index based on a summation of several questions tapping the same domain. Examples of unidimensional measures that measure physical functioning include the Katz Index of ADLs, Barthel Index of ADLs, and Comprehensive Older Person's Evaluation. Unidimensional measures that measure emotional functioning are Zung Self Rating Depression Scale, Zung Self Rating Anxiety Scale, and Beck's Depression Inventory. The Mental Status Questionnaire is an example of a unidimensional measure of cognitive functioning and the RAND Social Health Battery and the MOS Social Support Survey are examples of social functioning measures (Kane, 1997).

Multidimensional health status measures are also numerous. One of the most popular, as stated previously, is the MOS SF-36. This measure has been further shortened to another version called the MOS Short-Form 12 items (SF-12). Both measures assess eight subscales including physical functioning, role-physical, role-emotional, mental health, bodily pain, vitality, social functioning, and general health perception. Reliability coefficients range from .93 (physical functioning) to .78 (General Health) for the SF-36. Physical and mental health scores for the SF-12 correlate at .93 to .97 with the SF-36 version (Ware, 1993; Ware, Kosinski, & Keller, 1995). Other multidimensional health status measures include the Sickness Impact Profile, the Nottingham Health Profile, the Duke-University of North Carolina Health Profile, the Quality of Well-Being Scale, and the Dartmouth COOP Charts (Kane, 1997).

In addition to the generic measures of health status, there are disease- or condition-specific measures that have been tested with various patient population groups. For example, multidimensional measures of pulmonary specific health status include the Pulmonary Functional Status Questionnaire, the Asthma Quality of Life Questionnaire, the Pulmonary Functional Status and Dyspnea Questionnaire, and the Chronic Respiratory Disease Questionnaire (Titler, 1997).

SELECTION OF OUTCOME INSTRUMENTS

The selection of an outcome measure should be based on a clear sense of what is to be measured and why. This should include the definition and scope of both the outcome of interest and the instrument selected to measure it (Titler & Reiter, 1994). Once this is determined, the basic criteria for selecting a useful measure are that it is reliable (that is, it will provide the same results consistently), it is valid (that is, it measures what it says it does), and it can detect meaningful increments of change (Kane, 1997).

The issue of sensitivity to change should predominate, according to Stewart & Archbold (1992; 1993). They provided a list of seven questions to consider in selecting outcomes measures (Table 7–2). These questions addressed recommendations for the application of principles of reliability and validity in the context of sensitivity to change. In essence, Stewart & Archbold (1992; 1993) provided arguments for considering condition-specific measures, measures that detect change in the desired time frame, individualized measures, an evaluation of the sensitivity of specific items, use of a broad range of response options, the possible use of construct validity as an ap-

Table 7–2

Questions and Recommendations to Help Determine Outcome Measures and Their Sensitivity to Change

QUESTION	RECOMMENDATION
Is the conceptual link between the intervention and the outcome variable logical?	Be able to link the change in the outcome variable to the intervention and rule out the effects of other factors that may cause the change (have the outcome variable adequately specific).
To what extent is the outcome variable amenable to change?	Consider the extent to which the underlying attribute has the potential to change in the desired enduring or short-term fashion.
Is the content validity of the outcome measure adequate for detecting the effect of the proposed intervention?	Carefully examine the specific items on the measure and think about whether they, when taken singly and collectively, will capture the treatment effects. Identifying an existing individualized outcome measure may be especially helpful.
Does the evidence for the construct validity of the outcome measure argue for its potential to detect change as a result of the proposed intervention?	Review the literature, conduct a measurement assessment study, or obtain discrimination indices at the item level to determine whether the scale being considered is able to detect change.
Does the instrument used to measure the attribute have a potential distribution of scores that will allow detection of change?	Determine whether there is room for change to occur on the measure and whether the measurement units are adequately fine-grained to detect a treatment effect (broadening the range of response options for the items may improve sensitivity).
What type of reliability assessment is appropriate to consider for this outcome measure?	Report reliability estimates that reflect small degrees of measurement error and, when possible, aggregate measures to increase the true score component. Use empirical evidence of construct validity—whereas a reliable test is not necessarily valid, a valid test implies some degree of reliability.
How should the level of correlational stability over time be interpreted?	Interpretation of reliability estimates should consider the issue of sensitivity to change. High test–retest correlation may signal the measure of a highly stable attribute that is unlikely to change. Low test–retest correlation over longer intervals may provide evidence that the measure is sensitive to change.

Adapted from Stewart, B. J., & Archbold, P. G. (1992). Nursing intervention studies require outcome measures that are sensitive to change: Part one. Research in Nursing and Health, 15, *477–481 and Stewart, B. J., & Archbold, P. G. (1993). Nursing intervention studies require outcome measures that are sensitive to change: Part two.* Research in Nursing and Health, 16 77–81. *Copyright © 1993. Reprinted by permission of John Wiley & Sons, Inc.*

propriate reliability estimate, and careful interpretation of reliability estimates to consider sensitivity to change.

One of the considerations that are frequently discussed in the selection of outcome measures is whether to use a generic or condition-specific measure. Generic measures are comprehensive and assess overall effects. Condition-specific measures focus on symptoms and signs that reflect the status of a given medical condition. Therefore, they are likely to be more sensitive to subtle changes in the phenomenon under study. A basic rule is that the more global the outcome measure, the more distant it is from the specific effects of the immediate treatment and the more vulnerable it is to the effects of other intervening sources. Generic measures, on the other hand, tend to provide benchmarking opportunities that are more likely to be standardized with established validity and reliability. In addition, generic instruments have greater breadth and are, therefore, able to capture treatment effects across multiple domains (Kane, 1997).

Because each approach has strengths and weaknesses, the best alternative may be to combine the two approaches. In other words, a generic measure is used with the capability of adding condition-specific questions to expand more deeply into the domains of particular interest. This approach retains the comparability of the generic measurement and provides sensitivity and depth for the domains of greatest interest (Kane, 1997).

A final consideration in the selection of outcome instruments includes the practicality of the instrument. One must consider its length, readability, and cultural sensitivity (Brooten, 1997; Thoman & Titler, 1997). The number of questions an instrument has and the layout and readability of those questions can have an impact on response rate. This, in turn, has implications for the quality of the sample obtained. Issues of sampling bias are prevalent in surveys. Often, presentation of survey data results in questions regarding those who chose not to respond and how they may be different from those who did respond.

SUMMARY

In a short time, outcome evaluation has been transformed from a value-added process to an essential commodity. Patients, providers, and payers all recognize the importance of collecting and analyzing outcomes to help achieve the goals of high-quality, cost-effective care. This evaluation has the potential to add considerably to the empirical basis of health care practice. By improving these processes, the nation has the opportunity to use its resources more appropriately and raise the health status of the population as a whole. This chapter provides an overview of the outcomes movement and attempts to provide the clinician with the necessary knowledge to approach outcomes evaluation appropriately. Outcome measures, like any other powerful tool, must be handled carefully by persons skilled in their use. Attention to measurement issues and strategies necessary to select and use instruments appropriately is vital to this effort. As Kane (1997) suggested, "The best outcomes evaluation is likely to come from partnerships of technically proficient analysts and clinicians, each of whom is sensitive to and respectful of the contributions the other can bring" (p. 254).

REFERENCES

Anonymous. (1996). Medical outcomes trust. *Bulletin, 4*(5), 1.

American Nurses Association. (1995). *Nursing report card for acute care settings*. Washington, DC: Author.

Aydelotte, M. (1962). The use of patient welfare as a criterion measure. *Nursing Research, 11,* 10–14.

Brooten, D. (1997). Methodological issues linking costs and outcomes. *Medical Care, 35*(11), NS87–NS95.

Burns, N., & Grove, S. K. (1997). Outcomes research. In *The practice of nursing research: Conduct, critique, & utilization* (3rd ed., pp. 569–611). Philadelphia: W. B. Saunders.

Champion, H. R., Copes, W. S., Sacco, W. J., Lawnick, M. M., Keast, S. L., & Frey, C. F. (1990). The major trauma outcome study: Establishing national norms for trauma care. *The Journal of Trauma, 30*(11), 1356–1365.

Crane, S. C. (1992). A research agenda for outcomes research. In Patient outcomes research: Examining the effectiveness of nursing practice (NIH publication No. 93–3411, 54–62). Bethesda, MD: National Institutes of Health.

Davies, A. R., & Ware, J. E. (1991). *GHAA's consumer satisfaction survey and users manual.* (2nd ed.). Washington, DC: Group Health Association of America.

Donabedian, A. (1985). *The methods and findings of quality assessment and monitoring: An illustrated analysis.* Vol. 3. Ann Arbor, MI: Health Administrative Press.

Donabedian, A. (1966). Evaluating the quality of medical care. *Milbank Memorial Fund Quarterly, 44*(Suppl. 3), 166–206.

Goldberg, H. I. Cummings, M. A., Steinberg, E. P., Ricci, E. M., Shannon, T., Soumerai, S. B., Mittman, B. S., Eisenberg, J., Heck, D. A., Kaplan, S., Kenzora, J. E., Vargus, A. M., Mulley, A. G., & Rimer, B. K. (1994). Deliberations on the dissemination of PORT products: Translating research findings into improved patient outcomes. *Medical Care, 32*(Suppl. 7), JS9–JS110.

Greene, R., Maklan, C. W., & Bondy, P. K. (1994). The national medical effectiveness research initiative. *Diabetes Care, 17*(Suppl. 1), 45–49.

Greenfield, S., Kaplan, S. H., Sillman, R. A., Sullivan, L., Manning, W., D'Agostino, R., Singer, D. E., & Mathan, D. M. (1994). The uses of outcomes research for medical effectiveness, quality of care, and reimbursement in type II diabetes. *Diabetes Care, 17*(Suppl. 1), 32–39.

Griffiths, P. (1995). Progress in measuring nursing outcomes. *Journal of Advanced Nursing, 21*, 1092–1100.

Guadagnoli, E., & McNeil, B. J. (1994). Outcomes research: Hope for the future or the latest rage? *Inquiry, 31*, 14–24.

Haussmann, R. K., & Hegyvary, S. T. (1976). Monitoring the quality of nursing care. *Australian Nurses Journal, 5*(8), 29–32.

Hegyvary, S. T. (1991). Issues in outcomes research. *Journal of Nursing Quality Assurance, 5*(2), 1–6.

Hinshaw, A. S. (1992). Welcome: Patient outcomes research conference, In Patient outcomes research: Examining the effectiveness of nursing practice (NIH Publication No. 93–3411, pp. 9–10). Bethesda, MD: U. S. Department of Health and Human Services.

Horn, B. J., & Swain, M. A. (1978). Criterion measures of nursing care (DHEW Publication No. PHS 78-3187). Hyattsville, MD: National Center for Health Services Research.

Hover, J., & Zimmer, M. (1978). Nursing quality assurance: The Wisconsin system. *Nursing Outlook, 26*, 242–248.

Iezzoni, L. I. (1994). Using risk-adjusted outcomes to assess clinical practice: An overview of issues pertaining to risk adjustment. *Annuals of Thoracic Surgery, 58*, 1822–1826.

Jacox, A. (1994). Nursing-sensitive patient outcomes. In J. J. Fitzpatrick, J. S. Stevenson, & N. S. Polis (Eds.), *Nursing research and its utilization.* New York: Springer.

Jennings, B. M. (1995). Outcomes: Two directions—research and management. *AACN Clinical Issues, 6*(1), 79–88.

Johnson, M., & Maas, M. (1997). *Iowa outcomes project: Nursing Outcomes Classification (NOC).* St. Louis: Mosby.

Joint Commission for Accreditation of Healthcare Organizations. (1994). *A guide to establishing programs for assessing outcomes in clinical settings.* Oakbrook Terrace, IL: Author.

Joint Commission for Accreditation of Healthcare Organizations. (1997). *Nursing outcomes and outcomes measurement.* Oakbrook Terrace, IL: Author.

Jones, K. R., Jennings, B. M., Moritz, P., & Moss, M. T. (1997). Policy issues associated with analyzing outcomes of care. *Image: Journal of Nursing Scholarship, 29*, 261–267.

Kane, R. L. (1997). *Understanding health care outcomes research.* Gaithersburg, MD, Aspen Publishers.

Kelly, K. C., Huber, D. G., Johnson, M., McCloskey, J. C., & Maas, M. (1994). The medical outcomes study:

A nursing perspective. *Journal of Professional Nursing, 10,* 209–216.

Lamb, G. S. (1997). Outcomes across the care continuum. *Medical Care, 35*(11), NS106–NS114.

Lang, N. M., & Marek, K. D. (1990). The classification of patient outcomes. *Journal of Professional Nursing, 6,* 153–163.

Lohr, K. N. (1988). Outcome measurement: Concepts and questions. *Inquiry, 25,* 37–50.

Marek, K. D. (1989). Outcome measurement in nursing. *Journal of Nursing Quality Assurance, 4*(1), 1–9.

Mark, B. A. (1995). The black box of patient outcomes research. *Image: Journal of Nursing Scholarship, 27,* 42.

Mitchell, P. H., Heinrick, J., Moritz, P., & Hinshaw, A. S. (1997). Outcome measures and care delivery systems: Introduction and purposes of conference. *Medical Care, 35*(11), NS1–NS5.

National Committee for Quality Assurance (1996). HEDIS 3.0. Washington, DC: Author.

Nelson, E. C., Mohr, J. J., Batalden, P. B., & Plume, S. K. (1996). Improving health care, Part 1: The clinical value compass. *Journal on Quality Improvement, 22*(4), 243–258.

Nightingale, F. (1858). *Notes on matters affecting the health, efficiency, and hospital administration of the British army.* London: Harrison & Sons.

Reverby, S. (1981). Stealing the golden eggs: Ernest Amory Codman and the science and management of medicine. *Bulletin of the History of Medicine, 55,* 156–171.

Roper, W. L., Winkenwerder, W., Hackbarth, G. M., & Krakauer, H. (1988). Effectiveness in health care: An initiative to evaluate and improve medical practice. *The New England Journal of Medicine, 319,* 1197–1202.

Rubin, H. M., Gandek, B., Rogers, R., Kosinsky, M., McHorney, C., & Ware, J. (1993). Patient's ratings of outpatient visits and difference practice setting: Results from the medical outcomes study. *Journal of the American Medical Association, 280,* 835–840.

Schalock, R. L. (1995). *Outcome-based evaluation.* New York: Plenum Press.

Sonnefeld, S. T., Waldo, D. R., Lemieux, J. A., & McKusick, D. R. (1991). Projections of national health expenditures through the year 2000. *Healthcare Financing Review, 13*(1), 16.

Stewart, B. J., & Archbold, P. G. (1992). Nursing intervention studies require outcome measures that are sensitive to change: Part one. *Research in Nursing and Health, 15,* 477–481.

Stewart, B. J. & Archbold, P. G. (1993). Nursing intervention studies require outcome measures that are sensitive to change: Part two. *Research in Nursing and Health, 16,* 77–81.

Strickland, O. L. (1997). Challenges in measuring patient outcomes. *Nursing Clinics of North America, 32,* 495–512.

Tarlov, A. R., Greenfield, S., Nelson, E. C., Perrin, E., & Zubkoff, M. (1989). The medical outcomes study: An application of methods for monitoring the results of medical care. *Journal of the American Medical Association, 262,* 925–930.

Thoman, D., & Titler, M. G. (1997, September). *Methods and issues in outcomes management.* Paper presented at the Clinical Outcomes and Resource Management Conference, Iowa City, IA.

Titler, M. G. (1997, September). *Outcomes and resource measurement and management methodologies.* Paper presented at the Clinical Outcomes and Resource Management Conference, Iowa City, IA.

Titler, M. G., & Reiter, R. C. (1994). Outcomes measurement in clinical practice. *MEDSURG Nursing,* 3(5), 395–398.

U.S. Bureau of Census. Statistical abstract of the U.S.: 1997 (117th ed). Tables 153 & 698, pp. 112, 452, Washington, DC: Author.

U.S. Department of Health and Human Services. (1991). The feasibility of linking research-related data bases to federal and non-federal medical administrative data bases (AHCPR Publication No. 1991). Rockville, MD: Author.

U.S. Department of Health and Human Services. (1992a). Acute pain management: Operative or medical procedures and trauma: clinical practice guidelines. (AHCPR Publication No. 92-0032). Rockville, MD: Author.

U.S. Department of Health and Human Services. (1992b). Patient outcomes research: Examining the effectiveness of nursing practice (NIH Publication No. 93-3411). Bethesda, MD: Author.

University HealthSystem Consortium. (1997). Satisfaction Data Base [On-line]. Available: www.uhc.edu/about/overview.html #13.

University HealthSystem Consortium and the Picker Institute. (1998). *Patient Satisfaction Survey program.* Boston: Picker.

Ware, J. E. (1993). *SF-36 health survey manual and interpretation guide.* Boston: The Health Institute, New England Medical Center.

Ware, J., & Hayes, R. (1988). Methods of measuring patient satisfaction with specific medical encounters. *Medical Care, 26*(4), 393–402.

Ware, J. E., Kosinski, M., & Keller, S.D. (1995). *SF-12: How to score the SF-12 physical and mental health summary scales.* Boston: The Health Institute, New England Medical Center.

Ware, J. E., & Sherbourne, C. D. (1992). The MOS 36-item short-form health survey (SF-36). I. Conceptual framework and item selection. *Medical Care, 30,* 473–481.

Wennberg, J., & Gittelsohn, A. (1982). Variations in medical care among small areas. *Scientific American, 246*(4), 120–134.

Wennberg, J. E., Roos, N., Sola, L., Schori, A., & Jaffe, R. (1987). Use of claims data systems to evaluate health care outcomes: Mortality and reoperation following prostatectomy. *JAMA, 257*(7), 933–936.

Werley, H. H., & Lang, N. M. (1988). *Identification of the Nursing Minimum Data Set.* New York: Springer.

Williams, B. (1994). Patient satisfaction: A valid concept? *Social Science Medicine, 38*(4), 509–516.

Wood, L.W. (1990). Medical treatment effectiveness research. *Journal of Occupational Medicine, 32*(12), 1173–1174.

Zapka, J. G., Palmer, R. H., Hargraves, J. L., Nerenz, D., Frazier, H. S., & Warner, C. K. (1995). Relationship of patient satisfaction with experience of system performance and health status. *Journal of Ambulatory Care Management, 18*(1), 73–83.

Chapter 8

Program Evaluation

Heidi S. Lepper and Marita G. Titler

Program evaluation is becoming increasingly important in the modern health care system as economic resources for new clinical programs are shrinking and the viability and impact of existing programs are questioned. Nurses must understand and use methods to evaluate the effectiveness of clinical programs in order to make decisions that are appropriate for the future of American health care. Health care dollars that support new clinical programs (for example, pulmonary rehabilitation, cardiac rehabilitation, or home care for high-risk mothers) are not likely to be forthcoming if the proposal for a new program does not incorporate a well-devised evaluation plan. Similarly, existing programs whose patient–client populations are shrinking or that are deemed too expensive are at risk for being reduced or eliminated. Health care providers and nurse managers who are unable to produce information that illustrates the effectiveness of a program to elicit practice change, improve the quality of care, or reduce medical dollars spent are at greatest risk of having programmatic resources eliminated.

This chapter focuses on program evaluation from a clinical perspective. Methods de-scribed in this chapter are useful for nurses to use in evaluating a variety of clinical programs, such as discharge programs for new mothers; pulmonary, cardiac, or orthopedic rehabilitation programs; preoperative preparation of patients; and case management programs for the indigent elderly. Every nurse should know the essential components of a comprehensive clinical program evaluation and how to transform data into information for subsequent decision making. In this chapter, "clinical program" is viewed broadly to encompass entire programs that have various components (such as those previously listed) and programs that incorporate newly developed research-based practice protocols. The methods discussed herein can be applied to evaluate the various forms of changes in clinical practice.

In this chapter, particular attention is given to summative evaluation and the importance of well-defined and measurable outcome variables. Oftentimes, the sole focus of program directors is on the development, implementation, and process of the clinical program itself. Therefore, the long-term impact of the clinical program on patient care or its effectiveness to elicit practice change is neglected. For this reason, mastery of summative evaluation is particularly important in the modern climate of nursing quality improvement initiatives.

OVERVIEW OF PROGRAM EVALUATION

Three distinct phases encompass the process of program evaluation; they are (1) program planning, (2) program implementation, and (3) program success or effectiveness (Murray, 1992). The first two phases (program planning and implementation) are jointly termed *formative evaluation*, whereas the third is termed *summative evaluation*. In each of these evaluative phases, two types of data can be collected and examined, and the type of information obtained from each is inherently different. Data approaches are either *qualitative* or *quantitative*; the former is a nonnumerical or narrative approach (quality), whereas the latter is a numerical or statistical approach (quantity).

Formative Evaluation

The purposes of formative evaluation are to assess, monitor, and report on the development and progress of implementing a clinical program (King, Morris, & Fitz-Gibbon, 1987). Formative evaluations are conducted both before and during program implementation. A well-planned and executed formative evaluation helps ensure that the purpose of the program is well defined, its goals are realistic, and its variables of interest are measurable. In addition, formative evaluation focuses on the proper training of staff who will be involved in the program implementation. During this evaluation phase, data, which serve to monitor the activities of the project, are collected.

An example of formative evaluation is illustrated using a pulmonary rehabilitation program. During the initial implementation of a pulmonary rehabilitation program, it is important that during the planning phase of the program, a final decision is made about the overall purpose of the program and its component parts (Table 8–1). The knowledge and skills of the personnel regarding the components and purpose of the program need to be assessed. For example, a pulmonary clinical nurse specialist can provide oversight for program development and implementation, including working with physical therapists, respiratory therapists, and physicians in making decisions regarding program personnel qualifications, location for the program, referral base for patients, the time frame for program implementation, and the projected outcomes that serve to monitor the effectiveness of the program (see box).

Summative Evaluation

A summative evaluation, in contrast, focuses on measuring the general effectiveness or success of the program by examining the outcomes of the program. A summative evaluation includes information about whether the clinical program reached its intended goals, whether its purpose was upheld, and whether the intervention produced unanticipated outcomes; it even compares the effectiveness of the program with other similar interventions (King et al., 1987). This type of evaluation is conducted once the incorporation of changes suggested by formative evaluation are made and the program is completed. Summative evaluations compare the effectiveness of the different treatment programs, if more than one is implemented, or makes comparisons among persons in the "treatment" group (for example, those enrolled in the pulmonary rehabilitation program) and a natural comparison group (for example, those not enrolled in rehabilitation). Comparisons can also be made over time to determine the relative influence of the program at differ-

 Key Aspects of Formative Evaluations

- Delineate phases of the program and time frame for each phase.
- Assess staff perceptions of program implementation to aid in determining how well the program runs.
- Examine referral of patients into the program and whether patient enrollment is upheld.
- Obtain feedback about the program from patients.

Table 8–1

Example of Formative Evaluation in Pulmonary Rehabilitation Program

Planning Phase

Purpose of the Program: To improve activity level, to reduce symptoms, and to decrease health care resource use among patients with chronic obstructive pulmonary disease (COPD).

Components of the Clinical Program. To implement a pulmonary rehabilitation program in which physicians, clinical nurses, physical therapists, and occupational therapists collaborate to facilitate increasing activity tolerance among COPD patients through an outpatient rehabilitation program. The patients are required to learn and perform program exercises on an outpatient basis; perform these activities at home on their own or with the assistance of a friend or spouse; receive patient education about oxygen use, medication use, and management of symptoms; monitor their oxygen use; rate their ability to perform self-care behaviors; monitor their medication use; and rate their functional status on a continuing basis.

Program Protocol. Delineate the requirements of patients and the duties of staff to implement successfully the pulmonary rehabilitation program. This protocol should also include the plan for staff training and data collection and quality improvement methods. This protocol must also be clear to the staff involved in implementing the program. The patients must understand what is required for their participation in the rehabilitation program.

Implementation Phase

Evaluate Staff Training Program. Examine how staff are trained to follow the program protocol, to answer patient questions, and to ensure patient adherence to the program. Staff need to be trained in the correct methods of increasing activity tolerance among COPD patients, in educating patients on how to monitor their medication use and oxygen use, and in rating levels of functional status and ability to manage self-care behaviors.

Process Variables. Assess how well the program protocol is being implemented. Measure timeline and frequencies for patient recruitment into the program, determine whether number of staff involved in the program is sufficient, run focus groups or use interviews or diary data with patients and staff to determine whether there are any problems with the program implementation, and determine the barriers to efficient running of the program. Most importantly, determine the level of adherence of patients to their exercise requirements, their self-monitoring requirements, and their self-rating requirements. Also determine the level of adherence among staff to guidelines presented to them in the program protocol. By using direct observation techniques, the evaluator can determine how well the staff and patients are interacting during the outpatient phase of the program and how well the staff are collaborating with each other to increase activity tolerance among the participating patients and to track other process variables of interest.

---

ent stages. In other words, the summative evaluation also seeks to determine the long-term and lasting effects on patients for having participated in the program.

The two phases of an evaluation, formative and summative, can be further understood in terms of "process" versus "outcome." Process refers to *how* the program is run or *how* the program reaches its desired results. A formative evaluation is process-focused and requires a detailed description of the operating structure required for a successful clinical program. Outcome refers to the success of a program and the effects that it has on cost and quality of care. Outcomes can be individualized, whereby the effects of the program on each of the clients in the program are examined. The evaluator in this instance seeks to determine the im-

pact of the program on the personal lives of those involved. Outcomes can also be program-based, whereby the success of the program is examined on an organizational level and its overall impact determined. These program-based outcomes are often examined in terms of their fiscal impact or success as well as in comparison with the clinical program with other similar programs.

Use of Qualitative and Quantitative Data

Both qualitative and quantitative data are useful for program evaluations, although, oftentimes, one is chosen over the other. Qualitative data, which have rich and narrative quality, provide an understanding about the impact of the program for individuals enrolled in the program. The descriptive nature of qualitative data allows one to understand the operating structure of a program and the individualized outcomes of a successful program. On the other hand, quantitative data, which have a strictly numerical nature, provide statistical significance levels and power, and mathematical understanding of the factors involved in a program. In addition, quantitative data provide frequency counts and means or averages for the variables of interest. The statistical nature of quantitative data allows understanding of the overall programmatic outcomes and makes possible direct comparisons among clients and between program groups (if there are more than one). Most often, evaluators and clinicians have tended toward utilization of only one of these approaches, neglecting the beneficial provisions of the other. The two forms of data are not necessarily at odds with one another, but instead should be used in combination because each supplements the weaknesses inherent in the other. For qualitative data, direct observation and description are emphasized because these lead to a form of discovery or understanding of how program factors relate on an individual or client level. Quantitative data tend to rely upon standardized instrumentation and variable control and provide numerical figures that depict level of program success.

Triangulation is one way that both qualitative and quantitative data can be incorporated into a program evaluation. Denzin (1978) has described four forms of triangulation:

1. *Evaluator triangulation* is the use of several program staff members who have direct client interaction in order to reduce any bias that may be introduced by using a single staff member for the interactions.
2. *Perspective or theory triangulation* is the use of various perspectives to interpret the evaluator's results.
3. *Method triangulation* is the use of different methods on the part of the evaluator to evaluate the program.
4. *Data triangulation* is the collection of various types of data that seek to answer the same questions.

Data triangulation is the form most often used in program evaluations. To determine effectively the success of a clinical program, evaluators must measure and use several forms of data. For instance, the evaluator can gather information from patient medical records, self-reports made by staff and patients, self-reports made by the spouse of married patients, and direct observations. By combining various types of data that seek to answer the same questions, the weakness in each data source is supported by the strengths in another source. The most obvious drawback to using a triangulation method for program evaluation is its expense. The benefits of using at least more than one method, however, may be sufficient to warrant this added expense.

STEPS IN PROGRAM EVALUATION

The steps involved in a program evaluation are summarized in Table 8–2. Each of the steps are described in detail in the subsequent sections.

Selecting and Defining Variables of Interest

The first step in any program evaluation is to define carefully and accurately the independent (process) and dependent (outcome) variables to be measured. This step is likely the most daunting as well as the most important. Variable selection and definition must be precise enough not to be cumbersome for evaluation staff or for data analysis, yet to retain variables that are both meaningful and measurable. During formative evaluations, process variables are of primary interest, whereas during summative evaluations, outcome variables are of interest. Again, using the pulmonary rehabilitation example discussed previously, a process variable of importance is whether patients are learning how to exercise on their own while at home. An outcome variable in this example is defined as the level at which patients are still exercising 6 months to 1 year after completion of the formal program.

INDEPENDENT OR PROCESS VARIABLES

One of the most important independent or process variables that needs to be measured in program evaluations is level of pa-

Table 8–2

Examples of Evaluation Steps for Formative and Summative Evaluations

STEPS IN EVALUATION	FORMATIVE EVALUATION	SUMMATIVE EVALUATION
Selecting and defining variables of interest	Focus on process variables that determine how well the program is running. Are patients being recruited? Have staff been properly trained in the program protocol? Are staff members following program protocol? Are patients adhering to program requirements?	Focus on outcome variables that determine the effectiveness of the program. Were patients and staff satisfied with the program? Did patient health improve significantly? Were medical resources reduced as a result of the program? Are patients continuing the program on their own once the program is completed?
Measuring variables of interest	Focus on ways to measure how well the program is being run. Use the following: Focus groups to discuss problem areas and ways to improve the program Direct observation to measure how the staff are following protocol Staff diary data to measure problems that occur on a daily basis Interviews of patients to determine how well they are adhering to the program requirements	Focus on ways to measure the impact the program has had. Use the following: Self-reports of patients and staff to report on the progress of the patient in terms of health status, functioning, and symptoms Collateral reports from spouses of patients to get a second rating on the patient's improvements Biomedical data to determine changes in biological parameters of functioning Chart abstractions to measure health care resource use
Selecting a program evaluation design	Use descriptive designs or narrative accounts. Allow for a narrative account of how well the program is being run. Provide feedback from patients and staff on areas in need of improvement. Document patient adherence levels to the program requirements. Track process variables over the implementation of the program.	Use experimental, quasi-experimental, or sequential designs (when possible). Allow for a comparison among groups of patients that were assigned to receive the program or not to receive the program. Use random assignment to program groups whenever possible. Use overtime examinations, if resources permit. Allow for determination of impact that the program has had on patients' lives.

Table 8–2

Examples of Evaluation Steps for Formative and Summative Evaluations *Continued*

STEPS IN EVALUATION	FORMATIVE EVALUATION	SUMMATIVE EVALUATION
Data collection strategies	Use uniform collection procedures that do not disrupt the program implementation. Collected data must be coded with a uniform system that translates narrative data into meaningful groupings. For example, focus group comments can be grouped into comments about staff-related problems, patient-related problems, recruitment difficulties, and adherence difficulties. Program evaluators should not bias data collection strategies by holding preconceptions about how well the program is being run.	Use systematic procedures for collecting data across groups (if more than one) and across time. Collected data must be coded with a uniform system that translates the data into numerical values so that data analysis can be conducted. For example, responses to a question about health status that include poor, fair, good, and excellent need to be coded as 0, 1, 2, and 3. Across time data collection must follow the same procedures. For example, all patients either receive self-reports in the mail or from the program site. The procedures must not vary across patients.
Evaluating data analysis	Use both qualitative and quantitative approaches. Qualitative approaches provide narrative descriptions of the process variables. Allow for descriptive understanding of how well the program is running. Quantitative approaches provide frequency counts and means or averages for some of the variables of interest. For example, frequencies for patient recruitment can be computed for time periods in order to determine when lags in recruitment occurred and what the possible reasons are for the lag.	Use both qualitative and quantitative approaches. Qualitative approaches provide a narrative description of the impact that the program has had on individual patients. Quotes from patients to exemplify the personal impact can be used. Quantitative approaches provide the statistical comparison between groups (if more than one) or across time. Quantitative approaches can determine if the program was effective in increasing patient health status, increasing staff and patient satisfaction, and reducing the number of health care resources used. Quantitative approaches can also serve to make comparisons with other similar clinical programs.

tient adherence to any treatments or self-care regimens prescribed by the program. More than 25 years of research indicate that, on average, 40% of patients fail to adhere to the recommendations prescribed to them to treat their acute or chronic conditions (DiMatteo & DiNicola, 1982). The effectiveness of an intervention cannot be determined unless it is known how well patients adhere to the requirements of the intervention, which should be a sole focus of formative evaluations. Patient nonadherence has been found to be a causal factor in the time and money wasted in medical visits (Haynes, Taylor, & Sackett, 1979), and it must not be overlooked in determining how well a nursing intervention or new clinical program is being implemented. How well a program is implemented is intimately linked to level of patient adherence to the requirements of the program. For instance, if a program introduces barriers to adherence, such as by requiring time-intensive self-care routines, by introducing complex treatments with numerous factors to remember, by making it difficult to get questions answered, or by having uninformed or untrained staff, patient adherence will be diminished. As a complement to patient adherence is the issue of how well the nursing staff maintains or adheres to the program protocol. The integrity of an intervention or program is not upheld unless the staff assigned to carry it out are diligent in following procedures and protocol (Kirchhoff & Dille, 1994). In addition to the measurement of patient adherence, program evaluators need to ascertain the level at which staff members are adhering to the program.

The process variables important during formative evaluations include (1) how well patients are recruited into the program, (2) how well-trained and well-informed the staff are about the purpose and importance of the program, (3) the barriers (if any) to the implementation of the program, (4) the level at which the program site is conducive to conducting a well-run program, and (5) the perceptions held by staff and patients about the usefulness of the program. These factors generally are easier to correct than are the issues of patient and staff adherence. For this reason, evaluators need to spend a considerable amount of time in assessing and adjusting patient and staff adherence to program procedure and protocol.

DEPENDENT OR OUTCOME VARIABLES

Examples of dependent or outcome variables (Fitzgerald & Illback, 1993) that are measured by social scientists and health care services evaluators in determining the effectiveness of health care interventions include the following:

- Patient health status and daily functioning
- Patient satisfaction with providers and medical care received
- Health care provider satisfaction
- Medical cost containment

Evaluators and nurses alike should consider each of these variables as outcomes of a clinical program. The evaluator who conducts a program evaluation and who attempts to determine program effectiveness or success should pay particular attention to these four outcomes.

The first important outcome variable is that which defines and measures whether the intervention has allowed the patient to better his or her health or functional status. The outcome of importance is whether the research intervention has improved the quality of the patient's life and whether health goals have been achieved. If the intervention does not increase these outcome variables and the protocol or intervention has been followed (that is, patient and staff have adhered to the program), then the effectiveness of the program is questionable. Although expectations for health improvements may not be a focus of the program, client health status is an important outcome variable that needs to be examined. For this reason, measuring patient health status multiple times and in multiple ways through triangulation techniques over the course of the program, and even once the program is completed, needs to be a focus during summative evaluations.

As the empirical literature has made clear over the past 20 years, one of the most important outcomes of the health care delivery process is patient satisfaction. Increased patient satisfaction, as a result of the implementation of a new program, is another indicator of whether the intervention is effective. Research suggests that an intervention that decreases a patient's satisfaction with his or her health care may lead the patient to experience poorer health (Kaplan, Greenfield, & Ware, 1989), to adhere less well to treatments (Ong, DeHaes, Hoos, & Lammes, 1995), to keep fewer follow-up appointments (DiMatteo, Hays, & Prince, 1986), to litigate malpractice claims more often (Hickson et al., 1994), and to seek health care elsewhere (Ross & Duff, 1982) than a patient whose satisfaction is increased. Evaluators need to take into account changes in patient satisfaction with the program in particular, and with their health care in general, because any decrease in satisfaction can point to problems in the purpose, scope, and execution of the program.

Another outcome that is oftentimes overlooked is that of nursing staff satisfaction. Slevin, Somerville, and McKenna (1996) measured staff satisfaction during the evaluation of a quality improvement initiative and found that satisfaction among the nurses was related to better interpersonal care of patients. Level of satisfaction can pertain directly to the process and implementation of the intervention, or it can be more generally defined and include professional satisfaction. An intervention that introduces frustrations for the nursing staff will likely not be conducted in the fashion that was intended, will serve to diminish the quality of care delivered, and perhaps will influence the two outcomes previously discussed—patient satisfaction and health status. The staff who must implement the intervention on a daily basis and who must interact and negotiate with patients must be satisfied with the new program. Thus, evaluations of new interventions or programs also must address the impact that the program has on the staff involved and not simply the impact that it has on the patients.

Finally, of considerable importance to program evaluation is the outcome variable of cost containment or reduction. An effective program is one that improves the quality and delivery of care while maintaining, perhaps even reducing, medical costs to both the organization and the patient. This evaluation outcome, however, is generally long-term in nature and requires multiple follow-ups, which can pose a considerable burden for programs with limited resources. The data that may be available to assist in this aspect of outcome evaluation include information about any patient hospitalizations and related lengths of stay, emergency room visits, regular doctor office visits, sup-

plies and equipment costs, and personnel time. Program evaluators can work collaboratively with financial management personnel to acquire this necessary information.

Selecting Ways to Measure Variables

The next step in the evaluation process is to select the way in which each variable of interest will be measured. In making this decision, it is important to consider, first, the many ways in which variables can be assessed and measured (for example, self-reports, biomedical instrumentation, direct observation, or chart abstraction) and, second, the source from which the data will be collected (for example, patient, staff, or medical records). Measurement is an important element of program evaluation; without rigorous, reliable, and valid information, the data obtained and subsequent recommendations are questionable.

Program evaluators need to consider, if possible, the use of highly valid and reliable research instruments, rather than developing new instruments to measure the variables of interest. Many forms of instrumentation exist and many have been used in previous evaluations of new clinical programs (see box).

Several reference books contain compilations of a multitude of research instruments and normative data for measures (Robinson, Shaver, & Wrightsman, 1991; Stewart & Ware, 1992).

Fitzgerald and Illback (1993) delineate the various methods of obtaining information and corresponding data sources to consider in program evaluation. *Self-reports* from patients and from staff are likely the most widely used for acquiring information about the process and effects of an intervention. These measures are completed by participants and staff involved in clinical programs and they can often be completed at the individual's leisure. These measures can be either user-friendly, whereby the individual completes the questionnaire by circling his or her response to the various items, or research-friendly, whereby the individual transfers his or her responses onto a computer-scannable form. The main advantages of self-reports are their ease of use, cost-efficiency, limited coding requirements, and little need for highly trained staff to implement their use. The main disadvantage, in

➤ Benefits of Using Published Instruments to Gather Self-Report Information

- Gathered information has a greater chance of being reliable and valid. That is, the instrument measures what it intends to measure and has internal consistency.
- The program evaluator has a normative group by which to compare ranges, means, and standard deviations on the instrument to the sample being evaluated.
- The instrument is composed of items or questions that are understandable by the majority of respondents.
- The instrument has a response format that both fits with the stem of the question and is responded to with relative ease.

contrast, is the prevalent belief that self-report instruments elicit self-presentation tendencies (that is, individuals present themselves in a socially desirable manner or in a positive light). This view is often unfounded, in that many measurement experts hold the view that most people, most of the time, are accurate in their self-reported responses (Ware, Davies-Avery, & Donald, 1978; Stewart & Ware, 1992).

In addition to self-report inventories that the participant completes, *collateral reports* can be obtained. These reports rely upon the same instruments as those used for self-reports, however, with slight modifications in wording regarding the pronoun. These measures can provide additional information about the patient and can even provide a check on the patient's responses. Collateral reports are completed by an individual very close to the participant in the study (usually a spouse). These types of reports have not been used to a great extent in nursing research, although they have been used extensively in psychological research. These collateral measures have been found to be highly correlated with the self-report data and can serve either as a validity check on the self-report data or as an additional

source of variant information to be used in the program evaluation. For instance, if the collateral reports are consistently lower than self-reports in measures for health status, then the evaluator may feel compelled to question the level of honesty in which the responses were provided.

Use of *structured and unstructured interviews* is another method for acquiring information. Compared to the use of self-report questionnaires, interviewing either in face-to-face interactions or over the telephone adds a few benefits to the information obtained, yet also introduces a few drawbacks. The benefits of interviews include the ability to clarify any confusing questions or items for participants, to increase participant rates in the program, to obtain more complete information (that is, individuals are often more likely to leave questions blank on questionnaires), and to obtain narrative accounts that are not restricted by standardized questions and response formats. The main drawback to interviews, however, is the need for highly trained interviewers who are taught not to lead individuals into answers and who are not biased to the study (preferably interviewers should be blinded to the purpose of the program). Another drawback includes the reduced ability to acquire vast amounts of information, which self-report questionnaires have a greater ability to achieve.

Direct observation is an alternative method of measurement that does not rely upon the reports of the participants in the project. Observations, like interviews, require highly trained observers. To effectively obtain data, observers must record very specific and narrow pieces of information and may need to reduce the amount of time that a particular action is observed. For instance, a patient may be observed through the use of time-sampling techniques in which only the first 5 minutes or last 5 minutes of every hour are observed and recorded. In addition, direct observation can provide information only about observable behaviors and does not allow insight into the perceptions or attitudes of the participants.

A variation on interviews and direct observations is the use of *focus groups* (Packer, Race, & Hotch, 1994). The information obtained from focus groups is qualitative and is most beneficial when used during formative evaluations to assess areas that need to be further refined, changed altogether, or even eliminated. Focus groups were first used among marketing researchers and have been the method by which to obtain information about consumer preferences (Stewart & Shamdasani, 1990). The use of focus groups, however, is becoming a method used by program evaluators to understand patient preferences and expectations. For example, a focus group can be used to gather pertinent information from a group of patients who receive the clinical program or to provide feedback about how the program is proceeding. Focus groups can also be used (Morgan, 1988; Stewart & Shamdasani, 1990) to develop survey instruments specific to the program, to test hypotheses supported by the program, to learn how patients talk about the program or its directive, and to gather patients' perceptions about the program and its effectiveness and utility.

Stewart and Shamdasani (1990) have discussed the role of focus groups in program evaluation and defined the focus group technique as the collective interview of usually 8 to 12 individuals who are brought together as a group to discuss for an hour or 2 a particular topic. The group is generally directed by a trained moderator who keeps the discussion focused on the topic of interest; the moderator also enhances group interaction and probes for necessary details. Morgan (1988) points out that information acquired from group discussions is often more readily accessible than it would be from individual interviews, because individual members are cued or primed for giving information that they would not be in an interview. The topic of interest can vary depending on whether this technique is used during formative or summative evaluation of the success of the program.

Biomedical data include laboratory tests, blood pressure, heart and respiratory rates, or other types of data that require the use of a bioinstrument to collect data (for example, use of blood pressure monitor, heart rate monitor, or stress tests). Because of the expense of medical tests, their sole use in program evaluation may not be practical. If the program requires use of biomedical data collection as part of its protocol, however, the evaluator might be able to acquire this information. The type of biomedical information collected for program evaluations must provide information that is relevant to the program and its evaluation and that holds meaning outside of basic medical parameters. In other words, biomedical information is useless unless it can be translated into information that is directly meaningful in the determination of the effectiveness of the program (for example, if the goal of the program is to reduce hypertension, then the bioinstrumentation must demonstrate that blood pressure has been lowered among the program participants).

Medical record reviews or *chart abstractions* are another source of data to consider when conducting a program evaluation. Use of medical records as a data source requires development of a standardized evaluation form and coding scheme to use in abstracting data. These types of reviews need highly trained chart abstractors who are clear about the information to be gathered and the need to be systematic in the review process. Chart reviews oftentimes allow for the gathering of information that cannot be found by any other fashion. The main drawback to this method of measurement is that patient charts are not always complete or readable or do not contain accurate patient health histories. The main advantage of this method, on the other hand, is that the evaluator is relying upon an already developed set of data, no new data need to be collected, and retrospective data can be collected and used as part of the evaluation.

Using *diary data* is another method that can successfully measure the variables of interest. Diary data can be completed by either the health care provider or the patient; these data provide information that is immediate and time relevant. Data can be collected once a day (a nightly count of food consumed for that day), several times a day (when every prescription medication is taken), or even randomly (when a beeper goes off and the patient is required to write down the relevant information). The main disadvantage of using diary data is that patients and staff may not always take the necessary time to fill out the forms completely or accurately. Use of diary data, however, is a true advance in data collection when used in a triangulation method with the other forms of data discussed.

Selecting the Design

The third step in program evaluation is to select the method that will provide the in-

➤ Ways to Measure Variables

- *Self-reports* obtained from patients or staff
- *Collateral reports* obtained from family members
- *Structured or unstructured interviews* conducted by a trained interviewer
- *Direct observation* of the program implementation mechanisms
- *Focus groups* on benefits of and problems with the clinical program
- *Biomedical information* to substantiate progress of patient
- *Medical record* chart abstractions
- *Diary data* obtained from patients or staff

formation necessary to determine the effectiveness of a program. Numerous evaluation methods serve as both practical and efficient means to determine the effectiveness of new clinical programs and research-based interventions. For program evaluations to determine whether the outcomes of interest have improved, the program evaluation must be conducted with precision and stringency. The following discussion briefly describes evaluation methods or designs to consider using when conducting program evaluation. Each design differs in amount of time and financial expense to implement, the type of analysis plan necessary, the level of control that the evaluator has over the variables of interest, and the level of associated statistical power (Rossi & Freeman, 1989).

True, *randomized experiments* involve a comparison between one or more experimental groups that receive an intervention and a control group that does not receive the intervention. Participants in the experimental groups receive the research-based intervention or participate in the clinical program that is intended to effect a measurable outcome, whereas those in the control group serve as a comparison group. The key component to true experiments is the random assignment of patients to either the experimental group or the control group. This assignment process eliminates any individual differences among the groups before implementing the program. For this

reason, in experimental designs, the outcomes can be attributed to the program and not to differences among the participants of the program. Observed group differences in the selected program outcomes determine level of program success or failure. In other words, for the program to be deemed a success, it must have a significant, beneficial effect on the experimental group compared to individuals in the control group. If the clinical program is conducted in an experimental manner, program evaluators can decide to use this design in the evaluation by either assigning all of the participants to be evaluated or randomly selecting an equal number of participants from each group (experimental and control) for the evaluation.

In general, quantitative approaches to data collection are the most appropriate in experimental designs because these allow for statistical group comparisons. Before group comparisons are made, however, there is a need for a formative evaluation that should focus on how well the experiment is being conducted and whether random assignment to the groups is being upheld. The summative evaluation allows for comparisons to be made between the groups and to determine the true effectiveness of the intervention. Qualitative data are also helpful in experimental designs by illuminating the different perceptions held by those in the two separate groups. By providing a narrative description of the impact of the program on the individuals, the evaluator has further support for the effectiveness of the program.

Quasi-experiments involve the same intervention and comparison component as true experiments, except quasi-experiments differ in one critical way. Random assignment of subjects or participants to a "treatment" group is not feasible. For instance, a clinical program may have the goal of understanding gender differences in some health-related area. Because individuals cannot be randomly assigned to be in either the "male" or the "female" group, this design inherently involves a quasi-experiment. The evaluation process for quasi-experiments is similar to that for true experiments. The main difference, however, is observed during the summative evaluation. Because random assignment to treatment groups is not conducted, changes in outcome variables cannot be ensured to be the result of the intervention or clinical program. Differences among the individuals in the assigned groups (before group assignment) cannot be ruled out as producing observed changes in the outcome variables of interest.

One drawback to both experiments and quasi-experiments is the need for a control or natural comparison group. This need for an additional group can pose a limitation for research sites where patient participation is limited, recruitment of patients takes a great deal of time, or there is no natural comparison group available. In addition, some investigators have argued the ethical implications of providing some patients with care, or experimental care, and not providing equivalent care to other patients. For these reasons, a *cross-sequential design* might be the most practical. In the cross-sequential design, the program evaluator observes or assesses several different groups of patients over several time periods, but each group is observed initially in the same period (Rosenthal & Rosnow, 1991). This type of design allows the time of measurement and the patient group to be used as comparison groups, thus eliminating the need for a control group. In essence, a cross-sequential design simultaneously compares several different groups of patients on a set of variables observed during one time period. The evaluator is able to control for possible variations in how the program is conducted. If patients observed during the beginning of the program have different outcomes from those recruited later in the program, the evaluator can attempt to determine whether these differences are due to individual differences among the patients or to the program implementation differences.

Finally, *descriptive designs* are also useful in program evaluations. These designs track and describe key outcome variables over time and examine trends in data. Descriptive designs use a cross-sectional examination of reports of patients and staff, examine longitudinal trends in relationships among variables of interest, and provide narrative descriptions of the component parts of the program as viewed by patients and staff. These designs are particularly relevant for formative evaluations, because this phase of evaluation is focused on the process of planning and implementing the program as well as on *how* the program is being executed. Descriptions of the program can help to illuminate the areas related to problems in the execution, in particular the areas involved in adherence difficulties among the patients and the staff. For example, by examining the changes in functional status in a group of pulmonary rehabilitation patients over a 1-year period (by including measurements before the program, during the program, and after the program), the evaluator can determine to some degree the level of success of the program. If all of the patients are observed to have increases in their reports of functional status, and if this is corroborated by biomedical tests, staff reports, and diary data, then the program will likely be deemed effective. The true cause of the functional increases cannot be determined by such a design. The evaluator cannot guarantee that the program produced the better health of the patient.

Sample Size in Program Evaluations

When selecting a design for program evaluation, the evaluator must consider the necessary sample size for an effective evaluation. Sample size depends on several factors that must be taken into account. Among these factors are the expected effect size of the intervention (that is, whether the intervention produces a small amount or a large amount of change), the type of design used, and the analysis plan. For a further explanation of sample size and its related statistical power to detect significant effects, see Burns and Grove (1997), pp. 307–311.

Data Collection

The next step in evaluation is to establish a systematic procedure for data collection. For the data not to become contaminated (by bias or error), trained data collectors must be employed. The same procedures must be used for every participant in the program in order for the results of the evaluation to be trusted. Procedures for collecting the data to be used in the program evaluation should be the same for all individuals in the program, whether the data are collected from patients or from staff.

DATA COLLECTION QUALITY

The approach to data collection and its usefulness has always posed a dilemma in the evaluation of new clinical programs. Once the evaluator has decided upon data source, type, measurement, and collection strategy, the integrity of the data must be ensured at all levels. In all forms of data, similar problems become evident, in that each form requires precise units of measurement. Data collection procedures and data analysis are highly sensitive to variations, and one goal of the evaluator is to ensure the uniformity across the program. All collection procedures must be systematic, and potential bias on the part of the evaluator and the staff involved in the program must be eliminated.

DATA CODING

One of the most tedious components of the evaluation process is the coding and entering of all relevant data (Keppel & Zedeck, 1989; Lipsey, 1994; Coffey & Atkinson, 1996). The protocol for coding data needs to be well developed early in program planning, and, whenever possible, it should follow a standardized and published method. Because much of the data collected during an evaluation is narrative, the coding scheme for analyzing the accounts must be succinct, efficient, and meaningful. The accounts are usually sorted and divided into a manageable number of conceptual or programmatic categories. Oftentimes, not all of these categories are used in the evaluation of the program; nevertheless, a systematic coding scheme should be followed. Additionally, all self-report data, biomedical data, and chart data should be coded into numerical values that can be used in the computations for the final evaluations. Again, these coding procedures should be uniform across all participants (patients and staff reports) and across all forms of data. For instance, the anchor on all items or questions should consistently be zero or one, and should not vary throughout the coding scheme (for example, if the question has the first response as "poor," the code should be "zero"; if the question has the first response as "none of the time," the code should be "zero"; if the question has the first response as "never," the code should be "zero").

During data coding, the evaluator must also keep track of the direction in which questions are worded, or in which data from charts and bioinstruments are abstracted, so that these can be correctly re-coded. Mul-tiple questions that measure the same variable should be analyzed only when they are all coded in the same direction. Because many questions are asked in a negative manner to reduce response biases, these questions need to be re-coded to reflect the direction of the other questions in the same scale. Re-coding should follow with the direction of the positively stated questions and should reflect a higher score of the variable being measured (for example, a high score on a health status scale should reflect better health).

Analysis of Evaluation Data and Interpretation

Once all data are coded properly and entered into a database, the evaluator can take on the task of data analysis. See Chapter 26 for a thorough discussion of how to conduct a proper analysis.

The program evaluator has a cautious task in interpreting the results of an evaluation once it has been completed. The results can sometimes be confusing, but are oftentimes unassuming. Small effects are predominant in most evaluations; however, small effects do not mean that the effect is unimportant. Every evaluator should understand the size of effects for each of the various statistics and the relative importance given to each size. The effect size refers to the magnitude of the relationship between two variables; the smaller the related coefficient, the smaller the effect. The evaluator must keep in mind that the effect size coefficient is meaningful only in a statistical sense and does not reflect the meaning that the effect has on the lives of individuals (Cohen, 1988; Rosenthal & Rosnow, 1991).

Writing an Evaluation Plan and Report

Writing a *summative evaluation report* and disseminating the report to key stakeholders and administrators are essential final steps in program evaluation (see box) (see Chapter 28).

A full report describing each point with documentation supporting each of these points is helpful for the individuals directly responsible for the clinical program. A short *executive summary* is useful for administra-

➤ Ten Components of a Program Evaluation Report

1. The purpose of the report
2. The nature of the clinical program and its component parts
3. The setting of the program (for example, inpatient or ambulatory care or home settings)
4. The time frame for the program
5. The program staff resources used
6. The way in which data obtained during the formative evaluation were used to alter the program and improve its implementation process
7. The evaluation methods used, including the evaluation of the program process and outcome variables
8. Results of the data analysis
9. Recommendations for program revisions, refinement, and continuation
10. Summary of the overall effectiveness of the program in achieving its designed purpose

port and the subsequent executive summary of a new clinical program may seem like a daunting task, but this serves as a template for annual program reviews and funding updates.

SUMMARY

In summary, planning, conducting, and analyzing a well-devised and comprehensive clinical program evaluation is, at worst, time-consuming and, at best, creative and challenging. The effort put forth in an evaluation can be rewarded with fiscal reinforcement, community recognition, and a sound future for the program. Programs that are found to be effective in terms of increasing patient and staff satisfaction, increasing patient health status, and saving medical dollars are likely the ones that will receive continued or increased funding. The main purpose of the program evaluator is to examine and protect the integrity of the program at all levels, because, without maintaining integrity, the outcomes of the program are questionable.

REFERENCES

Burns, N., & Grove, S. K. (1997). *The practice of nursing research: Conduct, critique and utilization.* Philadelphia, PA: WB Saunders.

Coffey, A., & Atkinson, P. (1996). *Making sense of qualitative data: Complementing research strategies.* Thousand Oaks, CA: Sage Publications.

Cohen, J. (1988). Statistical power analysis for the behavioral sciences (2nd ed.). Hillsdale, NJ: Lawrence Erlbaum.

Denzin, N. K. (1978). *The research act.* New York: McGraw-Hill Publishing.

DiMatteo, M. R., & DiNicola, D. D. (1982). *Achieving patient compliance: The psychology of the medical practitioner's role.* New York: Pergamon Press.

DiMatteo, M. R., Hays, R. D., & Prince, L. M. (1986). Relationship of physicians' nonverbal communication skill to patient satisfaction, appointment noncompliance, and physician workload. *Health Psychology, 5,* 581–594.

Fitzgerald, E., & Illback, R. J. (1993). Program planning and evaluation: Principles and procedures for nurse managers. *Orthopaedic Nursing 12*(5) 39–45.

Haynes, R. B., Taylor, D. W., & Sackett, D. L. (Eds.) (1979). *Compliance in health care.* Baltimore, MD: Johns Hopkins University Press.

Hickson, G. B., Clayton, E. W., Entman, S. S., Miller, C. S., Githens, P. B., Whetten-Goldstein, K., & Sloan, F. A. (1994). Obstetricians' prior malpractice experience and patients' satisfaction with care. *Journal of the American Medical Association, 272,* 1583–1587.

tors and those individuals responsible for making decisions about whether to continue or to expand the clinical program, or to downsize its scope. Also critical in this executive summary is to document clearly the association between the program and the outcomes of interest, and to demonstrate clearly the benefits of the program, the cost saved, and the number of patients served.

The executive summary is usually written following completion of the final summative report that is designed to be a more comprehensive report of the program evaluation. The executive summary needs to be as succinct and clear in the outcomes of the program as possible. In addition, it is often best to illustrate the results with diagrams and charts. The evaluator needs to make the recommendations for the program clear and action-oriented so that the executive committee or those directly responsible for the program are clear about the purpose and results of the program, and the best actions to take regarding the future of the program. Writing the final summative re-

Kaplan, S. H., Greenfield, S., & Ware, J. E., Jr. (1989). Assessing the effects of physician-patient interactions on the outcomes of chronic disease. *Medical Care, 27,* S110–S127.

Keppel, G., & Zedeck, S. (1989). *Data analysis for research designs.* New York: W. H. Freeman and Co.

King, J. A., Morris, L. L., & Fitz-Gibbon, C. T. (1987). *How to assess program implementation.* Newbury Park, CA: Sage Publications.

Kirchhoff, K. T., & Dille, C. A. (1994). Issues in intervention research: Maintaining integrity. *Applied Nursing Research, 7,* 32–38.

Lipsey, M. W. (1994). Identifying potentially interesting variables and analysis opportunities. In H. Cooper & L. V. Hedges (Eds.), *The handbook of research synthesis* (pp. 111–123). New York: Russell Sage Foundation.

Morgan, D. L. (1988). *Focus groups as qualitative research* (Sage University Paper Series on Qualitative Research Methods, Vol. 16). Beverly Hills, CA: Sage Publications.

Murray, A. D. (1992). Early intervention program evaluation: Numbers or narratives? *Infants and Young Children, 4*(4), 77–88.

Ong, L. M., de Haes, J. C., Hoos, A. M., & Lammes, F. B. (1995). Doctor-patient communication: A review of the literature. *Social Science & Medicine, 40,* 903–918.

Packer, T., Race, K. E. H., & Hotch, D. F. (1994). Focus groups: A tool for consumer-based program evaluation in rehabilitation agency settings. *Journal of Rehabilitation,* Summer, 30–33.

Robinson, J. P., Shaver, P. R., & Wrightsman, L. S. (1991). *Measures of personality and social psychological attitudes.* San Diego, CA: Academic Press.

Rosenthal, R., & Rosnow, R. L. (1991). *Essentials of behavioral research: Methods and data analysis.* New York: McGraw-Hill Publishing.

Ross, C. E., & Duff, R. S. (1982). Returning to the doctor: The effects of client characteristics, type of practice, and experience with care. *Journal of Health and Social Behavior, 23,* 119–131.

Rossi, P., & Freeman, H. (1989). *Evaluation: A systematic approach,* (4th ed). Newbury Park, CA: Sage Publishing.

Slevin, E., Somerville, H., & McKenna, H. (1996). The implementation and evaluation of a quality improvement initiative at Oaklands. *Journal of Nursing Management, 4,* 27–34.

Stewart, A. L., & Ware, J. E., Jr. (1992). *Measuring functioning and well-being.* Durham and London: Duke University Press.

Stewart, D. W., & Shamdasani, P. M. (1990). *Focus groups: Theory and practice* (Applied Social Research Methods Series, Vol. 20). Newbury Park, CA: Sage Publications.

Ware, J. E., Jr., Davies-Avery, A., & Donald, C. A. (1978). Conceptualization and measurement of health for adults in the health insurance study. In *General Health Perceptions* (Vol. V). Santa Monica, CA: The RAND Corporation.

Chapter 9

Case Management Outcomes in the Community Setting

Jennie T. Nickel

Competitive forces within the U.S. health care system are reorganizing and restructuring the delivery of care. As hospitals and community-based providers merge into networks capable of assuming risks of managed care for groups of enrollees, needs for maximizing efficient use of staff and service resources have become critical. At the forefront of most network responses to such needs is the case manager.

The role of the case manager is to assess patient needs and to coordinate or authorize receipt of services across hospital, clinic, and other community organizations. Case managers work directly with individual patients while maintaining a population or group focus. For example, a nurse case manager based in a managed care organization may be assigned to monitor use of psychiatric services by enrollees. The case manager would work directly with individuals requesting psychiatric services to verify that services are indicated and would refer those needing services to appropriate care. At the same time, the case manager would monitor use of psychiatric services by all plan enrollees to keep costs within boundaries established by the organization.

Case managers are thus placed in the sometimes untenable position of balancing responsibilities of advocating for individual patient services against responsibilities of restricting total costs of care. Case managers are expected to ensure quality of care and high patient satisfaction with services, yet minimize use of high-cost services and achieve efficiency in use of organizational resources (Haslanger, 1995; Rosenberg, 1995).

Little is known about how such conflicting demands are carried out and whether case management ultimately yields positive or negative impacts on patient outcomes. Despite a lack of evidence validating effectiveness of case management, a recent survey of health maintenance organizations reported that 86% of respondents plan to implement or expand case management programs (Pacala et al., 1995). In the public sector, federal legislation has promoted the introduction of case management as a service under home and community-based Medicaid programs (Omnibus Budget Reconciliation Act of 1981; Consolidated Omnibus Budget Reconciliation Act of 1985). Hence, research and evaluation of the impact of case management and the most effective ways of providing case management are urgently needed. This chapter discusses issues involved in evaluation of case management. Although case management has recently emerged as a role within acute-care settings, the focus of this chapter is case management of community-based patients. The processes used in evaluating case management programs in the two types of settings are similar, however.

The first section of this chapter defines case management, assesses current research related to effectiveness of case management in community settings, and identifies unanswered questions about case management. The second section of the chapter focuses on methods of evaluating case management, looking at comparison strategies used in evaluation of case management programs, and analyzing in detail steps of the evaluation process as it applies to case management.

DEFINING CASE MANAGEMENT

The functions of case management have evolved in community agencies in a variety of forms over the past decades. The roles and functions of case management differ so widely across agencies and sites that specification of elements of the case management role is required before achieving any degree of communication. Table 9–1 summarizes

elements of the case management role with variations commonly seen within community settings.

Case management models in community settings vary with regard to (1) characteristics of site, (2) professional discipline of the case manager, (3) population served, (4) size of caseload, (5) intensity of service, (6) nature of services provided, and (7) funding. Case management may be conducted by an individual provider or through consultation with an interdisciplinary team, as a freestanding service within a specialized case management agency or integrated within a system of care. Responsibilities may be constrained to organizational boundaries or extend throughout the community. There are three models of case management typically seen in community settings:

1. Local agency model
2. State purchase authority model
3. Managed care model

These models are based on a classification system by Davidson, Penrod, Kane, Moscovice, and Rich (1991) and incorporate varying patterns of the elements listed in Table 9–1.

Local Agency Model

The case management model generally seen in local community health and service agencies involves coordination of patient services obtained within the agency and referral and advocacy for services outside the agency. Case managers provide the basic functions of case finding, needs assessment, care planning, and monitoring, and, if the case manager is a nurse, may provide direct nursing care. Planning for client services is often conducted in collaboration with a multidisciplinary care team. Even with a team, however, an individual case manager is generally designated—usually a nurse or a social worker.

Eligibility for case management services may be restricted to patients categorized as high need. For example, a local health department may provide case management services to all new mothers identified with risk factors for child abuse. Case managers provide relatively intense service to agency patients during crisis times with reduced intensity of services throughout the time

Table 9–1

Elements of the Case Management Role and Variations Common to Community Settings

ELEMENTS OF THE CASE MANAGEMENT ROLE	COMMON VARIATIONS
Characteristics of site	State and local public health agencies
	State and local mental health agencies
	Voluntary health agencies
	Home health agencies
	Hospice
	State and local human service agencies
	State and local departments for the aging
	Child and adult protective service agencies
	Managed care organizations
	Insurance companies
	Case management agencies
Professional discipline of the case manager	Registered nurse
	Social worker
	Physician
	Administrative/clerical staff
	Volunteer
Population served	Total group (for example, all enrollees, clients, or beneficiaries)
	High-risk or high-use groups (for example, frail elderly, chronically ill or disabled, psychiatric patients)
Size of caseload	15 to 25 (for example, terminally ill home care of persons with acquired immunodeficiency syndrome)
	200 to 300 (for example, authorization of services by insurance case managers)
Intensity of service	Frequency of contact—daily to infrequent
	Nature of contact—for example, home visits, telephone consultation, office/clinic interviews, record monitoring
Nature of services provided	Basic services
	Case finding
	Assessment of patient/family needs
	Assessment of family and community resources
	Development of a plan of care
	Implementation of services, including making referrals
	Monitoring of patient progress
	Monitoring of quality of services
	Evaluation of patient/family outcomes
	Optional services
	Direct nursing care
	Interdisciplinary teamwork
	Utilization review
	Authorization of services
	Budgetary control
Funding	Agency budget
	Annual capitation
	Fee for service

they are followed up by the agency. Duration of case management services tends to be intermittent and episodic, and restricted to the time of eligibility for agency services. Case managers operate within a fixed agency budget and typically have no authority (or very limited authority) to purchase services for patients. Because of the proliferation of this model within community agencies, patients who receive services from multiple agencies tend to have multiple case managers, and lack of coordination among the case managers is often a problem.

State Purchase Authority Model

State human services (Medicaid) offices and other state agencies (for example, departments of aging) often separate authorization of case management services from actual provision of services, contracting with public or private, non-profit case management agencies to conduct patient needs assessment and provide case management services for patients with complex service requirements. For example, there may be a contract for case managers to organize and monitor services for low-income Medicaid patients with multiple sclerosis during late stages of disease. The goal of such services is to maintain community-based living and avoid the high costs of nursing home or institutional placement. Because of the complex physical care decisions required, case managers are typically nurses.

Case management costs are funded through an agency contract with the state and the state agency maintains authority for approving high-cost services. Savings for the state in terms of averted institutional costs are expected to offset the costs of the case management programs.

Managed Care Model

The most recent case management model to emerge is based within managed care systems. Payment to providers is negotiated prospectively, for example, through a capitated system (designating a dollar amount for each person authorized to receive services from the agency for a 1-year period regardless of services required), or, alternatively, by setting a reimbursement amount for an episode of care. Because success in obtaining contracts from managed care systems depends on keeping prices competitive with other managed care groups, incentives are maximized for case finding and service containment across components of the provider network (including hospitals, physician organizations, and long-term care agencies). Case managers in capitated systems work to keep health costs of high-use enrollees within the contracted limits and may have expenditure caps for enrollees. Case management is thoroughly integrated across the various provider sites and may be structured through use of a variety of professional disciplines (nurses, physicians, and social workers) and at varying levels of intensity at each site (Grower, Hillegass, & Nelson, 1996).

In summary, case management models are highly variable in organizational and service features. Nurse case managers involved in evaluating their own practices or in transferring research findings to their practice need to be aware of the variations in model features. Because of lack of consistency in model classification, case managers must look carefully at case management model specifications to determine whether they are similar to their own practices. If the practice is found to be incongruent with overall models, findings may need to be analyzed with respect to specific elements of the models.

RESEARCH ON CASE MANAGEMENT OUTCOMES

Research on case management in the community setting has focused on high-need populations. Studies have been conducted with the frail elderly (Carcagno & Kemper, 1988; Eggert, Zimmer, Hall, & Friedman, 1991), the mentally ill (Goering, Wasylenki, Farkas, Lancee, & Ballantyne, 1988; Borland, McRae, & Lycan, 1989; Hodgkin, 1992; Mechanic, Schlesinger, & McAlpine, 1995), high-risk prenatals and infants (Mawn & Bradley, 1993; Erkel, Morgan, Staples, Assey, & Michel, 1994), patients with acquired immunodeficiency syndrome (Sowell et al., 1992; Nickel et al., 1996), and Medicaid enrollees (Miller & Gengler, 1993). Table 9–2 highlights the design and findings of selected studies that evaluate effects of community-based case management.

The studies outlined in Table 9–2 were selected based on criteria of strength of the research designs, relevance to nurses as case managers, and variety of populations involved. The case management interventions included in Table 9–2 studies represent local agency models without purchase authority, the one exception being the financial authority model included as one of two case management models in the Long Term Care Demonstration Project (Carcagno & Kemper, 1988; Phillips, Kemper, & Applebaum, 1988).

Populations included in these studies were all at high risk for complex psychological or physical care needs, and nurses were used as case managers in five of the six studies reported. All studies reported in Table 9–2 included some type of comparison group. Four of the studies compared case managed with control groups, two studies compared alternative models of case management, and one study compared case management to other treatment approaches. Five of the six studies reported control or comparison groups studied concurrently with the case management intervention group so that bias of changes in treatment situations over time would not impact findings. The one possible exception, the study of Goering and colleagues (1988), selected the control group before the case management group and did not state whether intervention times were concurrent. Four of the six studies used random assignment to groups, which is the preferred method of ensuring that subjects in the groups will be comparable on characteristics that might influence outcomes of the case management intervention.

Because agencies often include at least part of the basic elements of case management within their protocols and procedures of routine care, differentiation of services received by the case-managed group from the routine-care group is critical to the evaluation of case management as a unique intervention. These six studies have differentiated case management from routine care by designing case management protocols that provided increased intensity of assessment and monitoring of services in relation to the comparison group. This increased intensity is reflected by smaller caseloads for the case managers, more frequent client contact, continuation of case management services over a predetermined period of time

rather than restriction to a crisis episode, a proactive schedule of client contacts rather than reactions to client-initiated contacts, and use of face-to-face home visits in addition to telephone or office contacts. Case manager expertise in relation to the illness or condition (for example, patients with acquired immunodeficiency syndrome or mental illness) and knowledge of community services (for example, neighborhood model) are also emphasized.

Outcomes reported in these and other studies of case management tend to be relatively short term and to fit within the categories of health status, satisfaction with services, use of services, and costs of care. Findings of case management studies have been inconsistent in supporting improved functioning or health status, increased satisfaction of patients with care received, substitution of low-cost for high-cost services, and lower overall costs. The impact of case management on informal services received by patients has been studied by some researchers (Solomon & Draine, 1995) but results remain inconclusive. The effects of clinical guidelines in directing case management protocols in the community setting have not been assessed.

EVALUATING CASE MANAGEMENT

As research and evaluation of programs within this emerging practice role develop, nurses must be able to evaluate alternative studies related to these questions and apply findings relevant to their own practices. They may also be required to conduct evaluations of the impact of their own case management activities within their agencies or systems. Skills in evaluation of health outcomes for groups—the same skills that operate in research design—are thus essential to the competencies of case managers.

The remaining sections of this chapter detail issues in evaluating case management in the community setting. Alternative evaluation designs are presented and the evaluation process is analyzed, with some reference to the studies outlined in Table 9–2. The remainder of the chapter provides direction for conducting case management evaluation with methodological rigor.

Table 9–2

Selected Research Studies Evaluating Impact of Case Management

Case Management Model (CM)

STUDY FEATURES	CARCAGNO & KEMPER (1988)	GOERING ET AL. (1988)	EGGERT ET AL. (1991)	ERKEL ET AL. (1994)	JERRELL & RIDGELY (1995)	NICKEL ET AL. (1996)
Site	Community service agencies in 10 states	Psychiatric aftercare program—Toronto	Local agency and neighborhood, Rochester, NY	Public health agencies in two counties in South Carolina	Three psychiatric and drug outpatient treatment programs	Seven home care/infusion agencies, Columbus, OH
CM Discipline	Social workers with nurses as supervisors and consultants	Psychiatric nurse, social worker, occupational therapist	Community health nurse, social worker	Community health nurses	Mental health professionals and workers	Community health nurses, with interdisciplinary team
Population	Frail elderly	Psychiatric adults	Frail elderly	Medicaid-eligible newborns	Dual diagnosis: psychiatric/substance use adults	Late-stage human immunodeficiency virus–positive adults
Study groups	Two CM groups—one with financial authority Control group with routine care	CM group Control group with routine care	Two CM groups—traditional individual model and neighborhood team model	One county with CM; control county with routine care	Three treatment groups: 1. AA 12-step program 2. Behavioral skills training 3. CM	CM group Control group with routine care
Services provided	1. Basic CM model* 2. Basic CM model plus financial authority and expanded resources	Basic CM model with psychiatric expertise	1. Basic CM model 2. Basic CM model and neighborhood focus	Basic CM model	CM focus on community living	Basic CM model and expertise in human immunodeficiency virus

Comparison Strategy	Concurrent with random assignment†	Control group selected prior to CM—no random assignment	Concurrent with partial random assignment	Concurrent—with out random assignment	Concurrent with partial random assignment	Concurrent with random assignment
Sample Size	6326	164	476	98	132	57
Times of Reported Outcomes/Findings	12 mo, 18 mo	24 mo	24 mo	9 mo	6, 12, 18 mo	3 mo, 6 mo
Health status	No difference in functional status or longevity	Increase in occupational functioning and housing independence; reduced social isolation	No difference in functioning or mortality rate	—	Decreased psychiatric symptoms; decreased social functioning	Improved quality of life scores but not statistically significant
Satisfaction	Increased satisfaction with care and with life	—	No difference	—	Increased global satisfaction	No difference
Use of services	Increased use of community service; no difference in use of medical or informal services; fewer unmet needs	No difference in hospital readmissions or length of stay	Team model with reduced hospital days, reduced home health aide hours and higher nursing home use.	Increased number of child clinic visits and percent with age-appropriate immunizations	—	Reduced use of high-cost services‡
Costs	Increased total costs with CM	—	Team model with reduced average annual costs	Cost-effectiveness ratio one fifth that of control	—	No difference in average per diem cost‡

* Basic CM model included assessment of needs and resources, developing a plan of care, implementing the plan, monitoring progress, and evaluating outcomes.
† Carcagno and Kemper restricted evaluation to randomly assigned groups.
‡ Unpublished data from Nickel et al.

Unanswered Questions Related to Case Management Evaluation

Research is lacking for essential questions such as

1. What are the effects of varying models of case management on patient outcomes such as health status, satisfaction with services, use of services, and costs of care?
2. Which population groups benefit most from case management interventions?
3. Which elements of case management practice are most beneficial to patient outcomes?
4. What are the long-term effects of case management?
5. What are the effects of variation in informal and formal resources within the family and community?
6. What are the effects of the use of clinical guidelines and critical paths in monitoring care delivered in community settings?

Choosing a Comparison Strategy for Evaluation

The initial strategic question encountered in evaluating case management practice is "What will serve as the standard for comparison?" The choice of the comparison is critical because it is the degree of difference in outcomes between the case managed and comparison groups that constitutes the evidence for or against effectiveness of case management as an intervention. Alternatives are (1) a concurrent control group, established through random assignment, (2) a concurrent control group selected without random assignment, (3) outcome indicator standards established with data submitted by multiple participating agencies, and (4) service records for time periods preceding the introduction of case management. Figures 9–1 through 9–4 illustrate these basic strategies, highlighting time dimensions for the comparisons. Each of these alternatives must be considered in terms of strengths, weaknesses, and the availability and quality of required data.

CONCURRENT CONTROL GROUP WITH RANDOM ASSIGNMENT

A concurrent randomized control group (Fig. 9–1) results from selection of a client sample from the population, random assignment to either a case-managed or a control group, intervention and follow-up prospectively in time, and assessment and comparison of outcomes of the two groups at predetermined time points. This design provides the optimal control of patient and situational characteristics, including control of variation over time of case management practice or improved technology. Even though the National Long Term Care Dem-

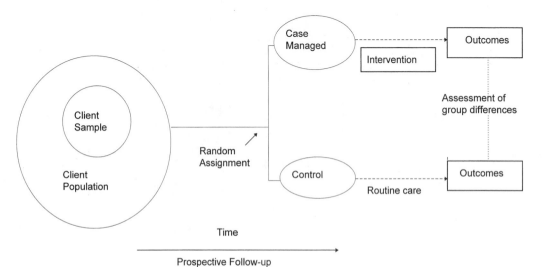

Figure 9–1
Evaluation strategy using concurrent control group with random assignment.

onstration Project (see Table 9–2) (Carcagno & Kemper, 1988) included both randomized and nonrandomized demonstration projects, evaluation of the project as a whole was limited to the randomized sites (Kemper, 1988). In practice, provider agencies may be reluctant to randomly assign patients to groups, thus committing one group to receiving a service that is intentionally withheld from the other. This reluctance is seen even though the merits of the intervention are undemonstrated.

A crossover design in which the groups alternate as intervention and control may be useful in avoiding such qualms. However, the question of how long the intervention phase should continue is often unclear, and carryover effects from the intervention to the control phase are likely to be a problem. A randomized control strategy with a delayed crossover of the intervention group might be acceptable.

CONCURRENT CONTROL GROUP WITHOUT RANDOM ASSIGNMENT

The second alternative, a concurrent non-randomized control group (Fig. 9–2), differs from the previous comparison strategy in that case-managed and control groups are drawn separately from the population, for example, from different geographical areas or from different clinical sites. This design

provides advantages of comparability of time periods and measurement of variables in both intervention and control groups. For example, Erkel and colleagues (1994) (see Table 9–2) implemented case management with Medicaid-eligible newborns in one county of South Carolina and compared outcomes with another county as control.

Disadvantages of this approach center around lack of control over differences in patient characteristics, such as socioeconomic status or disease severity. Erkel and colleagues noted that even though populations of the two counties were comparable in racial and socioeconomic characteristics, the case-managed county was rural and the control county was urban. They were unable to assess possible effects of the rural-urban difference on findings.

OUTCOME INDICATOR STANDARDS

The third alternative, use of outcome indicator variables such as measures of patient satisfaction and health status from pooled databases (Fig. 9–3), is an evaluation strategy that is gaining increasing attention, particularly within managed care environments. Outcome indicator standards are based on data using comparable measures aggregated across agencies.

Comparisons of results for a single network or agency to results reported by other

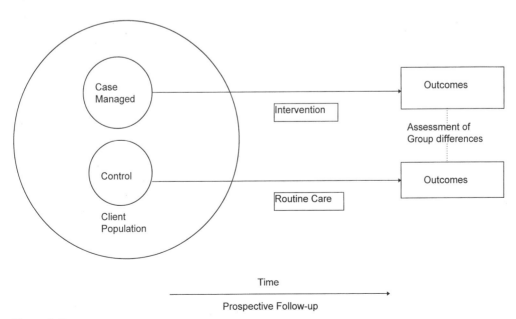

Figure 9–2
Evaluation strategy using concurrent control group without random assignment.

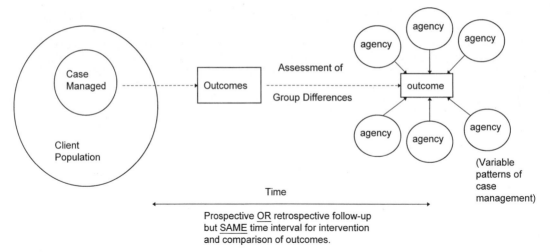

Figure 9–3
Evaluation strategy using outcome indicator standards established with data submitted by multiple participating agencies.

providers are again complicated by differences in patient characteristics and the nature and severity of illness. Also, the case management interventions may vary considerably across agencies and accuracy of provider reports is not ensured. Although this approach was not illustrated in Table 9–2 studies, it is increasingly referred to in the literature, and such "benchmarks" are likely to be extensively used in case management within managed care systems (Borok, 1995; Carroll, 1995). The Group Health Association of America (GHAA), a national managed care trade organization, developed the Consumer Satisfaction Survey (Davies & Ware, 1991) specifically for use as a comparable satisfaction measure across care providers. Similarly, the Health Plan Employer Data and Information Set (HEDIS) was recently developed by the National Committee for Quality Assurance as a listing of clinical indicators of quality of care for managed care enrollees (Corrigan & Nielsen, 1993). Alternative versions of HEDIS are available—a consumer version for use by providers in marketing services to employer purchasers of care and a second version for use by Medicaid enrollees in choosing between alternative managed care providers (MacPherson, 1996). Work is also in progress on outcome measures for Medicare patients (Hanchak, Harmon-Weiss, McDermott, Hirsch, & Schlackman, 1996) and for home care patients (Shaughnessy, Crisler, Schlenker, & Arnold, 1995).

Numerous provider agencies are reconfiguring patient data collection systems to ensure that the HEDIS indicators and GHAA satisfaction data are available. Case managers should be aware that even though the effects of agency case management activities may be reflected in HEDIS and GHAA satisfaction scores, case management as a program entity cannot be evaluated by global scores for the entire provider agency or managed care network.

RECORD REVIEW BEFORE AND AFTER INTRODUCING CASE MANAGEMENT

The fourth approach to choosing a comparison strategy (Fig. 9–4), use of service records before and after introduction of case management activities, does not provide an accurate evaluation of case management practice in a rapidly changing service environment. Because the time period of data collection for outcome measures in this design is not the same for the case-managed and comparison groups, differences that are observed are likely to be the result of factors other than the case management intervention, for example, changes in client or provider mix, and changes in treatment technology. Retrospective comparisons such as this also tend to be restricted by missing or noncomparable data in service records. Furthermore, documentation of illness under prospective payment systems is often slanted to maximize reimbursement and

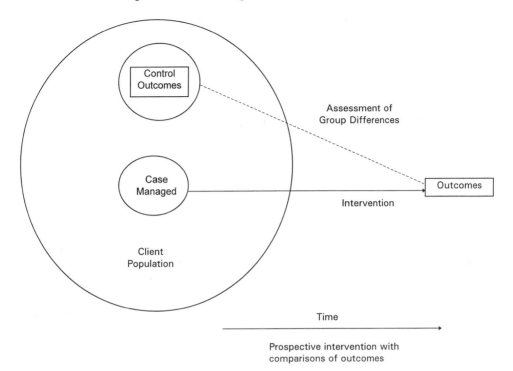

Figure 9–4
Evaluation strategy using service records for time periods preceding introduction of case management.

thus is not a valid indicator of severity of illness among patients served.

In summary, in choosing a comparison strategy for case management, the advantages of randomized assignment to groups make some form of this evaluation strategy preferable if at all possible. If use of an alternative strategy is required by practice circumstances, the case manager should carefully analyze potential problems and strive to offset these pitfalls in the evaluation designs.

STEPS OF THE EVALUATION PROCESS

The evaluation of case management is structured with progressive steps parallel to steps of both program evaluation and research processes. Considerations in program evaluation are in Chapter 8. Other helpful chapters are Chapter 13, for information on obtaining approval for a project, and Chapter 25, for planning data collection and conducting a study. Considerations in the evaluation of case management outcomes include patient population, case management implementation issues, outcome

measures, situational factors, integrated information systems, data analysis, and conclusions.

Patient Population

In addition to identification of the case management model, evaluation of case management requires specification of the patient population. Characteristics likely to affect outcomes of health, satisfaction, and service use and costs include patient age, socioeconomic characteristics, and nature and severity of illness. For example, if the case-managed patients are older, of lower socioeconomic status, or in poorer health than the comparison patients, the positive effects of case management may not be evidenced because of the greater service needs of the case-managed group. Percentages of new patients are also an important factor, because new patients tend to require more intensive case management services than established patients. Numbers of cases assigned to a case manager may vary from 15 to 20 to 200 or more depending on the intensity of case management services provided. Haslanger (1995) has observed that the research supports the statement, "You get what you pay for." That is, case management is more likely to be effective with smaller caseloads, resulting in greater intensity of case management services.

Characteristics of patients withdrawing from participation over the duration of the evaluation period must be monitored closely. Greater loss of severely ill patients during the project (for example, as a result of death) in either the case-managed or the comparison group results in inaccuracies of improved health indicator average scores for the surviving group members. Also, withdrawal from participation of dissatisfied program enrollees within the case-managed or comparison group raises average satisfaction scores for that group. Bias in indicators of satisfaction can yield false interpretations of outcomes. Case management evaluation strategies that incorporate prospective follow-up of patients should include plans for minimizing withdrawal of patients in the case-managed and comparison groups and for gathering information for analysis of bias resulting from unavoidable patient loss.

Numbers of patients included in the evaluation must be sufficient to allow valid statistical comparisons of outcomes. Case managers planning evaluations should check with a statistician to ensure adequacy of projected numbers of patients. Estimates of required subject numbers are based on the anticipated frequency of specific outcome events (for example, hospital or long-term care admissions), the difference in average scores of clinical or service measures important to detect (for example, differences in scores from health status or patient satisfaction questionnaires), the level of error acceptable in estimations of group differences, and the statistical models to be used in analyses of outcomes. Professional assistance in these determinations is likely to be necessary for valid analyses.

Case Management Implementation Issues

Estimation of the duration of the intervention time required to demonstrate effects is another essential step in planning evaluation. Start-up learning time is required for newly established programs. Although two

of the studies summarized in Table 9–2 involved follow-up to 24 months, case management research to date has focused on short-term effects of case management interventions on cost, satisfaction, and clinical outcomes. Virtually no information is available on long-term effects of case management (Mechanic et al., 1995). Because effects of case management in preventing disease complications or reducing risk for other medical or social problems are generally realized over the long term, preventive outcomes have not been studied to any extent.

Because the practice of case management remains a "black box" with regard to understanding which of the elements of practice are critical to bringing about desired outcomes, clear documentation of the nature and frequency of case management intervention activities is important. Such documentation provides the data necessary for identifying and factoring out effects of specific components or activities of case management practice. Clinical practice guidelines and critical pathways common to acute care settings (Zander, 1988; Lynn-McHale, Fitzpatrick, & Shaffer, 1993) are only beginning to appear in community-based case management practice (Goodwin, 1992). In addition to the unavailability of such guidelines, patent and copyright laws protecting the new guidelines entering the market impose monetary barriers to financially stressed agencies looking to use clinical practice guidelines in case management interventions. Innovations such as clinical practice guidelines hold considerable promise for enabling evaluation of case management interventions through standardizing the case management process in community settings.

Outcome Measures

Outcome measures for evaluation of case management practice typically center on measurement of patient health status, satisfaction with services, use of services, and costs of services. More information on outcome measurement is in Chapter 7. A summary of types and possible specifications of outcome measures is included in Table 9–3. Each of these outcome measures presents unique challenges in measurement.

Table 9–3

Outcome Measures Commonly Used in Evaluation of Case Management Health Status

Health Status
General health status indexes such as Medical
   Outcomes Study SF-36 or SF-12*
Disease-specific health status indexes†
Physiological signs and symptoms
Psychosocial symptoms
Functioning in activities of daily living
Functioning in instrumental activities of daily
   living
Work disability status
Complications of disease or medical care
Longevity and mortality

Satisfaction with Services
Group Health Association of America or other
   satisfaction scales (Gold & Wooldridge, 1995)

Use of Services
Hospital admissions or readmissions
Nursing home admissions or readmissions
Emergency department visits
Outpatient clinic visits
Physician visits
Home care visits (by professional discipline)
Noncompliance with scheduled visits
Patient reports of unmet service needs
Use of community support services (for
   example, housing, home-delivered meals,
   adult day care, respite services)

Costs of Services
Total costs
Costs per unit of time
Costs per service (for example, hospital,
   physician, home care)
Cost-effectiveness ratios (ratio of differences in
   group costs per difference in group outcome
   unit)

---

*The SF-36 and SF-12 can be ordered from
   Medical Outcomes Trust
   20 Park Plaza, Suite 1014
   Boston, MA 02116-4313
   Phone (617) 426-4046
   FAX (617) 426-4131
†Information about a number of general and dis-
ease-specific health status indexes and how to obtain
these indexes has been compiled by McDowell and New-
ell (1987) and Spilker (1990).

HEALTH STATUS

Health status is a broad concept, generally assumed to contain elements of clinically diagnosed illness, physical or emotional symptoms of distress, patient
functioning in work activities or activities of
daily living, and social interrelations within
the family or community. Whereas death
may be considered as a "measure of health,"
unless the patient group is extremely large,
death will likely occur too infrequently to
serve as a valid outcome for comparison.
Also, research findings indicate that patient
preferences for health outcomes relate more
to "health status" or "quality of life" than to
mere extension of survival time (Levine,
1990).

Achieving consistency in measurement of
health status indicators is a major challenge
in evaluation. Approaches to measurement
include use of group health indicators in
administrative databases as well as use of
individually administered health status
questionnaires. The first approach is illustrated by HEDIS indicators such as percentages of immunized 2-year-old children and
percentages of diabetic patients receiving
retinal examinations (Corrigan & Nielsen,
1993). The second approach requires use of
an instrument that is tested for reliability
and validity with a variety of populations
and that is appropriate across diagnostic
categories, across institutional and community sites, and across a wide spectrum of
ages. The SF-36 and SF-12 health status
questionnaires from the Medical Outcome
Study (Kravitz et al., 1992) come close to
meeting these criteria and are used in a
wide range of research and clinical settings.
However, the SF-36 and SF-12 have been
developed for use with adult populations.
Standard questionnaires for measurement
of health of children and infants are less
well developed; the instrument by Stein and
Jessop (1990) is one of the most useful instruments across childhood age groups.

PATIENT SATISFACTION

Like health status, patient satisfaction
has proved a difficult concept to measure.
Global satisfaction with life in general and
health care in general tends to carry over
into evaluations of specific care episodes.
The GHAA Consumer Satisfaction Survey
is rapidly becoming the standard in the field
(Davies & Ware, 1991). The 1991 edition of
this instrument measures satisfaction with
a variety of service components, including
access to care, costs of care, technical quality, communication, choice, paperwork, and
information provided. Gold and Wooldridge

(1995) provide a comparison of instruments most commonly used for surveying patient satisfaction with health services, including the GHAA Consumer Satisfaction Survey. Westra and colleagues (1995) have reported development of a satisfaction instrument specifically for home care.

USE OF SERVICES

Use of services is an essential outcome for case management systems, with patterns of use indicating whether high-cost inpatient, emergency room, and long-term institutional services are being reduced or replaced by lower-cost outpatient services. Indicators for use of services include frequency of admissions or visits to service sites, length of stay, and readmissions within 30 days of discharge (sometimes used as a proxy for complications). Use of hospital or nursing home admissions as an outcome requires a large number of subjects in the study group if admissions occur relatively infrequently. In addition to actual use of services, patient perceptions of adequacy of access to services are often assessed in order to detect unmet needs.

COSTS OF SERVICES

Costs of service constitute the "bottom line" in the evaluation of case management practice and are directly linked to the measures of services used. Actual costs rather than charges or reimbursement levels should be used in calculations because the latter are subject to pricing and negotiating strategies. Costs incurred by the case management program must be offset by savings in services averted if a cost-benefit for case management is to be realized. For example, failure to demonstrate cost savings for case management in the Long Term Care Demonstration Project (Table 9–2) (Carcagno & Kemper, 1988) was attributed to overall good health of the subjects. Because subjects were at low risk for nursing home admissions, cost savings for the program were not realized. Also, case management cost reductions may not be observed with groups that are not experiencing initially high costs. Specification of the perspective of cost analysis must be identified—a societal perspective takes in all costs to society whereas an agency perspective disregards costs shifted to entities outside the organization.

Costs incurred beyond a 1-year duration should be adjusted for inflation so that dollar values are comparable (Warner & Luce, 1982). A detailed discussion on cost is in Chapter 11.

In summary, health status, patient satisfaction, use of services, and costs of services are the primary *outcome* measures for any case management program. Additional *process* factors related to delivery of care, such as professional qualifications of the case manager, patterns of staffing, continuity of providers, and decision-making patterns within the agency may be important in interpreting outcomes observed (Hammermeister, Shroyer, Sethi, & Grover, 1995).

Situational Factors

In addition to outcome measures, evaluation of case management practice should incorporate situational factors that may impact effectiveness of the case management intervention. Such factors include health promotion behaviors of the patient, involvement of family and friends in patient care, availability of health and social service services within the geographical area, and financial resources for services (for example, supplementary insurance for Medicare enrollees). Information on situational factors related to case management outcomes should be compared for intervention and control or standard groups and, if groups are found to be dissimilar, effects of such factors must be controlled in analyses.

Integrated Information Systems

Because evaluation of case management is based on outcome data, the quality of the underlying patient database is critical. Methods of data collection on health care needs and services provided to patients are undergoing revolutionary change. Computer systems are rapidly being developed that link patient data systems within organizations (for example, data on clinical outcomes and operational costs), link data across providers of integrated managed-care systems, and link hospital and public health outpatient services in certain geographical regions. Such systems as CHIN (Weaver, 1995; Work & Pawola, 1996) and IRIS (Ruffin, 1995) illustrate the leading edge in integrated patient information systems. These systems enormously enhance ability to connect patient acute-care, home care, and outpatient services and facilitate more in-depth assessment and quality improvement of patient services (Custer, 1993; Borok, 1995; Brennan, 1995; Wagner, 1995).

Data Analysis

Methods of data analysis for the evaluation of case management center on detection of significant differences in outcomes between the case management and control groups or between the practice being evaluated and reported standard indicators. Differences may be assessed by comparing percentages of the case management and control groups experiencing a certain outcome or by comparing average scores of the two groups on a questionnaire or clinical test. For example, if the SF-12 is used to measure health status outcomes, differences in average total scores for the case managed and control groups should be assessed.

If individuals are enrolled for varying lengths of time in the case management and control groups, such differences in time of opportunity to experience the outcome must be controlled. This can be done by designating the follow-up time starting at a baseline of zero (when subjects enter the study) and counting duration of time on case management from the baseline time, for example in months. Outcomes can then be analyzed by looking for differences in outcomes for case-managed and comparison groups at 1 month, 3 months, 6 months, and so on. Differences in costs can be analyzed for the case-managed and the comparison groups based on a specified time period of observation, for example, as average costs per day or per month. Total cost comparisons are not appropriate unless durations of follow-up for the case-managed and control groups are equivalent. For example, if control subjects tend to drop out of the study early, costs are reduced simply because the time period for assessing costs is shorter.

Regardless of the analytical method used, estimates of effects must be adjusted for patient and situational factors that impact outcomes and that differ between the intervention and control group or between the intervention and standard (Iezzoni, 1994).

Such factors may be controlled by conducting analyses with subgroups of patients. For example, if gender is related to use of a given service and the intervention group contains a significantly higher percentage of females than the control group, then differences in intervention and control use of the service should be compared separately for males and females (compare outcomes for male case-managed versus control subjects; then compare outcomes for female case-managed versus control subjects). Alternatively, multivariate statistical models can be used to control for group differences in specific variables. Because either positive or negative effects may result from case management effects, statistical tests should be specified for detection of effects in either direction, for example, a gain in health status as well as a loss in health status.

Conclusions

If the evaluation of case management is conducted within an agency or system structure, findings should be summarized in a three- to four-page executive summary, with details of the evaluation and analysis attached. Quantitative findings may be supplemented by direct quotes from patients or staff. Implications of findings specific to operations for the agency of analysis should be included. Case managers should be alert to which case management issues are relevant to agency executives or boards and address evaluation findings relevant to such issues in the evaluation report.

Case Study

Kathy Barnes is supervisor of case management services at a local home care agency and has assumed responsibility for evaluation of the effectiveness of this unit's activities.

In this home care agency, nurse case managers are assigned to chronically ill elderly patients identified as being at risk for nursing home placement. Six case managers are employed by the agency, each with a caseload of 25 to 30 patients. Case management services are contingent on receiving services from the agency—patients who are discharged, transferred to another agency, or admitted to home care lose their eligibility for these services. Actual case management services include comprehensive assessment, care planning, monitoring of services, facilitation and coordination of Medicare-reimbursed services, and occasional direct care.

Kathy categorizes case management at her agency as within the local agency model without purchase authority. She reviews the research literature on effectiveness of this case management model with frail elderly populations and finds evidence suggestive of improved satisfaction with life and fewer unmet needs but potentially higher costs and no evidence of improved health status (Carcagno & Kemper, 1988).

After consideration of alternative comparison strategies for evaluation, Kathy chooses to evaluate her agency's case management program using a "concurrent control group without random assignment." She contacts the administrator of a home care agency within the same chain but in another city and initiates the process for considering use of this agency's clients as the control group. The control agency provides home care to a similar patient population but caseloads are larger (50 to 75 patients per nurse), the nursing role focuses on supervision of home care aides, and the agency does not provide specific case management services. Kathy recognizes that, with this nonrandomized design, findings are vulnerable to biases from lack of comparability of the client caseloads and availability of resources. She verifies that client ages, types of diagnoses, and socioeconomic characteristics are comparable as are the types of community resources available to clients. Comparability of the clients served by the two agencies is further ensured by restricting the evaluation to individuals aged 65 years and older who are newly admitted to each of the agencies within the first 6 months of the upcoming year and who exhibit dysfunction in at least two activities of daily living and are thereby at risk for nursing home placement.

Kathy hypothesizes that the group of case-managed clients, when compared to the control group, will exhibit significantly better health status (as measured by the MOS SF-12), greater satisfaction

with services (as measured by the GHAA Consumer Satisfaction Survey), reduced use of high-cost services (measured by hospital and nursing home admissions, readmissions, and length of stay), and lower per diem costs of services (agency costs as well as costs to Medicare and Medicaid). She reviews the number of patients at both agencies who would meet eligibility requirements for the evaluation and consults a statistician to ensure that the projected numbers of clients and the time of follow-up will be adequate to detect hypothesized differences on the various outcome measures. She also projects a participation rate based on reports of similar evaluations in the literature and provides this to the statistician for use in calculating the required sample size for the evaluation.

Kathy develops the packet of data forms to be used with each client, obtaining permission from the organizations holding copyrights to the SF-12 and the GHAA. She designs forms to collect information on client demographic characteristics, implementation of the intervention, and situational factors such as the presence and involvement of family members in patient care, availability of supplementary insurance, and family economic resources. She then submits the plans for the evaluation to the human subjects committee for the agency chain. Once approval is received, she pilot tests the procedures and forms for subject recruitment and data collection. She holds training sessions for data collectors of the two agencies.

During the course of the evaluation, Kathy continually monitors adherence of procedures followed to those specified in the evaluation plan, checks the completeness of the data, and monitors the quality of data entry. On completion of the study, she works with the statistician in conducting comparisons of outcomes of the two groups. Once findings are complete, she presents both written and oral reports to the corporation executives, who are especially interested in this comparison of the effectiveness of the two alternative service delivery models within this same home care agency chain. Because Kathy has applied rigorous methodology throughout her evaluation of the case management program, her findings hold

➤ Steps Used in Evaluating Case Management Services Illustrated in Case Study

1. Identify type of case management model, for example, local agency model.
2. Review research literature, in this case, on the effectiveness of case management model in the frail elderly population.
3. Determine alternative comparison strategy for evaluation, for example, a concurrent control group without random assignment such as a home care agency within the same chain in another city.
4. Identify case management implementation issues. Differences between the groups including larger caseloads in the control agency, nursing roles that focus on supervision of home care aides, and an agency that does not provide specific case management services.
5. Decide outcome measures, such as health status, satisfaction with services, cost of services, readmission and length of stay, per diem cost of services.

6. Plan and implement the steps for the evaluation project. For example, review the number of eligible patients, consult with statistician to project required sample to detect differences between the two groups, obtain permission to use tools from copyright holders, and design data collection form.
7. Consider situational factors, such as presence and involvement of family members in patient care.
8. Obtain approval from institutional review board to conduct the project.
9. Implement evaluation by performing pretest procedures and recruitment of subjects, conducting training sessions for data collectors, and monitoring adherence to procedures.
10. Monitor data collection, ensuring completeness of data and quality of data entry.
11. Analyze data—consult with statistician.
12. Disseminate findings—prepare oral and written reports.

---

up to scrutiny and critique by the executives and serve to provide sound guidance in decision making by the organization. The box illustrates the steps Kathy used to evaluate case management services.

analytical skills to reports of case management research and by conducting evaluation within case-managed clinical practice, nurses have a key role to play in advancing effective use of case management for promotion of community-based patient care.

SUMMARY

Despite inconclusive evidence as to its effectiveness, case management is rapidly being integrated into service delivery systems. Nurses are among the professional disciplines most frequently chosen to provide case management services and they must be equipped with knowledge and skills needed for rigorous evaluation of the case management service. Among the competencies required is knowledge of variations of elements of case management models, comparison strategies for evaluation, and steps of the evaluation process as they apply to case management. Through application of these

REFERENCES

Borland, A., McRae, J., & Lycan, C. (1989). Outcomes of five years of continuous intensive case management. *Hospital and Community Psychiatry, 40*(4), 369–376.

Borok, L. S. (1995). The use of relational databases in health care information systems. *Journal of Health Care Finance, 21*(4), 6–12.

Brennan, C. P. (1995). Managed care and health information networks. *Journal of Health Care Finance, 21*(4), 1–5.

Carcagno, G. J., & Kemper, P. (1988). The evaluation of the National Long Term Care Demonstration: 1. An overview of the Channeling Demonstration and its evaluation. *HSR: Health Services Research, 23*(1), 1–22.

Carroll, W. J. (1995). Case management: Balancing cost containment and utilization controls with quality outcomes. *Journal of Long-Term Home Health Care, 14*(3), 43–48.

Corrigan, J. M., & Nielsen, D. M. (1993). Toward the development of uniform reporting standards for managed care organizations: The Health Plan Employer Data and Information Set (Version 2). *Journal of Quality Improvement, 19*(2), 566–575.

Custer, M. L. (1993). Enhancing case management through computerized patient files. *Clinical Nurse Specialist, 7*(3), 141–147.

Davidson, G. B., Penrod, J. D, Kane, R. A., Moscovice, I. S., & Rich, E. C. (1991). Modeling the costs of case management in long-term care. *Health Care Financing Review, 13*(1), 73–81.

Davies, A. R., & Ware, J. E., Jr. (1991). *GHAA's Consumer Satisfaction Survey and User's Manual.* Washington, DC: Group Health Association of America.

Eggert, G. M., Zimmer, J. G., Hall, W. J., & Friedman, B. (1991). Case management: A randomized controlled study comparing a neighborhood team and a centralized individual model. *HSR: Health Services Research, 26*(4), 471–507.

Erkel, E. A., Morgan, E. P., Staples, M. A., Assey, V. H., & Michel, Y. (1994). Case management and preventive services among infants from low-income families. *Public Health Nursing, 11*(5), 352–360.

Goering, P. N., Wasylenki, D. A., Farkas, M., Lancee, W. J., & Ballantyne, R. (1988). What difference does case management make? *Hospital and Community Psychiatry, 39*(3), 272–276.

Gold, M., & Wooldridge, J. (1995). Surveying consumer satisfaction to assess managed-care quality: Current practices. *Health Care Financing Review, 16*(4), 155–173.

Goodwin, D. R. (1992). Critical pathways in home healthcare. *Journal of Nursing Administration, 22*(2), 35–40.

Grower, R., Hillegass, B., & Nelson, F. (1996). Case management: Meeting the needs of chronically ill patients in an HMO. *Managed Care Quarterly, 4*(2), 46–57.

Hammermeister, K. E., Shroyer, A. L., Sethi, G. K., & Grover, F. L. (1995). Why it is important to demonstrate linkages between outcomes of care and processes and structures of care. *Medical Care, 33*(Suppl 10), OS5–OS16.

Hanchak, N. A., Harmon-Weiss, S. R., McDermott, P. D., Hirsch, A., & Schlackman, N. (1996). Medicare managed care and the need for quality measurement. *Managed Care Quarterly, 4*(1), 1–12.

Haslanger, K. D. (1995). Is case management of any value? What is the evidence? *Journal of Long-Term Home Health Care, 14*(2), 37–43.

Hodgkin, D. (1992). The impact of private utilization management on psychiatric care: A review of the literature. *Journal of Mental Health Administration, 19*(2), 143–157.

Iezzoni, L. I. (1994). *Risk adjustment for measuring health care outcomes.* Ann Arbor, MI: Health Administration Press.

Jerrell, J. M., & Ridgely, M. S. (1995). Comparative effectiveness of three approaches to serving people with severe mental illness and substance abuse disorders. *The Journal of Nervous and Mental Disease, 183*(9), 566–576.

Kemper, P. (1988). The evaluation of the National Long Term Care Demonstration: 10. Overview of the findings. *HSR: Health Services Review, 23*(1), 161–174.

Kravitz, R. L., Greenfield, S., Rogers, W., Manning, W. G., Zubkoff, M., Nelson, E. C., Tarlov, A. R., & Ware, J. E. (1992). Differences in the mix of patients among medical specialties and systems of care: Results from the Medical Outcomes Study. *Journal of the American Medical Association, 267*(12), 1617–1623.

Levine, R. J. (1990). An ethical perspective. In B. Spilker (Ed.), *Quality of life assessment in clinical trials.* (pp. 153–162). New York: Raven Press.

Lynn-McHale, D. J., Fitzpatrick, E. R., & Shaffer, R. B. (1993). Case management: Development of a model. *Clinical Nurse Specialist, 7*(6), 299–307.

MacPherson, M. (1996). Measure by measures. *Hospitals and Health Networks, 70*(6), March 20, 53–56.

Mawn, B., & Bradley, J. (1993). Standards of care for high-risk prenatal clients: The community nurse case management approach. *Public Health Nursing, 10*(2), 78–88.

McDowell, I., & Newell, C. (1987). *Measuring Health: A Guide to Rating Scales and Questionnaires.* New York: Oxford University Press.

Mechanic, D., Schlesinger, M., & McAlpine, D. D. (1995). Management of mental health and substance abuse services: State of the art and early results. *The Milbank Quarterly, 73*(1), 19–55.

Miller, M. E., & Gengler, D. J. (1993). Medicaid case management: Kentucky's Patient Access and Care Program. *Health Care Financing Review, 15*(1), 55–69.

Nickel, J. T., Salsberry, P. J., Caswell, R. J., Keller, M. D., Long, T., & O'Connell, M. (1996). Quality of life in nurse case management of persons with AIDS receiving home care. *Research in Nursing and Health, 19*(2), 91–99.

Pacala, J. T., Boult, C., Hepburn, K. W., Kane, R. A., Kane, R. L., Malone, J. K., Morishita, L., & Reed, R. L. (1995). Case management of older adults in health maintenance organizations. *Journal of the American Geriatrics Society, 43*(5), 538–542.

Phillips, B. R., Kemper, P., & Applebaum, R. A. (1988). The evaluation of the National Long Term Care Demonstration: 4. Case management under channeling. *HSR: Health Services Research, 23*(1), 67–81.

Rosenberg, C. (1995). Controversies in case management. *Journal of Long-Term Home Health Care, 14*(3), 37–42.

Ruffin, M. (1995). Developing and using a data repository for quality improvement: The genesis of IRIS. *Journal of Quality Improvement, 21*(10), 512–520.

Shaughnessy, P. W., Crisler, K. S., Schlenker, R. E., & Arnold, A. G. (1995). Outcome-based quality improvement in home care. *CARING Magazine, 14*(2), 44–49.

Solomon, P., & Draine, J. (1995). Consumer case management and attitudes concerning family relations among persons with mental illness. *Psychiatric Quarterly, 66*(3), 249–261.

Sowell, R. L., Gueldner, S. H., Killeen, M. R., Lowenstein, A., Faszard, B., & Swansburg, R. (1992). Impact of case management on hospital charges of PWA's in Georgia. *Journal of the Association of Nurses in AIDS Care, 3*(2), 24–31.

Spilker, B. (Ed.). (1990). *Quality of life assessments in clinical trials.* New York: Raven Press.

Stein, R. E. K., & Jessop, D. J. (1990). Functional Status II(R): A measure of child health status. *Medical Care, 28*(11), 1041–1055.

Wagner, E. H. (1995). Population-based management

of diabetes care. *Patient Education and Counseling,* *26,* 225–230.

Warner, K. E., & Luce, B. R. (1982). *Cost-benefit and cost-effectiveness analysis in health care: Principles, practice, and potential.* Ann Arbor, MI: Health Administration Press.

Weaver, C. G. (1995). CHINs: Making the important decisions. *Healthcare Financial Management,* June, 58–64.

Westra, B. L., Cullen, L., Brody, D., Jump, P., Geanon, L., & Milad, E. (1995). Development of the home care client satisfaction instrument. *Public Health Nursing, 12*(6), 393–399.

Work, M. R., & Pawola, L. (1996). Information systems for integrated healthcare delivery. *Healthcare Financial Management,* January, 27–30.

Zander, K. (1988). Managed care within acute care settings. *Health Care Supervisor, 6*(2), 27–43.

Chapter 10

Managing Variances of Care

Magdalena A. Mateo, Cheryl Newton, and Eileen McMyler

The emphasis on efficient and cost-effective delivery of care has led to the use of standardized practices through the use of protocols that may be in the form of clinical guidelines, standardized orders, or critical paths. The elements of these protocols are derived from the literature and from practices that have been reported to successfully predict the desired outcomes from the patient and organization perspectives. Because these protocols are used to predict the course of a patient's condition and required care, it is essential to identify variances as they occur. Immediately after identifying variances, it is necessary to determine the variance source and institute measures to rectify the variance and to collect data about variances over time so that trends are monitored and addressed to avoid future occurrences of variances.

Research methods are useful in managing variances of care. Developing guidelines for practice, identifying variances that are important to monitor, developing methods for monitoring these variances, determining the sources of variances, and identifying ways of preventing the occurrence of variances are vital steps in effective management.

A variance is any deviation, positive or negative, from a critical pathway or clinical protocol (Mateo & Newton, 1996). It is the difference between the planned process of care for a homogeneous group of patients and the actual care provided (Zander, 1997) or what actually happened, such as not meeting a goal (Hronek, 1995).

Variances may be categorized into patient/family, health/illness, caregiver/clinician, and hospital/environment (Zander, 1991; Hampton, 1993). Patient/family variances may result when there is difficulty with compliance from the patient or family, when there is knowledge deficit regarding the disease process or treatment, or when there is inability for a caregiver to care for the patient. Health/illness variance occurs as a result of a patient's current medical status or a complication from a procedure that may result in increased length of stay (LOS). Caregiver/clinician variances are those over which the health team has the most control, whereas hospital/environment variances are attributed to inefficiencies in the system. Table 10–1 lists types of variances and examples.

In applying the concept of variance in the emergency department (ED), Dagher and

Table 10–1

Types of Variances and Examples

TYPES OF VARIANCE	EXAMPLES OF VARIABLES THAT MAY AFFECT OUTCOME
Patient/family	Readiness for education, sources of patient education materials such as the Internet, life experiences
Health/illness	Acuity
Caregiver/clinician	Education preparation, competency, knowledge and adherence to protocols, multidisciplinary collaboration
Hospital/environment	Institutional initiatives such as continuous improvement projects with the focus on the discharge planning process

Lloyd (1991) reported variances related to structure and process. Structure variances comprise perceived differences between the institution's services and what the patient feels should be the standard in the ED— access, physical environment, perception about the condition and appearance of medical equipment, ED policies and procedures, and effectiveness. Process variances result when there is a lack of standardization in the way staff implement policies and procedures.

OBTAINING INFORMATION FOR USE IN STANDARDS FOR PRACTICE

Numerous sources are used in developing clinical guidelines, protocols, and critical pathways. These include the literature, clinical databases, and information obtained through the benchmarking process.

Literature

Literature includes articles in journals or on-line, publications of organizations such as the Agency for Health Care Policy Research (AHCPR), or position papers from specialty groups such as the American Thoracic Society. Articles primarily written as synthesis or review of research are helpful because criteria for review are used, thereby enabling readers to obtain an overview of findings. When reviewing individual research publications, it is vital to consider scientific merit, relevance, and feasibility to practice. Other useful guidelines are presented in Chapter 17.

Experts in a designated field of research

and practice (for example, pain management) have written a number of AHCPR publications. Research findings are summarized and practice applications are explicit and relevant.

World Wide Web publications are readily available through the Internet in an increasing number because of the technological advances and the growing market. The accessibility of information makes it tempting to use; however, it is important to be cautious. The following should be considered before using information from the World Wide Web (Ackerman, 1997).

- Source of data. Are the sources and the credibility of the author and the organization evident?
- Author credentials. Are author credentials included and verifiable?
- Review process. Has the information met some type of institutional criteria for quality?
- Disclaimer about the information. Are the purpose, scope, limitation, and currency of the information provided?

Databases

Computerized clinical databases are rich sources of data on processes and outcomes of nursing care. Wuerker (1997) reported the availability and increasing sophistication of numerous databases in which fiscal data and service use in many areas can be linked. Examples of databases are psychiatric case registers, data from health maintenance organizations, and the National Child Development Study in Great Britain. There are issues related to using databases. These issues relate to obtaining permission to use the data, structuring the data for use because there may be redundancy, and analysis. Nail and Lange (1996) described the processes for obtaining and using databases:

- Locating and accessing the databases—determining the focus of the inquiry, identifying relevance of the database, obtaining access, and ensuring confidentiality of subjects
- Assessing the content, quality, and usability of the data
- Retrieving and analyzing the data—establishing criteria for inclusion of data, obtaining permission to access desired data, designing the database according to the goals of the user, and conducting data analysis

Benchmarking

Benchmarking is a process used to identify "best practices" by comparing the processes of one organization with those of similar institutions (Czarnecki, 1996). Choosing the right organizations for benchmarking is crucial in obtaining usable data (see box). A written questionnaire or telephone interview may be used to collect data from organizations that are known to be managing variances. Demographics of the organization, questions on processes used to manage variances, and initiatives that might influence outcomes of practice are items that need to be included in the data collection tool (Mateo, Matzke, & Newton, 1998). Refer to Chapter 19 for information on developing survey questions.

IMPLEMENTING A SYSTEM FOR MANAGING VARIANCES

The establishment of a system for managing variances includes several phases. These are determining the patient population, selecting from existing tools or developing tools for monitoring, conducting gap analysis, initiating standardized data collection and management procedures, and establishing a format for reporting outcomes.

Determine the Patient Population

Determining the patient population to be monitored is foremost. The basis for making

➤ Selecting Benchmarking Partners

- Keep an open mind. The best partners may not be those that seem to be obvious choices, for example, an industry that is not in health care.
- Have a clear understanding of the information you want to know. Two types of information that may be useful are specific organizational characteristics (number of employees, bed occupancy) and information related to the focus of the project (transfer of patients from a service to another service).
- Determine how your organization defines "best practices."
- When reviewing organization information, use objective criteria to evaluate and verify databases, online sources, and information.

From Powers, V. J. (1997). Selecting a benchmarking partner: Five tips for success. *Quality Digest*, October, 37–41.

the decision includes the frequency that care is provided for a group of patients and the predictability that if the prescribed interventions are implemented in a standard way, positive outcomes are achieved. There has to be an adequate number of patients to warrant the development of standardized tools. Furthermore, there must be sufficient data to be collected and analyzed.

Select Monitoring Methods

It is beneficial to use a multidisciplinary approach when establishing methods for managing variances. Variances can be manually tracked by using a flowchart. A graphic multidisciplinary variance and co-morbidities tracking system allows for individual and group patient variance analysis (Tidwell, 1993). Process mapping can be used to identify the aspects of care in which a variance may occur, for example, in the admission or consultation process (Dagher & Lloyd, 1991).

There are numerous decision support systems that can be used to integrate operational, clinical, and financial information. It is important that a decision support system is able to integrate clinical outcomes as part of the standard analysis (Nunnelly, 1996). Operating system, platform, architecture, use, functionality, and services are considerations in choosing a decision support system. An example of an automated decision support system is the Transitions Systems (Transitions Systems, Inc., 1998), which can be used to integrate essential clinical, financial, and operational information from different sources. This interactive system allows organizations to use real-time information to guide decisions during the patient care process. TSI has a method for alerting other systems so that care can be redirected. On-line information about TSI is available at http://www.tsidss.com.

Using methods for determining variances at the time of occurrence is important in improving efficiency and reducing costs. Real-time intervention has the most potential for producing desired outcomes because the occurrence of an unwanted event that results in a variance is prevented (Rosenstein & Propotnik, 1997).

Conduct a Gap Analysis

When the desired methods for managing variances are identified, gap analysis is suggested. Gap analysis is a technique used to determine the adequacy of existing systems for meeting desired outcomes (Parasuraman, Zeithaml, & Berry, 1991). In variance management, gap analysis can be used to identify the current method for identifying variances, prospective or retrospective; develop a vision of desired method; and determine the method for capturing information. After the desired method is identified, it is important to determine whether there is a gap in resources between currently used and desired methods for managing variance. For example, if a computerized system is being used, are the staffs who are primarily responsible for monitoring variances familiar with computer applications? If the response to this question is "no," then plans must be implemented to ensure that competency in the use of computer programs is gained.

Initiate Standardized Data Collection Methods

After the tools and timeline for collecting data are chosen, it is vital to initiate standardized data collection methods. It is necessary to conduct a pilot on the data collection methods to validate its feasibility. Debriefing data collectors on the forms and methods is necessary to determine changes that are required for the process. Periodic assessment of the data collection process is essential for the reliability and validity of data.

A process for examining the events that led to a variance has to be documented to identify the actual source for the occurrence of a variance (Mateo & Newton, 1996). For example, when a patient's discharge is delayed, thereby resulting in the addition of a day to the LOS, the delay may be initially attributed to a late discharge order (caregiver/clinician variance). After further examination, the actual delay is linked to a delay in release of test results because of a computer problem (hospital/environment variance).

Establish Report Format

A uniform format for reporting variances allows the notation of trends over a period of time and the identification of sources of variance. It is also vital to identify the staff who will be provided with the report so that the information is relevant. When staff nurses are the recipients of the report, the emphasis has to be on the clinical aspects of the patient care and their role in preventing variances as well as understandable fiscal information. On the other hand, administrative staff require the inclusion of a wider scope such as financial aspects and processes throughout the organization and the community because they apply to referrals and consultation.

APPLYING VARIANCE MONITORING TO OUTPATIENT SURGERY AREAS

Outpatient surgery (OPS), ambulatory surgery, and same-day surgery refer to the same phenomenon: patients are admitted for their procedures, have the procedure, and are discharged to home on the same day. If the OPS area is hospital-based rather than a free-standing surgical center, procedures requiring more than 23-hour observation are considered a hospital admission.

Discharge Criteria

Currently, outpatient surgery departments or ambulatory surgery centers use discharge criteria to evaluate whether a patient is physically ready to go home. The criteria used by most organizations are usually similar (Parnass, 1993; Patterson, 1994a, 1994b; Chung, Chan, & Ong, 1995). These criteria include the patient's ability to void, ambulate, breathe without difficulty, and understand discharge instructions. In addition, the patient is alert and oriented, has sensation appropriate for the type of anesthesia performed, and has minimal pain and little or no nausea or vomiting. There is no excessive bleeding for the procedure performed and no signs of impaired circulation. Stephenson (1990) proposed essential and desirable categories for patient readiness for discharge following same-day surgery (see box).

Patients admitted for outpatient surgery are going to have their procedure or surgery, recovery, and discharge on the same day; therefore, events or things that result in an extension of a patient's stay in the hospital could be considered as variances. Canceled surgery, increased LOS, or admissions as a 23-hour observation or inpatient status because the patient was unprepared for surgery or unable to meet the discharge criteria are undesired OPS admission outcomes. When one thinks of variances as occurrences that alter the expected outcome of going home on the day of surgery, these could be considered variances.

Clinical Pathway in the Outpatient

Clinical pathways are not routinely used in the outpatient surgery setting. However, pathways that are seen in the OPS setting are those that started for a specific inpatient population and resulted in an outcome of decreased LOS for that patient population (Bran, Spellman, & Summitt, 1995; Palmer, Worway, Conrad, Blitz, & Chodak, 1996). Because clinical pathways used in the outpatient surgery setting have been

> ## ➤ Proposed Essential and Desirable Categories for Patient Readiness for Discharge Following Day Surgery

- Mental state—recovery from effects of premedication and anesthetic on mental abilities
- Mobility—mobilization and related problems of dizziness or faintness
- Pain—postoperative pain
- Eating and drinking—oral intake, nausea, vomiting
- Elimination—voiding, urine retention
- Information—need for predischarge information
- Social—need for transportation and support within the home

From Stephenson, M. E. (1990). Discharge criteria in day surgery. *Journal of Advanced Nursing, 15*(5), 601–613.

those used in the inpatient setting, variances would be the same. Variances may be related to patient/family, health/illness, caregiver/clinician, or hospital/environmental (Mateo & Newton, 1996), although there are limited data to support as much. Because clinical pathways are not implemented on all outpatient procedures, variances are not being tracked on all outpatient surgery patients.

Hospital-based surgical centers that are developing pathways have similar goals: decreased LOS, decreased cost of care, adequate pain management, and patient ability to follow discharge instructions (Patterson, 1994a, 1994b; Leosh, Wohlford, Dean, & Schwab, 1997). As the cost of medical care continues to increase and the switch to outpatient care continues, new outcome measures may be considered, such as those mentioned by Kleinbeck and Eells (1997): "confirmed ability to manage self-care, perceived satisfaction with service, functional status, and return to productivity or employment."

Tracking Outcomes

How are undesirable outcomes in the OPS population that are not on a clinical path-

Table 10–2
Applying the Research Process to Managing Variances

COMPONENTS OF THE RESEARCH PROCESS	STEPS IN MANAGING VARIANCES
Formulating the research problem	Determining the occurrence of positive or negative variances in homogeneous patients
Reviewing related literature	Using the literature to identify clinically and financially relevant outcomes
Identifying variables	Identify possible explanations for variances
Determining the methods	Who are the patients to be monitored? What data will be used to determine outcomes? How will the validity and reliability of data collection be monitored?
Doing a pilot study	Conducting a pilot of data collection methods
Collecting the data	Tracking progress of patients in meeting desired course of care
Analyzing the data	Identifying the sources of variances, trends
Interpreting results of the study	Interpreting results
Reporting findings—audience format	Reporting findings—audience, format

way measured or tracked? It is standard for ambulatory surgical areas to make a postoperative telephone call to patients. The follow-up telephone call could be used to track variance from discharge criteria or new outcome measures besides patient satisfaction data. As with any survey or follow-up telephone call, the tool used reflects the data obtained. The follow-up telephone call template would have to be designed to track increased LOS and other outcome measures. Hospital statistics may also be used to track outcome measures such as extra time in the recovery room or a change in patient status from outpatient to inpatient.

It is important to use the data to determine how events affect practice. For the clinical pathways that have been incorporated into outpatient surgical areas, it has been evident that for the patient to progress according to the pathway, preoperative testing and education is vital. Systems need to be in place to ensure that preadmission work can be arranged (Patterson, 1994a, 1994b; Bran, Spellman, & Summitt, 1995).

SUMMARY

Variances are a major source of cost. The research process can be used to identify components of standards of practice by doing a literature review, selecting data collection tools, analyzing data, and reporting findings on an ongoing basis (Table 10–2). Although variance management has been initially associated with case management, its applications are being examined in various settings such as the ED, outpatient surgery, and home care.

Preventing variances is accomplished by closely monitoring a patient's progress by collecting real-time data. This is possible when a multidisciplinary approach is used in addressing issues with a computerized system that integrates information from various organizational data.

REFERENCES

Ackerman, M. J. (1997). You can't believe everything you read on the WEB. *Journal of Medical Practice Management, 13*(2), 88–89.

Bran, D. F., Spellman, J. R., & Summitt, R. L. (1995). Outpatient vaginal hysterectomy as a new trend in gynecology. *AORN Journal, 62*(5), 810–814.

Chung, F., Chan, V. W., & Ong, D. (1995). A postanesthetic discharge scoring system for home readiness after ambulatory surgery. *Journal of Clinical Anesthesia, 7*(6), 500–506.

Czarnecki, M. (1996). Using benchmarking in the hospital environment: A case study. *Best Practices and Benchmarking in Healthcare: A Practical Journal for Clinical and Management Applications, 1,* 221–224.

Dagher, M., & Lloyd, R., J. (1991). Managing negative outcome by reducing variances in the emergency department. *Quarterly Review Bulletin, 17*(1), 15–21.

Hampton, D. C. (1993). Implementing a managed care framework through care maps. *Journal of Nursing Administration, 23*(5), 21–27.

Hronek, C. (1995). Redesigning documentation: Clinical pathways, flowsheets, and variance notes. *MEDSURG Nursing, 4,* 157–159.

Kleinbeck, S. V., & Eells, K. R. (1997). Monitoring postdischarge ambulatory surgical recovery: Costs and outcomes. *Surgical Services Management, 3*(6), 33–35.

Leosh, J., Wohlford, S., Dean, R. J., & Schwab, W. W. (1997). Developing a critical pathway for outpatient ACL reconstruction. *Surgical Services Management, 3*(6), 23–26.

Mateo, M. A., Matzke, K., & Newton, C. (1998). Designing measurements to assess case management outcomes. *Nursing Case Management, 3*(1), 2–6.

Mateo, M. A., & Newton, C. (1996). Managing variances in case management. *Nursing Case Management, 1*(1), 45–51.

Nail, L. M., & Lange, L. L. (1996). Using computerized clinical nursing databases for nursing research. *Journal of Professional Nursing, 12,* 197–206.

Nunnelly, J. (1996). Decision-support software clarifies cost, revenue division. *Health Management Technology, 17*(7), 44–50.

Palmer, J. S., Worway, E. M., Conrad, W. G., Blitz, B. F., & Chodak, G. W. (1996). Same day surgery for radical retropubic prostatectomy: Is it an attainable goal? *Urology, 47*(1), 23–28.

Parasuraman, A., Zeithaml, V., & Berry, L. (1991). Gap analysis. In C. Lovelock (Ed.), *Service Marketing* (2nd ed.). London: Prentice-Hall.

Parnass, S. M. (1993). Ambulatory surgical patient priorities. *Post Anesthesia Care Nursing, 28*(3), 531–545.

Patterson, P. (1994a). ORs streamline patient care, control resource utilization. *OR Manager, 10*(7), 1,6–7.

Patterson, P. (1994b). Perioperative case managers redesign processes. *OR Manager, 10*(7), 8–10.

Powers, V. J. (1997). Selecting a benchmarking partner: Five tips for success. *Quality Digest, October,* 37–41.

Rosenstein, A. H., & Propotnik, T. (1997). Case management. *Journal of Healthcare Resource Management, 15*(2), 11–16

Stephenson, M. E. (1990). Discharge criteria in day surgery. *Journal of Advanced Nursing, 15*(5), 601–613.

Tidwell, S. L. (1993). A graphic tool for tracking variances and comorbidities in cardiac surgery case management. *Progress in Cardiovascular Nursing, 8*(2), 6–19.

Transitions Systems, Inc. (1998). Integrated Decision Support & Healthcare Information Systems [computer software]. Boston, MA: TSI Services.

Wuerker, A. K. (1997). Longitudinal research using computerized clinical databases: Caveats and constraints. *Nursing Research, 46,* 353–355.

Zander, K. (1991). The core of cost/quality care. *The New Definition, 6*(3).

Zander, K. (1997). Use of variance from clinical paths: Coming of age. *Clinical Performance & Quality Health Care, 5*(1), 20–30.

Suggested Readings

Burden, N. (1992). Telephone follow-up of ambulatory surgery patients following discharge is a nursing responsibility. *Journal of Post Anesthesia Nursing, 7*(4), 256–261.

Clement, R., & Sangermano, C. (1992). Twenty-three hour recovery: Observation versus hospitalization. *Seminars in Perioperative Nursing, 1*(4), 261–167.

Chung, F. (1993). Are discharge criteria changing? *Journal of Clinical Anesthesia, 5*(6 Suppl. 1), 64–68.

Fetzer-Fowler, S. J., & Huot, S. (1992). The use of temperature as a discharge criterion for ambulatory surgery patients. *Journal of Post Anesthesia Nursing, 7*(6), 398–403.

Honish, P. K., Rivera, L. M., & Shattler, P. (1995). Timely discharge for the patient undergoing outpatient surgery. *Oncology Nursing Forum, 22*(1), 148.

Marley, R. A., & Moline, B. M. (1996). Patient discharge from the ambulatory setting. *Journal of Post Anesthesia Nursing, 11*(1), 39–49.

Schreiner, M. S., Nicolson, S. C., Martin, T., & Whitney, L. (1992). Should children drink before discharge from day surgery? *Anesthesiology, 76*(4), 528–533.

Chapter 11

Cost as a Dimension of Outcomes

Robert J. Caswell

Anyone who has worked in health care for more than a few minutes has probably already been harangued about cost and the absolute necessity of controlling it. Those outside the immediate setting are also bombarded with messages about health care cost, usually about how it is "spiraling" (even though that is not a very helpful image), threatening both the budgets of households and the viability of firms in the global economy. Despite this constant attention, cost is not always well understood, particularly its complexity in health care. This chapter discusses both the basic concepts of cost and some of the practicalities of identifying, measuring, and evaluating cost in the clinical setting. First, the fundamental idea of cost is discussed, then a variety of terms used by economists and financial managers, including some of the jargon that can be confusing to the uninitiated, are defined. The next section deals with the primary ways in which cost is evaluated in the clinical setting, specifically as one of the dimensions of the outcomes of health care. The approaches include cost-effectiveness analysis (CEA), which has become one of the most widely used tools in managed care (or at least the principle is widely invoked, even if the actual technique is not always apparent). Finally, there is a brief discussion of some of the issues and practical concerns that affect assessment of cost in clinical settings.

WHAT IS COST?

Cost Versus Price

The words *cost* and *price* are frequently interchangeable in everyday speech, but they represent different ideas in economics. When a person goes into a store and asks how much an item costs, he or she is really asking for a price. Although the words may be interchangeable, the concepts are not: *price* represents the amount that must be paid in order to gain ownership or use of something, whereas *cost* measures the resources that are used. For example, the *price* of this book is whatever was paid in order to buy it from its previous owner. The *cost* of this book is the paper and ink required to print it, the labor of those who were involved in writing, printing, transporting, and marketing it, and so on. The distinction between price and cost is particularly important in health care, in which prices can be extremely complex and far removed from the apparent buyer. What is the price of a coronary artery bypass graft performed on a person insured under both Medicare and a private supplemental policy? One might reasonably ask, "the price to whom?" It is even possible for the *price* to the recipient of care to be zero—hospitals and other providers frequently care for patients as charity cases, providing treatment to the patients without any intention of billing them. (This is different from a "bad debt," in which a patient is billed but does not pay). It is *not*, however, possible for the *cost* to be zero, because real resources are consumed in providing the service.

Even though price and cost are emphatically not the same thing, they are not unrelated. The party that incurs the cost would be very interested in whether the price received is sufficient to pay for the resources used. In the example of "free" hospital care, it is unlikely that the price to all parties will be zero; for instance, the price not paid by a particular patient may cause the prices to other patients to be higher as the provider attempts to collect enough to pay for all costs—the real resources consumed. Similarly, even though true cost is measured in resources, it is not unusual to encounter price (or *expenditure*) used as a proxy measure. When data on cost are difficult to obtain, price is often used to represent the cost of an action from the point of view of the patient or payer (for example, Stone and Walker [1995] define cost as "the economic impact of charges"). It is the responsibility of the researcher to distinguish clearly what measure is being used and to what extent it may depart from the real cost of the resources.

Opportunity Cost

The fact that cost is conceptually a measurement of resources leads to one of the most important ways of thinking about cost. *Opportunity cost* defines the cost of any particular use of resources as the loss of the alternative uses of the same resources. The time during which a person reads this chapter has an opportunity cost, in that the person has lost the opportunity to use that time for competing purposes (for example, sleeping, watching television, walking the dog). To make a good decision, resources should always be put to their most valuable use. Thus, the authors of this book thank its readers for deciding that there is no other more valuable alternative use of time than reading this book.

The concept of opportunity cost is powerful. Persons who are paid on a piecework basis (for example, physicians paid fee-for-service) may choose to take short vacations or constantly look at their watches during meetings. Persons who are paid by salary may be equally skilled, but the opportunity cost of spending more time at a particular activity is quite different.

Cost Is in the Eye of the Beholder

Cost may not be the same when measured from different points of view. The most common cause for costs to appear different is variation in the level of inclusiveness or aggregation. For example, persons who smoke generally have higher health care costs than those who do not. It is also true that the health care costs attributable to smoking can be reduced when smokers quit smoking, even at relatively older ages. Therefore, wouldn't it save money for all taxpayers if older persons quit smoking, thus using fewer services paid for by Medicare? The answer depends on point of view. If smoking cessation leads to a longer life span, it may be that the health care costs resulting from needing care for more years will more than offset the savings resulting from reducing the costs attributable to smoking. Thus, if the objective is simply to reduce each individual's total expenditures in the Medicare program, it might be better to encourage smoking and hope people die sooner. In a broader concept of cost, including the lost productivity of persons who are ill, the costs to others in the society incurred from passive smoke or fires, and the psychological cost of watching family members suffer from lung disease, then encouraging smoking cessation would be quite appropriate. Cost can be measured meaningfully only after deciding on the boundaries that are relevant to the decision or evaluation at hand. The work of LaGodna and Hendrix (1989) illustrates this principle: the authors compute the cost of impaired nurses from the separate points of view of the nurse, the employer, and the profession. Although their estimates are rough, the elements of cost that are included in each are distinct (for example, lost income, hiring cost, investigation and adjudication).

CONCEPTS OF COST MEASUREMENT AND BEHAVIOR

Direct Versus Indirect Cost

In almost every complex activity, some of the cost can be attributed easily to the output of that activity itself. When a laboratory test is done, it is clear that the chemicals used, the time of the technician, and the time of a pathologist to examine the results are all direct resource costs incurred to perform the test. However, how should one consider the cost of employing a laboratory manager, of routine cleaning of the laboratory, or of having excess capacity available so that urgently needed tests can be done immediately? These are all examples of *indirect* cost; they are not attributable directly to any particular output of the laboratory but are nevertheless necessary for the overall activity to be done. That is, the true cost of a particular output such as a simple urinalysis would be understated if only the

direct costs were considered. However, because the indirect costs are not attached to specific outputs, they must be *allocated* in some way.

Cost allocation has become a critical activity for health care organizations as they struggle to understand the true costs of their activities in order to manage those costs and to set prices that are both competitive and adequate. There are many examples of such allocation problems in nursing; it is easy to attribute the cost of nursing to a specific patient when identifiable procedures are being performed, but much less so in general care and especially in activities of coordination and management. The usual approach to indirect cost allocation is to arrive at an *allocation basis*, which serves as a sort of proxy for the relationship between the indirect cost and the outputs. For example, it is common to allocate the cost of housekeeping on the basis of the number of square feet in an area, possibly weighted by some other factor such as special procedures for infectious disease (see box).

Explicit Versus Implicit Cost

The principle of opportunity cost described earlier—such as the cost of a person's time in reading this chapter—is a reminder that not all costs involve a payment transaction. *Explicit* costs are those for which there is an actual expenditure, such as the salary and retirement benefit cost of hiring an employee. *Implicit* costs are those that need to be recognized in a decision, even though there is no actual payment made. Although there are many kinds of implicit costs, two are seen frequently: foregone earnings and depreciation. There is an implicit cost of foregone earnings, for example, when a per-

> ➤ **Typical Allocation Bases for Indirect Cost**

WHEN ALLOCATING COST FROM THIS INDIRECT COST CENTER:	IT MIGHT BE DIVIDED AMONG OTHER AREAS ON THE BASIS OF:
Housekeeping Department	Relative size of each area in square feet
Nursing Administration	Number of patient days in each area
Personnel Department	Number of employees or paid hours in each area
Admissions Department	Number of admissions or discharges in each area
Clinic Management	Number of patient visits in each area

son paid fee-for-service uses time for other unpaid purposes. Perhaps less obviously, it arises whenever one makes a decision about how to finance a large purchase. If a clinic pays cash for an X-ray machine, the finance charge on a debt is avoided, but the opportunity to earn interest on the cash is also lost. These lost interest earnings are an implicit cost of cash financing. This same reasoning can be extended to much more complex decisions. The other best-known implicit cost is depreciation, which simply means that something may lose value over time through either actual deterioration or obsolescence. If a diagnostic device must be replaced approximately every 5 years, then it is reasonable to think that there is an implicit cost of using the device equal to approximately one fifth of the replacement cost per year, in addition to the explicit cost of operating the device. If the owner of the device recognizes this implicit cost and sets aside the money for depreciation at this rate (even though it is not due to anyone as a payment), then at the end of the 5 years, there will be a fund from which the needed replacement can be purchased.

Cost Variability with Output

If the number of patients in a neonatal intensive care unit doubles, does the cost of providing nursing care double, more than double, or less than double? This sort of question is particularly important for planning and budgeting purposes, and is the subject of a very large body of the research on cost in health care. Some costs do not change at all as the quantity of output changes, at least as long as the change is not too large. For instance, the cost of utilities (for example, light, heat), insurance, and nursing administration might not change at all as the number of patients in the neonatal intensive care unit varies. These costs would be described as *fixed costs*. Conversely, any costs that do change as the quantity of output changes, such as supplies or overtime hours, would be *variable costs*. Using these two definitions, a simple relationship can be described:

Total Cost = Fixed Cost + Variable Cost
or, symbolically, $TC = FC + VC$

Describing a cost as fixed or variable depends on the time span that is relevant. If the cost is in a particular patient care area during the next shift, almost all costs are fixed because it is too late to make any meaningful changes in them. If the time span stretches to several months or years, then most or all of the costs become variable because radical changes could be made in the way the work is accomplished, including using new technologies, hiring a different mix of staff, or building a new building. In most situations, some costs are fixed and some are variable, although there is clearly a continuum depending upon how easily the cost can be changed. Figure 11–1 illustrates the components of total cost. Fixed cost is represented by the horizontal line, showing the same level of cost no matter what quantity of output there is (even if there is no output at all). The variable cost is indicated by the rising line above fixed cost, showing that cost increases as the quantity of output increases, although not necessarily at a constant rate.

Total Cost Versus Unit Cost

For some management and budgetary purposes, it is enough to know the total cost of all the activity in an organization or some relevant part of it. For example (although this is oversimplified), the hospitals in the Department of Veterans Affairs system are given an annual budget allocation and are expected to meet their care responsibilities

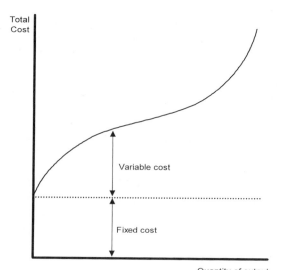

Figure 11–1
Components of total cost.

within that budget. One could argue that, from the point of view of the agency granting the funds, all that matters is that the cost not exceed what was authorized in total. However, many decisions require information on the cost per unit of output. *Unit* in this case means whatever is used to measure the quantity of output. In nursing, the unit might be a specific procedure, a patient visit, or a patient day in an inpatient setting (not to be confused with the idea of a "nursing unit" as a geographical space or a way of organizing care in a hospital or other facility). It is important that the units used to measure work be meaningful representations. In a setting in which all the patients are similar, cost per patient visit could be a reasonable measure, even though it would be an inappropriate measure for an emergency department that treats both trauma and runny noses.

The most common measure of unit cost is the *average cost*, which can be calculated from the simple equation for total cost ($TC = FC + VC$). If both sides of the equation are divided by Q, the quantity of output (for instance, neonatal intensive care patient days), each of the variables become a measure per unit of output (that is, cost per neonatal intensive care patient day):

$$\frac{TC}{Q} = \frac{FC}{Q} + \frac{VC}{Q}$$

Or, Average Total Cost = Average Fixed Cost + Average Variable Cost

Average fixed cost (FC/Q) will decline as the quantity of output gets larger, because the fixed cost in the numerator will stay the same and the quantity in the denominator will grow. This pattern is what financial managers sometimes describe as "spreading the overhead." That is, the fixed cost is spread over more and more units as output grows. It cannot be predicted what will happen to average variable cost, and therefore to average total cost, as output grows. The discovery of these relationships is yet another of the heavily researched topics in health care cost. Figure 11–2 shows typical shapes for these relationships, in which average variable cost and average total cost decline at first as output grows, possibly resulting from specialization and better use of resources, and then increase, probably as capacity is approached and constraints due

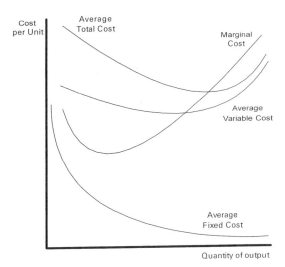

Figure 11–2
Cost per unit of output.

to fixed circumstances are felt (for example, business outgrows a particular area and another space that is less well suited must be used).

One of the most important uses of unit cost measurements is in making predictions about the impact of change. For instance, in an underutilized inpatient area with extra beds available, what is the additional cost of caring for just one more patient? It could be the same as the average cost for patients already receiving treatment, but it usually is not. This is because more fixed cost would not be incurred and additional variable cost might depend on how many existing patients there are, the capabilities of the staff, and so on. The appropriate measure for this situation is called *marginal cost*, referring to the change in cost per unit of change in output. As previously stated, average total cost is simply total cost divided by the amount of output (TC/Q); marginal cost is similar, but is calculated as the *change* in total cost divided by the *change* in output:

$$\text{Marginal Cost} = MC = \frac{\Delta TC}{\Delta Q}$$

Because the quantity of output could be changing in either direction, marginal cost represents either the additional cost per unit of increased output (for example, the additional cost of one more patient day in cardiology) or the reduction in cost per unit of decreased output (one less patient day in cardiology). The managerial and policy uses of marginal cost are many, but the most common is estimating the response of cost to a fluctuating workload. In the short run, many costs are fixed, and the marginal cost of changes in workload may be considerably less than the average cost per unit of work. From a practical point of view, this simply means that the existing staff may just "work harder" to cover a small increase in workload, so that total cost does not go up by much. Note that this reasoning also applies when the workload is decreasing: the marginal cost saved by a downward fluctuation in workload may be small, because there is no opportunity to adjust the fixed costs. Marginal cost has also been used to analyze broader issues such as estimating the savings from closing hospital beds or diverting patients to an alternate setting (Williams, 1996).

EVALUATING COST AS A DIMENSION OF OUTCOMES

The researcher's reason for measuring cost could be the "Mount Everest principle" (because it's there) but is more likely to be motivated by a desire to *evaluate* cost as an outcome of a decision or intervention. It is usually assumed, at least by economists, that in ordinary market transactions (for example, buying a pizza), the purchaser is fully capable of understanding the decision and makes an implicit evaluation—if the item is a good value for the price, it is bought; otherwise, it is not. In the case of health care, there may be many complicating factors that prevent or distort the simple operation of the market, such as inadequately informed purchasers, "spillover" effects of various kinds (for example, when purchase of care benefits someone else as well, such as with immunizations), or concerns about the fairness of pure market allocation (should the wealthiest always get the most?). In the special case of government sponsorship or subsidy, the element of coercion (a person may not choose whether to pay taxes) and the lack of market constraints present a special need for economic evaluation.

Researchers frequently want to analyze whether a particular decision seems appropriate in some sense, given the cost that was (or will be) incurred. A variety of evaluative approaches may be used, depending on the nature of the question being asked and the realistic opportunities for data collection. The researcher should note that titles of articles in the literature are not a reliable guide to the technique being used; although such terms as *cost-benefit* and *cost-effectiveness* have specific meanings, they are sometimes used in a rather loose and inaccurate manner.

➤ Choosing the Correct Cost Concept

Research Question	Most Appropriate Cost Concept*	Principal Issues
What is the cost (of this action, program, intervention)?	Cost identification analysis (estimation of total, average, and/or marginal cost)	Point of view (inclusiveness) Indirect cost allocation
Is this worth doing (or, how much of this is worth doing)?	Cost-benefit analysis	Valuation of nonmonetary benefits Discount rate
Which alternative way of doing this is the best?	Cost-effectiveness analysis or cost-utility analysis	Subjective or objective evaluation of principal outcomes and side effects Discount rate

*The determination of which cost concept is most appropriate can depend on many things, but the choices indicated are likely to be helpful in the majority of circumstances.

Cost Identification

At the simplest level, the evaluation of cost is a careful aggregation of cost, incorporating all the elements that are relevant from the viewpoint of the evaluator. The technique in this case is straightforward: first, define the boundaries of the viewpoint that has been chosen (for instance, is cost borne by the patient's family relevant in the evaluation?); second, identify each of the components of cost (for example, supplies, employee turnover); third, perform the measurements and sum the costs. This frequently involves the researcher in problems of *valuation*, if some of the relevant costs are not obvious or do not have clear monetary units. Valuation would address such concerns as the proper cost to assign to a lengthened response time of nursing resulting from some kind of reorganization of duties, or the cost of using capital equipment (Hundley et al., 1995). The issues involved in valuation are explained in a later section.

Many applications of the cost identification approach involve comparison of alternatives that are assumed to have identical, or at least very similar, outcomes other than cost. In these situations, cost identification is essentially a shortcut version of CEA. Cost identification is also appropriate when it has already been determined that a course of action is desirable, but the question is whether it is financially feasible. The sorts of results reported in the literature range from crude averages (Regan, Byers, & Mayrovitz, 1995) to detailed attempts to adjust for factors affecting cost (Mauskopf, Paul, Wichman, White, & Tilson, 1996).

Cost-Benefit Analysis

In theory, cost-benefit analysis (CBA) comes the closest of any of the evaluation methods to reproducing the logic of the ordinary market decision by asking the question, "Does the benefit of this action exceed the cost?" This is precisely the question that economists believe is asked implicitly every time someone makes a decision concerning a use of resources in the marketplace (for example, buying a tube of toothpaste—is it worth what it will cost me to get it?). In simple everyday transactions, this sort of logic is intuitive and not difficult for the consumer;

as the complexity of the evaluation increases (for example, a variety of benefits and costs spread over long time periods), so does the difficulty of relying on implicit calculation and intuition.

In the context of health care, CBA is used when the goal is to determine the net value of an action or the appropriate level of expenditure on a particular intervention: "How do the benefits of this program compare to its costs?" or, "How do the benefits and costs of this program change as the level of program activity is changed?" Thus, at least in principle, CBA can be used to answer questions such as, "Is this worth doing at all?" or, "How much more of this is worth doing?"

CBA requires that all benefit and cost values, regardless of what they represent, be expressed in monetary terms. This allows the calculation of a net value (benefit minus cost). Stating *cost* in monetary terms is usually straightforward, but in the case of health programs it can sometimes be difficult to put the *benefits* into dollar units. For instance, if the purpose of the program is to save lives by lessening the severity of myocardial infarctions (for example, by a drug therapy), what is the appropriate *monetary* value of the benefit?

The basic equation of CBA is the calculation of a net present value (NPV):

$$NPV = \sum_{i=1}^{t} \frac{B_i - C_i}{(1 + r)^i}$$

where i = a particular time period, one of t, the total number of time periods included in the analysis
B_i = benefits in time period i
C_i = costs in time period i
r = the appropriate discount rate (see explanation below)

NPV is discussed in terms of *net* costs because costs are subtracted from benefits, and as a *present value* because the evaluation is made from the point of view of the current time, even though the costs and benefits may extend well into the future (in the case of immunizations, perhaps decades). The summation sign (Σ) indicates that the net benefit (benefit minus cost) is added over all time periods included in the analysis. A positive NPV means that over the relevant time span, the value of the benefits exceeds the value of the costs (and the reverse is true for a negative NPV). Although there are many possible complications, the most important being a limited budget, one could generalize simply by saying that anything with a positive NPV is "worth doing," and the higher the NPV, the better the activity is.

The *discount rate* is essentially an interest rate, used to estimate the impact of time on the decision (note that this is a special use of the word *discount*, which can also have its usual meaning of a price reduction; one must rely on the context to know which is correct). For instance, a cost of $100 that will not be incurred until 5 years in the future is clearly different from a cost of $100 in the present. One way to think of the present value of that future $100 cost is to determine how much money would currently have to be set aside in an investment in order for the accumulated interest to raise the value of the investment to $100 in 5 years to meet the cost. The higher the interest rate, the lower the needed investment (the present value of the future amount) and vice versa. The same reasoning can be applied to benefits: a promise to receive $100 in the future is not the same as receiving $100 in the present. The NPV equation is an application of the ordinary compound interest formula that would be used to calculate the future value of a savings account. It depends on the present value, the interest rate, and the amount of time the investment is allowed to grow:

$$FV = PV(1 + r)^i, \text{ where}$$

$$FV = \text{future value}$$

$$PV = \text{present value}$$

$$r = \text{the interest rate}$$

$$i = \text{the number of time periods into the future}$$

If you want to calculate instead how much money you would need in the present to achieve a particular future value (say $100 in 5 years), the equation can be rearranged to look much like the cost-benefit equation:

$$PV = \frac{FV}{(1 + r)^i}$$

Thus, if the appropriate discount rate is 6%, a cost or benefit of $100 that occurs in 5 years is worth slightly less than $75 in the present:

$$PV = \frac{\$100}{(1 + .06)^5} = \$74.73$$

Cost-Effectiveness Analysis

Unlike CBA, CEA allows the measure of outcome or benefit to be left in nonmonetary units. This means that CEA is sometimes more straightforward to undertake, because there may be natural measures of effectiveness (for example, years of life saved). It also means that CEA is more readily applied in circumstances in which the purpose of the analysis is to compare ways of achieving the same kind of outcome: the alternatives may be compared directly in terms of cost per unit of effectiveness achieved (or the inverse, effectiveness per dollar spent). Clearly, CEA is not appropriate for the comparison of programs with widely variant purposes. For example, it is hard to understand how to compare the cost-effectiveness of two programs if the outcome of one is dental caries avoided by fluoridating water and the outcome of the other is lives saved by immunization. However, it would be appropriate to compare the cost of saving lives (or the number of lives saved per dollar spent) in two different methods of implementing immunization. CEA can be used when the purpose is to decide whether something is worth doing, but only if there is a standard of some kind against which the result can be tested (for example, is it worth spending X dollars per additional cancer detected in a screening program?).

Generally, CEA is used when the goal is to allocate health related investments in order to maximize health effectiveness of a particular kind. It attempts to answer the question, "Which of the known ways of achieving the outcome we want produces the most of that outcome per dollar spent on the program?" CEA is particularly widely used in technology assessment (for example, assessing use of drugs, medical devices, or certain procedures) to determine whether it is appropriate to switch to a new way of doing something.

In the case of cost-effectiveness of alternative treatment programs, the analysis would be set up as shown, with the resulting ratios compared as a guide to selection (the notation being used is that of Weinstein and Stason, 1977):

$$CE \text{ ratio} = \Delta C / \Delta E$$

$$\Delta C = \sum_{i=1}^{t} \frac{\Delta CRx_i + \Delta CSE_i - \Delta CM_i + \Delta CRx\Delta LE_i}{(1 + r)^i}$$

$$\Delta E = \sum_{i=1}^{t} \frac{\Delta Y_i + \Delta YM_i - \Delta YSE_i}{(1 + r)^i}$$

where Δ represents a change in the level of a variable, and

C = cost

E = effectiveness

CRx = cost of the treatment program

CSE = cost of treating side effects of the program

CM = cost avoided because of reduced morbidity

$CRx\Delta LE$ = (net) cost incurred because of treatments that will become necessary owing to an increase in life expectancy

Y = years of life or other measure of program effectiveness

YM = quality added to years of life because of reduced morbidity

YSE = years of life lost owing to side effects

Each of the cost and effectiveness measures is discounted to the present and summed in the same way as was done in CBA. Although the equations may look formidable, the reasoning is intuitive. The numerator includes all the measures indicating how the program under analysis changes cost, and the denominator contains all the measures of how the program has an impact on the outcome or effect. The ratio is then interpreted as a cost per unit of outcome.

Cost-Utility Analysis

Cost-utility analysis (CUA) is actually a type of CEA in which the effectiveness mea-

sure reflects *subjective* valuation as well as objective outcome. For instance, a person facing extensive chemotherapy might not evaluate the additional life span gained as being worth as much as the same life span without the side effects of the treatment, because of the impact of the side effects on the perceived quality of life. In standard CEA, side effects are important because they may diminish the objective effectiveness of the program or require additional treatment; for instance, a screening program might result in a small number of injuries that require treatment and thus add to cost. CUA is concerned about this impact but would add any positive or negative *subjective* evaluation by those being screened (for instance, some persons might prefer not to know that they have a condition if there is no effective treatment available). CUA may also consider varying response to the seriousness or acceptability of certain symptoms (Danese, Powe, Sawin, & Ladenson, 1996). There is no new arithmetic to learn in CUA, which follows the CEA calculations. However, there is extensive literature on the ways to elicit utility (subjective value) judgments from individuals in order to modify the effectiveness measures appropriately. A good survey can be found in Richardson (1994).

ISSUES IN COST MEASUREMENT AND ANALYSIS

The Impact of Time on Value

As explained previously, the discounting process reflects both the subjective preference to have things in the present rather than later, and the real effect of interest rates. The choice of the discount rate can have a substantial impact on the decision, especially if costs and benefits occur in a very different pattern over time. A common pattern in some health programs would be to have all costs up front, but with benefits delayed or spread over several years. The choice of discount rate can raise troubling intergenerational issues—for example, the higher the discount rate applied to future benefits, the more likely one is to favor programs that achieve results quickly, and thus to reject programs that are primarily preventive or aimed toward the young (see box).

➤ Impact on Project Evaluation of Varying the Discount Rate*

		Undiscounted Benefits and Costs in Each Time Period† (Years from Current Period)				Present Value at Different Discount Rates		
		0	1	5	10	0%	3%	6%
Project A	Benefit	0	0	0	200,000	200,000	148,819	111,679
	Cost	100,000	0	0	0	100,000	100,000	100,000
	Net present value					100,000	48,819	11,679
Project B	Benefit		0	50,000	100,000	0	150,000	134,804	121,896
	Cost	100,000	0	0	0	100,000	100,000	100,000
	Net present value					50,000	34,804	21,896

* Shaded cells indicate higher net present value.
† The calulations assume that benefits and costs occur *only* in the time periods shown. Project A has higher total benefits than Project B ($200,000 versus $150,000), but the benefits occur later. At a high discount rate, Project B looks better than Project A.

Inflation

In addition to the influence of time on values as discussed previously, time may create a complication in the measurements resulting from the phenomenon of persistently increasing prices. A one-time increase in a price is not inflationary; there must be an expectation that the price will continue to increase and that such increases will be generally spread throughout the economy. In the context of research on cost, inflation becomes important if the time periods under study extend fairly far into the future (or into the past). If so, it may be that any measures with monetary value will need to be adjusted so as not to be misleading. For instance, expenditure for a typical day in the hospital has increased manyfold over the period since the introduction of Medicare and Medicaid in the mid-1960s. Some of that increase in expenditure represents a real change in utilization, but some is nothing more than the change in prices attached to equivalent units. Depending on the purpose of the research, it may be appropriate to remove the effect of inflation by expressing all the monetary magnitudes in "constant dollars" of one particular time period.

This conversion to constant dollars is carried out by dividing the unadjusted monetary values by an index number that expresses the relationship between prices in the period being adjusted and in some other period chosen as the base. For example, if

the Consumer Price Index is chosen as the measure of price change, the base currently used in the CPI is the average of prices in the years 1982–1984, and the general price index for all urban consumers in July 1996 is 157. That is, prices measured by this index increased approximately 57 index points or 57% between 1982–1984, when the index was at its base value of 100, and July 1996. Thus, if a particular price in July 1996 was $1258, then it can be calculated to be $1258 divided by 157, or $801.27 in the dollars of the 1982–1984 period. As this example illustrates, the arithmetic of inflationary adjustment is simple. What is not so simple is the choice of an appropriate index to represent inflation in a particular setting, especially that of health care. This complex topic has been treated extensively in the literature (for example, see Newhouse [1989], and Getzen [1992]).

Geographical Variability

Research done in a single location does not need to consider geographical variability, but any research that compares sites may need to account for variation in prices and costs resulting from such things as urban and rural location. It would not be surprising to find that caring for a patient of a particular type is more expensive in Boston than in a small town in Ohio, because of differences in labor costs, rent, and so on.

These variations are no different in principle from the inflationary changes previously discussed. Adjusting for geographical variation requires index numbers that measure change related to spatial location rather than the passage of time. This has been a major issue in public programs such as Medicare, which must pay for the same services in highly diverse locations. The data available for measuring regional variation are not as well developed (and are subject to more disagreement over interpretation) as the data for recognizing change in prices in a single place. The researcher is likely to have very little recourse but to use the available index values, knowing that there is controversy (for example, see U.S. Department of Health and Human Services [1995]).

Valuation

Valuation is required in two basic situations. The first, and somewhat easier, is in deciding the appropriate cost measurement for a durable resource such as capital. This is usually handled, in part, as an allocation question, with the monetary cost per unit of service (for example, an hour of magnetic resonance imaging equipment time) determined by a depreciation allowance. The more difficult situation involves the need to measure intrinsically nonmonetary things such as human life or well-being in monetary terms, a task that is not unique to health care programs. It is present in many legal situations, such as for compensation for workplace injury. One important difference is that, in many legal settings, the value that is relevant (at least for the purposes of the court, although the injured party might not agree) is some measure of the person's worth in the labor market, such as expected lifetime income with appropriate adjustments for uncertainty and discounting. The problem with applying this sort of reasoning in health care programs is that it would place the highest value on saving the life or health of the wealthiest persons—so the top priority would probably be given to diseases of corporate executives, professional athletes, and media figures. Note also that the effect of any discrimination in the labor market would remain systematically in the evaluation of the health program; for example, if women are paid less than men, then the analysis would continue this bias.

Because of this problem, it is more common to use measures other than income. There are several creative alternatives. For instance, if one examines the differences in wages demanded by persons with different levels of risk in their work, one can calculate an implicit value that workers assign to the possibility of injury or death. It is also possible to ask the question directly, usually in the form of willingness to pay to avoid a known risk. The problem with this approach is obviously that the person may view the question as entirely hypothetical, in which case the answer may be quite different from what would be given if the person actually faced the risk. As a final example, one can calculate implicit values demonstrated by policy decisions. If X dollars are spent on a program of a particular type with a known set of outcomes, what value appears to be placed on life or health within that program? Although this is not very finely tuned, it can at least give a comparative standard. These difficulties of CBA sometimes lead to "mixed" analyses, with CBA applied to monetary outcomes and CEA applied to others (Finkler, Kovner, Knickman, & Hendrickson, 1994).

In many cases, the benefit or effectiveness measures may represent outcomes that should be modified in some way to account for variation in quality of life, as suggested by CUA. For instance, a laryngectomy may extend the life of a throat cancer patient, but the evaluation of the quality differential of that longevity might vary from patient to patient, depending on the value placed on ease of oral communication. Similarly, many therapies have relatively severe side effects, which should be taken into account in evaluating outcomes. The most important point is that a complete analysis should make some attempt to determine whether such quality adjustments are likely to have a significant impact on the evaluation—for example, an otherwise cost-effective alternative that has significant negative side effects may be less desirable than others after adjustment for change in the quality of life.

SOME PRACTICAL CONCERNS IN RESEARCH ON COST
Sources of Cost Data

There are three basic approaches for obtaining cost data in health care organizations. The majority of organizational providers are participants in Medicare and Medicaid, and thus there is generally a legally mandated uniform cost-reporting system in place. Second, most health care providers are also engaged in major internal cost-finding and cost-accounting efforts in order to negotiate reasonable payment under managed care contracts or to establish their own prices. Finally, the researcher can collect data unique to the task at hand. The uniform data collected for public programs have the advantages of low cost, because the data have already been assembled, open access as public documents, and relatively straightforward comparability from institution to institution because of the accounting standards. However, the cost reports are designed to answer the operational needs of the payment programs and thus frequently aggregate or omit items that would be useful to the researcher asking a focused question. If the organization has undertaken a comprehensive cost-accounting program for its own decision making, the researcher may find that these internal reports contain much greater detail; the trade-off is that the data may lack external comparability and are proprietary, which may require more cumbersome approval to gain access. The researcher who engages in specialized data collection needs organizational approval and can maintain external comparability only if there is a protocol for this purpose within the research design.

Price Versus Cost Revisited

One of the most common confusions in research on cost in health care is the myriad ways that financial data are described. As discussed previously, *price* and *cost* refer to different concepts in economics, and this is certainly true in health care. To add to the confusion, there are multiple versions of price data, depending on the payer: very few pay the nominal fee-for-service charges quoted by the provider, because there is almost certain to be a contractual agreement that specifies some sort of discount from these charges or an alternative payment system altogether such as capitation (a fixed payment per patient to the provider, regardless of the quantity or cost of services provided). It is thus essential that the researcher ensure that the data being used in

fact represent cost rather than one of these price variables. If it is necessary to use some form of price or expenditure as a proxy for cost, it is important to ensure that the price concepts being used are consistent. Otherwise, it is clearly possible that apparent cost variation in comparisons might simply reflect differences in bargaining ability for discounts rather than true differences in cost. It is also true that some payers do not recognize certain elements as acceptable cost, and there may therefore be more than one system of accounting in place for costs. One of the most common examples of this is the cost of education in the hospital; these costs are certainly incurred, but they are sometimes difficult to disentangle from the actual treatment cost of particular patients. Although it may be intuitively obvious, it is

➤ The Jargon of Health Care Payment

CHARGE

The nominal and largely fictional price for a service, which is generally relevant only for a few cash-paying buyers.

CONTRACTUAL ALLOWANCE

The reduction in charge made to a particular payer, usually by negotiation or competitive bidding. The true price is the charge less the contractual allowance.

REIMBURSABLE COST

The components of cost permitted by a party whose payment is based in some way on cost, which is now usually a relatively small proportion of payers.

WRITE-OFF

Charges that cannot be collected for a reason other than a contractual allowance. Includes two components: bad debts (billed, but payment not collected) and charity care (not billed, and no intention to collect).

➤ Example of Indirect Cost Allocation

Indirect cost area: Human Resources Department
Cost to be allocated: $400,000
Cost allocation basis: Number of employees in the area receiving the allocated
                            indirect cost

Areas Receiving Indirect Cost	Number of Employees in Area	Percent of Total Employees	Cost Allocated to Area	Output of Area*	Allocated Cost per Unit of Output
Inpatient Unit 1	23	46%	$184,000	12,000 patient days	$15.33
Inpatient Unit 2	16	32%	$128,000	5,000 patient days	$25.60
Outpatient Unit 1	4	8%	$32,000	9,000 visits	$3.56
Outpatient Unit 2	7	14%	$56,000	14,000 visits	$4.00
TOTAL	50	100%	$400,000		

* These are crude measures for the purpose of the example.

important for the researcher to understand precisely what is and is not included in the cost data being used (see box on page 142).

Allocating Cost to Activities

Cost allocation can have two related meanings. The first, mentioned previously, is the assignment of indirect costs, such as nursing management, to the final units of output for which a cost estimate is desired (for example, cost per case or per patient day). Traditionally this has meant assigning the cost of "nonrevenue departments," for which no separate charge was made, to "revenue departments," whose output was given a price. The myriad ways of paying for care have blurred this distinction, but it is still important to know the full cost of an activity.

Indirect costs are usually allocated according to a measure of activity or workload. For instance, the cost of the human resources department might be allocated to the patient care departments on the basis of the number of employees in each department (see box). Many standard procedures are available for these allocations, including those used by the government for determining cost in the Medicare program.

The other meaning of cost allocation is the estimation of relative resource requirements for different outputs within a depart-

ment. The three principal methods are the ratio of cost to charges (RCC), relative value units (RVUs), and activity-based costing (ABC). RCC is acknowledged to be a rough estimate based on the assumption that resource use is proportional to price. RVUs have been widely used in nursing, usually in the form of some sort of severity adjustment to the basic unit of work (Barhyte & Glandon, 1988; Flarey, 1990; Ballard, Gray, Knauf, & Uppal, 1993; Wong, Gordon, Cassard, Weisman, & Bergner, 1993; Moss, O'Connor, & Windle, 1994). It is usually conceded that ABC, which examines cost at a micro level and attempts to link cost allocation to "cost drivers" for each service, gives the most accurate results (Llewellyn et al., 1994; Fox, Ehreth, & Issel, 1994; West, Balas, & West, 1996; Wise et al., 1996).

SUMMARY

There is a great amount of research literature on the costs of health care, exploring an enormous variety of descriptive and analytical cost-related questions. However, many of the basic tasks in all these studies are the same: deciding upon a consistent point of view in measuring cost, keeping price and cost as separate concepts, and using appropriate measures of cost for the question at hand. The fact that there are so many research options suggests the importance of sensitivity analysis, in which the assumptions or approaches are varied in order to observe the impact on the results. Sensitivity analysis can discover huge differences in cost estimates—one study reports a 60% variation depending on the options chosen (Wilson, Prescott, & Aleksandrowicz, 1988). Such a possibility for variation creates a serious responsibility for the researcher to proceed with care and document scrupulously so that the interpretation of the findings is clear.

REFERENCES

Ballard, K. A, Gray, R. F., Knauf, R. A., & Uppal, P. (1993). Measuring variations in nursing care per DRG. *Nursing Management, 24,* 33–36, 40–41.

Barhyte, D. Y., & Glandon, G. L. (1988). Issues in nursing labor costs allocation. *Journal of Nursing Administration, 18,* 16–19.

Danese, M. D., Powe, N. R., Sawin, C. T., & Ladenson, P. W. (1996). Screening for mild thyroid failure at the periodic health examination: A decision and cost-effectiveness analysis. *JAMA, 276,* 285–292.

Finkler, S. A., Kovner, C. T., Knickman, J. R., & Hendrickson, G. (1994). Innovation in nursing: A benefit/cost analysis. *Nursing Economics, 12,* 18–27.

Flarey, D. L. (1990). A methodology for costing nursing service. *Nursing Administration Quarterly, 14,* 41–51.

Fox, S., Ehreth, J., & Issel, L. M. (1994). A cost evaluation of a hospital-based perinatal case management program. *Nursing Economics, 12,* 214, 215–220.

Getzen, T. E. (1992). Medical care price indexes: Theory, construction & empirical analysis of the US series 1927–1990. In R. M. Scheffler and L. G. Rossiter (Eds.), *Advances in health economics and health services research. 13,* (pp. 83–128).

Hundley, V. A., Donaldson, C., Lang, G. D., Cruickshank, F. M., Glazener, C. M. A., Milne, J. M., & Mollison, J. (1995). Costs of intrapartum care in a midwife-managed delivery unit and a consultant-led labour ward. *Midwifery, 11,* 103–109.

LaGodna, G. E., & Hendrix, M. J. (1989). Impaired nurses: A cost analysis. *Journal of Nursing Administration, 19,* 13–18.

Llewellyn, J., Giese, R., Nosek, L. J., Lager, J. D., Turco, S. J., Goodell, J., Coleman, J., McQuone, M. J., Collier, P. A., Minard, D., Cottrell, J. H., Stralow, J., & Gautney, L. (1994). A multicenter study of costs and nursing impact of cartridge-needle units. *Nursing Economics, 12,*208–214.

Mauskopf, J. A., Paul, J. E., Wichman, D. S., White, A. D., & Tilson, H. D. (1996). Economic impact of treatment of HIV-positive pregnant women and their newborns with zidovudine: Implications for HIV screening. *JAMA, 276,* 132–138.

Moss, M. T., O'Connor, S. A., & Windle, P. E. (1994). A perioperative acuity measurement system. *Nursing Management, 25,* 64A–B, F, H.

Newhouse, J. P. (1989). Measuring medical prices and understanding their effects. *Journal of Health Administration Education, 7,* 19–26.

Regan, M. B., Byers, P. H., & Mayrovitz, H. N. (1995).

Efficacy of a comprehensive pressure ulcer prevention program in an extended care facility. *Advances in Wound Care, 8,* 49–55.

Richardson, J. (1994). Cost utility analysis: What should be measured? *Social Science and Medicine, 37,* 7–21.

Stone, P. W., & Walker, P. H. (1995). Cost-effectiveness analysis: birth center vs. hospital care. *Nursing Economics, 13,* 299–308.

U.S. Department of Health and Human Services, Health Care Financing Administration, Office of Research and Demonstrations (1995). *Medicare Geographic Practice Cost Index.* Report to Congress 1995.

Weinstein, M. C., & Stason, W. B. (1977). Foundations of cost-effectiveness analysis for health and medical practices. *New England Journal of Medicine, 296,* 716–721.

West, T. D., Balas, E. A., & West, D. A. (1996). Contrasting RCC, RVU, and ABC for managed care decisions. *Healthcare Financial Management, 50(8),* 54–61.

Williams, R. M. (1996). The costs of visits to emergency departments. *New England Journal of Medicine, 334,* 642–646.

Wilson, L., Prescott, P. A., & Aleksandrowicz, L. (1988). Nursing: A major hospital cost component. *Health Services Research, 22,* 773–796.

Wise, L. C., Bostrom, J., Crosier, J. A., White, S., & Caldwell, R. (1996). Cost-benefit analysis of an automated medication system. *Nursing Economics, 14,* 224–231.

SUGGESTED READINGS

Allred, C. A., Arford, P. H., Michel, Y., Dring, R., Carter, V., & Veitch, J. S. (1995). A cost-effectiveness analysis of acute care case management outcomes. *Nursing Economics, 13,* 129–136.

Centerwall, B. S., & Criqui, M. H. (1978). Prevention of the Wernicke-Korsakoff syndrome: A cost-benefit analysis. *New England Journal of Medicine, 299,* 285–289.

Comried, L. A. (1996). Cost analysis: Initiation of HBMC and first CareMap. *Nursing Economics, 14,* 34–39.

Eckhart, J. G. (1993). Costing out nursing services: Examining the research. *Nursing Economics, 11,* 91–98.

Eisenberg, J. M. (1989). Clinical economics: A guide to the economic analysis of clinical practices. *JAMA, 262,* 2879–2886.

Hillner, B. E., & Smith, T. J. (1991). Efficacy and cost effectiveness of adjuvant chemotherapy in women with node-negative breast cancer. *New England Journal of Medicine, 324,* 160–168.

Jackson, L. A., Schuchat, A., Gorsky, R. D., & Wenger, J. D. (1995). Should college students be vaccinated against meningococcal disease? A cost-benefit analysis. *American Journal of Public Health, 85,* 843–845.

Joyce, T., Corman, H., & Grossman, M. (1988). A cost-effectiveness analysis of strategies to reduce infant mortality. *Medical Care, 26,* 348–360.

Mark, D. B., Hlatky, M. A., Califf, R.M., Naylor, C. D., Lee, K. L., Armstrong, P. W., Barbash, G., White, H., Simoons, M. L., Nelson, C. L., Clapp-Channing, N.,

Knight, J. D., Harrell, F. E. Jr., Simes, J., & Topol, E. J. (1995). Cost effectiveness of thrombolytic therapy with tissue plasminogen activator as compared with streptokinase for acute myocardial infarction. *New England Journal of Medicine, 332,* 1418–1424.

Saywell, R. M. Jr., Lassiter, W. L. III, & Flynn, B. C. (1995). A cost analysis of a nurse-managed, voluntary community health clinic. *Journal of Nursing Administration, 25,* 17–27.

Seitz, C. H., & Edwardson, S. R. (1987). Nursing care costs for stroke patients in a rehabilitation setting. *Journal of Nursing Administration, 17,* 17–22.

Skydell, B., & Arndt, M. (1988). The price of nursing care. *Nursing Clinics of North America, 23,* 493–501.

West, D. A., Hicks, L. L., Balas, E. A., & West, T. D. (1996). Profitable capitation requires accurate costing. *Nursing Economics, 14,* 162–170, 150.

Wong, R., Gordon, D. L., Cassard, S. D., Weisman, C. S., & Bergner, M. (1993). A cost analysis of a professional practice model for nursing. *Nursing Economics, 11,* 292–297, 323.

Zbrozek, A. S., Agbara, E., & Head, M. (1994). Mannitol injections: With or without filter needles? A cost-effectiveness analysis. *Nursing Economics, 12,* 196–200.

Conducting Research

Chapter 12

Research Facilitation

Karin T. Kirchhoff and Magdalena A. Mateo

Although most nurses value the importance of research in practice, few are actually involved in conducting research. Organizations continue to seek ways of promoting activities that foster the conduct and use of research in practice, particularly at a time when there is increased emphasis in evaluating outcomes of care from the consumer and provider perspectives. Examples of activities that promote research are including research as an integral aspect of organizational goals, establishing a research committee, defining staff responsibilities for research, and using components of the research process in developing and evaluating innovations in practice. This chapter presents organizational strategies for promoting the integration of research in practice.

BARRIERS TO INTEGRATING RESEARCH INTO PRACTICE

Identifying factors that deter nurses from achieving research-based practice is essential. Champagne, Tornquist, and Funk (1997) used a BARRIERS instrument to identify barriers to using research. The four subscales of the instrument are (1) characteristics of the nurse—research values, (2) characteristics of the setting—perceived barriers, (3) characteristics of the research—methods and conclusions, and (4) characteristics of the research presentation. Respondents who reported that their primary job responsibility is clinical rated the top 10 barriers related to characteristics of the setting. Not having enough authority to make changes and not enough time are the two major barriers identified. These categories of barriers for research use could also be used in describing barriers for the conduct of research.

Nurses reported that they lacked the confidence to participate in designing and conducting research (Butler, 1995). Barriers that have been identified include difficulty in accessing research publications and lack of knowledge about research (Logan & Davies, 1995).

STRATEGIES FOR FACILITATING RESEARCH

Establishing ways for collaboration among staff nurses, advanced practice nurses, and nursing faculty can promote the development of an inquisitive mind set among staff. A mentoring program focusing on research can be initiated as part of an organization's strategy to provide career development. Examples of activities include review of research-based practice guidelines, protocols, or critical paths for feasibility and relevance. Having staff nurses actively participate in developing guidelines is a good way to introduce them to applications of research to practice.

Characteristics of the Nurse

ORIENTATION TO RESEARCH

Orientation to research may occur when staff are new employees or when staff become involved for the first time in the conduct and use of research. Orientation to the research process may include the use of peers or collaboration with staff in advanced nursing roles or nursing faculty.

Including the importance of research in practice is highlighted when new employees are informed about their role. When there are multiple applicants for a single position, a choice can be made to select the nurse with some commitment to research. Orientation programs need to include specific ideas on how employees are expected to support the research mission. Examples of roles that staff could assume include responding to product evaluation surveys, attaining the desired outcomes by ongoing monitoring of patient care, or using research literature in developing patient care guidelines or critical paths.

Orientation to research also occurs when a nurse is participating in research for the first time. Nurses expressing interest can be encouraged to speak to staff who have successfully participated in research as a way to acquire a realistic perspective about the required commitment (Mateo, 1992). Then, the interested worker can decide whether it is feasible to pursue a research experience.

It is important to orient staff to ways of communicating research findings to their colleagues on the unit, other disciplines, and at conferences to instill the value that dissemination of findings is an integral step in research.

RESPONSIBILITIES OF STAFF

Leadership in an organization has responsibility to create an environment in which creative thinking is rewarded and questioning is encouraged. In this environment, nurses feel free to question their practice, look for ways to improve care, and challenge tradition. Valuing of nursing research is evident when it is included in the departmental philosophy and objectives (Kirchhoff & Titler, 1994).

Managers can do things that take little time but that are seen as important rewards to staff nurses. When a staff nurse receives a letter from his or her manager that acknowledges that nurse's role in conducting a study, that letter is treasured. Mentioning ongoing research or research use at unit meetings provides positive feedback to the involved nurses.

Annual evaluations should include discussion of research activities in which the nurse has participated. The staff nurse may choose to keep a portfolio of professional activities, including research. Examples of scholarly activities that contribute to the development of research skills should be included when setting goals for the next evaluation. This includes participating in research projects, assisting in identifying potential subjects for a study, reviewing data collection protocols, recruiting subjects for a study, assisting with the orientation of staff to research, responding to surveys, or participating in focus groups. Participation of staff in focus groups is vital for organizations because they can provide administrators with substantial information on a selected topic (Crawford & Acorn, 1997).

Characteristics of the Setting

RESOURCES FOR RESEARCH

There are numerous ways organizations show support for research. In some organizations there is a director of nursing research, whereas other organizations combine this role with other responsibilities such as continuous improvement or education. Academic health centers with a college of nursing may have a faculty with a joint appointment (Kirchhoff & Mateo, 1996). Having a designated person for research facilitation helps in the research productivity in terms of funded projects, publications, and presentations (Mateo & Kirchhoff, 1995).

Stonestreet and Lamb-Havard (1994) described the following six categories of organizational strategies for promoting research-based practice. The primary levels of accountability were designated to the individual, unit or service, and department or institution.

- Establish the expectation—direction and commitment
- Develop the knowledge base—facilitation of knowledge of the research process and utilization
- Disseminate research findings—strategies for communicating study findings
- Provide support structures—systems to support conduct and use of research
- Provide tangible resources—funding, time, access to literature
- Facilitate change in practice—an environment and system that thrive on change

One of the roles of nurse practitioners is integration of research in practice. The availability of a microcomputer for direct data entry by the nurse practitioner during client interaction or from records in the clinical facility makes the integration of the research role manageable (Matteson & Hawkins, 1993). Direct entry by using software programs allows for flexibility in data management, eliminates the need for paper data collection tools, and eliminates the step of data entry from data sheets, which may be a source of error.

CONSORTIUM ARRANGEMENTS

A consortium, an arrangement among local or national organizations to share resources, has been successfully used in research efforts. The consortium enhances collaboration among staff from participating organizations and conserves resources. This collaboration allows staff to gain access to subjects when a study can be conducted across settings.

RESEARCH COMMITTEE

Many clinical settings have a research committee to facilitate the conduct of research by both their own staff and students, faculty, or clinicians at other settings. Research facilitation is done through various committee charges (see box). This committee has the potential for slowing down access to the agency; the process needs to be reviewed regularly for the degree of facilita-

➤ Frequently Reported Charges of Research Committees

- Facilitation of conduct and use of research
- Determination and facilitation of the research agenda of the institution
- Assurance of the scientific merit of projects
- Dissemination of study results and information on ongoing and completed studies
- Manuscript review
- Resource allocation
- Presentation of research education

tion offered to investigators. The research committee frequently sees its major function as ensuring scientific merit, but that function is frequently met by the student's thesis committee or by faculty peer review. More importantly, feasibility should be attended to and the overuse of certain populations (for example, laboring mothers or infants in the neonatal intensive care unit) should be evaluated.

Reviewers must be clinicians and have some advanced research training to be credible to those reviewed. Assigning two or more members as primary reviewers for a study assigns special responsibility to a few for leadership in the discussion. Orientation of new members and periodic review for all members is helpful to keep the original purpose of the committee to the forefront.

Dissemination of results of studies conducted in the agency is another useful function of the committee. These could be in poster or paper format and offered on a special day or during Nurses' Week. On a regular basis, a newsletter could provide information on ongoing and completed studies. On a local area network accessible to the staff, a listing of ongoing and approved studies keeps up the interest of the staff in the future results. This list could also serve as a resource for identifying mentors or collaborators.

The research committee could also serve as an internal review group for manuscripts intended for submittal for publication. Even persons who do not have clinical expertise in the topic of the manuscripts have useful comments.

Research committees have also assumed the responsibility for allocating resources and for determining and facilitating an organization's research agenda (Vessey & Campos, 1992; Stonestreet & Lamb-Havard, 1994). Resources may include funding for studies, scholarships to attend a research conference, or access to research literature through the local area or the Internet. Staff could be invited to submit an essay of the benefit that can be gained from attending a research conference in the areas of patient care, professional practice, and development of skills. As part of the entry to the contest, applicants should include a plan for sharing their experience with staff. Using predetermined criteria, scholarship could be awarded to the person who is best able to articulate the benefits that can be accrued from attending a research conference. Access to a MEDLINE search on the patient care unit promotes the use of the literature in seeking information that could help in solving clinical problems. The strategic plan can be used to determine the institution's research agenda. The committee could issue a call for proposals to fund studies that relate to the organization's strategic goals such as investigation of care delivery models, reduction of costs, or recruitment and retention of diverse staff.

In some settings, unit-based research committees are initiated. Unit-based research committees often serve as a vehicle to facilitate the development of the staff's research knowledge.

RESEARCH MENTORSHIP PROGRAM

A research mentorship program may be initiated. A formal program has the advantages of giving progressive opportunities for developing research skills through collaboration and the facilitation of practice-relevant research experiences. Govoni and Pierce (1997) described the following seven C's of collaboration between clinical nurse specialists and staff nurses: cohesion, contribution, communication, commitment, compatibility, consensus, and credit (see Chapter 15).

A list of staff and nursing faculty who could serve as mentors can be developed along with their areas of research interest

so that this is readily available to staff. See Chapter 6 for information on mentorship.

Characteristics of the Research

Although nurses have developed problem-solving skills, the steps in the research process and the terms used by researchers may seem foreign and not understandable. The most productive way to overcome this barrier is to facilitate the nurse's education for the next degree. When this is not feasible, alternatives include attendance at research education programs or research meetings and participation in research (see Chapter 6).

Issues in evaluating research for use include the appropriateness of the conclusions and the fit of a single study into the group of studies on that topic. Education of the nurse and assistance from those with advanced skills (clinical nurse specialists, nurse practitioners, or nurse researchers) are ways of overcoming this barrier.

Some studies are not ready for clinicians to read or use. For example, the results of laboratory studies testing interventions under controlled conditions may not generalize well. They could be tests of theories or tools. The studies most relevant to clinicians are those about clinical research topics in which nursing practices are tested under real conditions or in which information about their patients or clients is provided.

Characteristics of the Research Presentation

Some speakers have a clearer presentation style than others and some have a better understanding of their methods and can give cogent presentations. Research meetings that plan for a critique of the reports or interpretive comments have the possibility of a wider understanding by the audience.

Applicability of the results to the nurse's practice setting is the draw to attend certain sessions. Those in attendance appreciate clear, understandable presentations that include applications to practice.

SUMMARY

The characteristics of the nurse and the setting have a major impact on whether re-

search is facilitated. Selection and orienta-
tion of the staff are critical functions.
Administrators have a major influence on
the setting and available resources. Distri-
bution of resources reveals the values of the
leaders.

   Characteristics of the research and how it
is presented tend to be more external to the
setting and are heavily influenced by the
researchers (faculty, students, and staff in a
research function). Focusing on all of these
aspects will facilitate both the conduct and
use of research.

REFERENCES

Butler, L. (1995). Valuing research in clinical practice: A basis for developing a strategic plan for nursing research. *Canadian Journal of Nursing Research, 27,* 33–49.

Champagne, M. T., Tornquist, M. A., & Funk, S. G. (1997). Achieving research-based practice. *American Journal of Nursing, 97,* 16AAA–16DDD.

Crawford, M., & Acorn, S. (1997). Focus groups: Their use in administrative research. *Journal of Nursing Administration, 27*(5), 15–18.

Govoni, A. L., & Pierce, L. L. (1997). Collaborative research among clinical nurse specialists and staff nurses. *The Journal of Continuing Education in Nursing, 28,* 181–187.

Kirchhoff, K. T., & Mateo, M. A. (1996). Roles and responsibilities of clinical nurse researchers. *Journal of Professional Nursing, 12*(2), 86–90.

Kirchhoff, K. T., & Titler, M. G. (1994). Responsibilities of nurse executives in conducting and using research in the practice setting. In R. Spitzer-Lehman (Ed.), *Nursing Management Desk Reference.* Philadelphia: W. B. Saunders.

Logan, J., & Davies, B. (1995). The staff nurse as research facilitator. *Canadian Journal of Nursing Administration, 8*(1), 92–110.

Mateo, M. A. (1992). Socializing nurses to using research: Strategies that work in the clinical setting. *Journal of Nursing Administration, 22*(12), 10–11.

Mateo, M. A., & Kirchhoff, K. T. (1995). Productivity of nurse researchers employed in clinical settings. *Journal of Nursing Administration, 25*(10), 37–42.

Matteson, P. S., & Hawkins, J. W. (1993). Facilitating the nurse practitioner's research role: Using a microcomputer for data entry in clinical settings. *Journal of the American Academy of Nurse Practitioners, 5,* 125–129.

Stonestreet, J. S., & Lamb-Havard, J. (1994). Organizational strategies to promote research-based practice. *AACN Clinical Issues in Critical Care Nursing, 5*(2), 133–146.

Vessey, J. A., & Campos, R. (1992). The role of nursing research committees. *Nursing Research, 41,* 247–249.

Chapter 13

Gaining Support for the Study

Marquis D. Foreman

A preliminary yet essential step for conducting research is gaining the support of a clinical setting. The process of gaining support could have various results: (1) the study could be favorably and readily facilitated through the organizational and bureaucratic requirements for conducting research, (2) the study could be subject to overt or covert obstacles, ultimately resulting in sabotage, or (3) the study could fall into some state between these two extremes. The importance of attending to this process is evident; however, the process often receives too little attention from the principal investigator (PI) and is sometimes delegated to a research assistant. In addition, the process of gaining support is time-consuming. McHugh and Johnson (1980) reported that gaining the support of an organization for a study can take as long as 1 year. Adequate time must be allocated in the timetable of the project to successfully complete this process.

Gaining support of a clinical setting for a study should be guided by the principle that resources provided by a clinical setting are as important as the research plan itself. A clinical setting provides tangible resources (access to subjects or assistance in collection of data) and intangible resources (continued enthusiasm for a study in the face of a slow accrual of subjects). In negotiating access to and support of a clinical setting for a study, the investigator and the clinical setting become partners in the pursuit of knowledge.

Gaining the support of a clinical setting for a study is a dynamic process and involves four phases: (1) garnering support, (2) gaining entry, (3) gaining access, and (4) maintaining support. The process varies according to whether the researcher is an "outsider" or "insider" to the organization and whether the researcher is a "professional," a member of the nursing staff conducting research, or a student conducting research as a degree requirement. The process also is colored by various characteristics of the organization. Each phase of the process and recommendations for successfully gaining the support of a clinical setting for a study are presented in the following discussion.

GARNERING SUPPORT

Garnering support is the exploratory phase in gaining support of a clinical setting for a study. The objectives herein are to determine whether the demands of conducting the study and of operating the organization are congruent, and whether it is possible to establish a working partnership among interested parties. The activities for accomplishing these objectives include (1) contacting the potential data collection sites, (2) examining the requirements for conducting the study and the organizational policies, (3) establishing commitment, and (4) finalizing the research plan.

Contacting the Potential Data Collection Sites

Abbott (1981) and McHugh and Johnson (1980) recommended that the initial contact with a clinical setting be through the department of nursing and, preferably, with the person responsible for research (a clinical nurse researcher, chair of nursing research committee, or clinical nurse specialist). That person is most likely to have a clear understanding and appreciation of the proposed study. Initial contact should occur by telephone to determine whether further dialogue between the investigator and clinical setting is indicated. It should focus on the purpose of the study, the population to be studied, any potential problems, what is expected of the clinical setting for involvement in the study, and what the clinical setting can expect in return from the investigator. If additional dialogue is warranted (evidenced by an adequate number of the target population and expressed interest on the part of the clinical setting), a meeting should be arranged to discuss the research plan and timeline in detail.

Examining Requirements

In preparation for this meeting, certain factors that apply for all researchers must be addressed. Regardless of a stated commitment to research, the first priority in a practice setting is always service (Williams, 1989). Researchers and service personnel alike share a desire to improve patient care services. While the investigator is evaluating the potential of the clinical setting, the clinical setting is likewise evaluating the behavior of the researcher (Oda, 1983). If handled correctly, all of this can produce a partnership that yields mutual benefits for research and practice in the pursuit of knowledge. However, health care resources (those supporting the conduct of research as well as those in patient care services) are scarce. Within the context of these realities, the investigator should prepare for the meeting with the organization by developing a thorough draft of the proposal, with the focus being the procedure for data collection. The researcher should examine the relationship between the research procedure and patient care services, specifically, how one will affect the other positively and negatively. McHugh and Johnson (1980) recommended observing the delivery of patient care services in the areas used for data collection to ensure compatibility between nursing care policies and procedures and research protocol.

The purpose of the proposal meeting is to assess the feasibility of implementing a study in the given clinical setting. The investigator and the representative of the clinical setting must realize that compromise is required to complete the specific study successfully in a particular setting. The degree to which compromise can be achieved without adversely affecting the integrity of the research method or the quality of patient care services, however, must be considered. For example, Flaskerud and Janken (1978) reported on negotiations with a clinical site in which persons in the clinical site attempted to change the focus of the study. Further attempts at developing a research relationship were terminated.

Additional questions must be addressed to clarify participation of the nursing staff in the study. It must be established whether release time from job responsibilities will be granted to conduct the study (including time to search the literature, write the proposal, and collect the data), whether the study has to be conducted on personal time, or whether the study will be conducted using some combination of these protocols. Answers to such questions not only determine study feasibility but also influence the selection of the study design, data collection procedures, and timeline. The availability of resources for literature searches, typing services, and photocopying services for forms, data collection instruments, and reports should be discussed.

Other factors to be considered during this initial phase include (1) the presence of concurrent research projects that could interfere with, compete with, or contaminate the study; (2) the climate for research at the potential settings that could either facilitate or impede the study (Sayner, 1984), such as interpersonal relationships, patients' rights, support of the administration, task orientation of the staff, and availability of tangible resources for research; and (3) the existence of institutional or departmental philosophies that extol the importance of research for the achievement of goals and objectives. Direct statements about the importance and benefits of research are not necessarily evidence of a positive environment toward research.

Meetings such as those described should reveal the expectations of the clinical setting and the investigator and should make each aware of the other's intent. Initial meetings can determine whether the demands of conducting the study and of operating the organization are congruent, and whether a partnership is warranted and feasible.

Establishing Commitment

To assist in establishing the commitment of an organization to a study, the investigator should make explicit the benefits that the organization can realize as a result of participation. Although direct, or tangible, benefits for participation in research are numerous (see box) (Oberst, 1985; Blichfeldt, Deane, & Lancaster, 1987; Smeltzer & Hinshaw, 1988), there are also indirect, or intangible, benefits (see box) (Blichfeldt, Deane, & Lancaster, 1987; Smeltzer & Hinshaw, 1988). Convincing the clinical setting that there are benefits from participation enhances the probability of successfully completing the study.

Finalizing the Research Plan

After all negotiations are completed and both parties agree to the requirements for successfully implementing the research plan, the proposal should be revised to include any negotiated alterations. Two additional points should be considered in finalizing the proposal. First, the procedure for data collection must minimize the demands on and consumption of resources from the clinical setting. It is much more likely for the study to be successfully implemented and completed if this can be guaranteed. Second, the direction of the proposal must maximize the benefits for both parties.

➤ **Direct Benefits for Participation in Research**

1. Improvement in the quality, efficacy, effectiveness, and cost effectiveness of patient care services.
2. Improvement in nurse satisfaction, and, as a result, improvement in the retention of staff.
3. Generation of income by financial remuneration for resources used in the conduct of the study or exchange of professional services (for example, inservice or continuing education of staff, provision of equipment and supplies needed by the unit, and journals or other references for the unit).
4. Provision of opportunity for staff promotion.
5. Solution of a frustrating patient care problem.
6. Provision of objective documentation that nursing services make a difference in patient care outcomes.

GAINING ENTRY

The second phase in gaining support for a study includes obtaining formal support and approval. This phase occurs once it has been

➤ **Indirect Benefits for Participation in Research**

1. Improvement in professionalization of the staff.
2. Intellectual stimulation.
3. Improvement in collaborative and multidisciplinary relationships.
4. Improvement in the critical thinking and problem-solving abilities of the staff.
5. Contributions to the profession and the knowledge base for practice.
6. Sensitization to a practice problem area.

agreed that the requirements for conducting the study and the policies for operating the organization are compatible. This agreement constitutes a partnership. Activities at this point are similar for nurse researchers, members of the nursing staff conducting research, or students conducting research as a degree requirement. They include (1) identifying the organizational and departmental mechanisms (the policies and procedures for gaining access to research subjects) and (2) obtaining "formal" approval to pursue these avenues.

Identifying Policies and Procedures

Issues other than the formal research application process need to be addressed in the identification of the organizational and departmental mechanisms for gaining access to research subjects. In addition to filling out the required forms, the definition of PI should be considered. An internal faculty or staff member, however, could "sponsor" the proposal and serve as a proxy PI. Generally, it is understood that a proxy PI is merely a formality and does not convey "ownership" of the ideas in the proposal or of the data generated. On occasion, proxy PIs have attempted to dictate conditions in the study and to demand authorship on publications resulting from the study. It is necessary, therefore, to discuss the roles, responsibilities, and expectations of actual and proxy PIs.

Application to an organization for approval to conduct a study can be greatly influenced by the previous experiences of the organization with research. Positive experiences help expedite progress of a proposal through the "bureaucratic jungle." Negative experiences, however, lead to cumbersome procedural obstacles or to the withdrawal of the organization from participating as a data collection site (Oda, 1983). Knowledge of the previous experience of an organization can help in developing strategies for successful application.

The investigator should inquire about any necessary support, other than financial, for the application process. Is the investigator expected to obtain a physician's approval to approach patients for participation in a study, or is notification that a study is to occur adequate? Similarly, must the heads of all departments affected by the study be

informed about the study, or must they actively approve and sanction the conduct of the study? Whose signatures are required on what forms and for what purposes? Are the signatures merely required or are formal letters of support necessary? If a formal letter is required, can the investigator facilitate this process by providing a prepared letter for signing? Such strategies are viewed as being considerate of the resources of the clinical site and add to the credibility of the researcher. Although it is the responsibility of the clinical setting to clearly and precisely delineate the application procedure, this process can be facilitated greatly by anticipating some of the aforementioned issues.

Obtaining "Formal" Approval

The process of obtaining approval varies among clinical settings. Some organizations favor a committee structure consisting of two review bodies: (1) a nursing research committee (Kirchhoff & McGuire, 1985) to examine scientific merit and resource consumption issues and (2) a human subjects review committee (also known as the institutional review board [IRB] or the hospital research committee) to examine issues related to the protection of subjects from the risks of participating in research.

If a committee structure exists, either a nursing research committee or an IRB, the investigator must also consider the following:

1. Frequency of the committee meetings. Some organizations in which the conduct of clinical studies is infrequent schedule meetings on an as-needed basis. Also relative to frequency is whether, if both a nursing research committee and an IRB exist, a proposal for review can be submitted to both simultaneously, or must approval from one be obtained before submission to the other. This must be factored into the timeline for the study, possibly adding several months to the process (Hodgman, 1978).
2. Composition of the review committees membership. It cannot be assumed that all review committees include at least one nurse member. It is important to know whether a nurse

member sits on the committee, because this could influence how the proposal is written (Williams, 1989).

3. The presence of site-specific idiosyncrasies (for example, the need for a proxy PI, letters of support). Although these issues might seem trivial, such things can slow the process of approval while the committees seek out additional information, or they can become obstacles to the study. By dealing directly and proactively with these issues, the investigator establishes credibility and demonstrates professionalism (Hodgman, 1978).

NURSING RESEARCH COMMITTEES

Nursing research committees were initiated for the review of (1) the scientific merit of a proposal for which an investigator is seeking support from the nursing services and (2) the nature and magnitude of the resources required of nursing services to implement the proposed research (see box).

The nature and magnitude of resource consumption can range from being minimal (for example, a request merely for access to subjects for the study) to being significant (for example, nursing service staff are expected to implement various elements of an intervention as well as to collect data regarding the feasibility and efficacy of the intervention).

INSTITUTIONAL REVIEW BOARDS

IRBs (also called human subject review committees) exist to provide fair and impartial reviews of research proposals to protect human subjects from any unnecessary risks associated with participation in research. IRBs are required by the federal government of any institution receiving federal funding (National Institutes of Health, 1991). Institutions that do not receive federal funding, that are small, or that produce a limited volume of research might have no formal review structure, or they might have an agreement with another larger institution to provide for them the required oversight.

In large organizations, or where there is a large volume of research conducted, there may be two IRBs: a biomedical committee and a social-behavioral committee. In the absence of federal funding and a formal re-

view structure, the review may be done informally by an administrator of the institution. In this instance, the investigator should, however, obtain a review from an external human subjects committee to provide documentation of adherence to federal guidelines concerning the protection of human subjects from risks.

Some professional groups or national health organizations may be willing to conduct research reviews in the absence of an IRB or when an investigator is conducting research independent of a sponsoring body. In any case, the guarantee of protection of human subjects from undue risks is a joint responsibility of the investigator and the data collection site. Failure to comply with federal regulations regarding the protection of human subjects from research risks can result in withdrawal of current federal funding and loss of eligibility for future federal funding (National Institutes of Health, 1991).

Federal policy (National Institutes of Health, 1991) also stipulates the composition of the IRB. An IRB must consist of a minimum of five members with varying backgrounds to ensure a complete and adequate review of the research activities commonly conducted by the institution. Furthermore, an IRB may not consist entirely of members of one profession, gender, or racial group. Collectively, the IRB must be sufficiently qualified through the experience and expertise of its membership; the diversity of their personal backgrounds, for example, inclusive of racial, gender, and cultural heritage; and their knowledge of and sensitivity to prevailing community attitudes (Office for Protection from Research Risks, 1993, pp. 1–3). If the particular IRB routinely reviews research involving vulnerable subjects, then the composition of the board must include individuals knowledgeable and experienced with such vulnerable populations. Also, the IRB must include at least one member whose primary concerns are scientific, one whose primary concerns are in nonscientific areas, and one who is not otherwise affiliated with the institution or a family member of one who is. One of the members should be able to discuss issues emanating from the perspective of the community and its values. Lastly, an IRB may invite additional individuals with special areas of expertise to participate in the review and discussion of research proposals to en-

Sample Form for Review of Consumption of Clinical Resources

NURSING RESEARCH ACCESS FORM
(Please complete for each unit accessed)

Title of study: _____

_____

Principal investigator: _____

Business phone: _____ Home phone: _____

Department/Agency: _____

IRB APPROVAL: Approved date/Number: _____

1. MEDICAL CENTER UNIT(S) INVOLVED

2. CLINICAL FEASIBILITY

• Can the study be conducted without disruption to unit routine?

Yes [ ]   No [ ]   If no, please explain

• Are the target subjects likely to be available?

Yes [ ]   No [ ]   If no, please explain

[ ] I have read the application or proposal and support the conduct of this study on my unit.
[ ] I do not think it is feasible to conduct this study on my unit. (Please explain).

_____   _____
Signature of Head Nurse   Date

_____   _____
Signature of Director of CPD   Date

_____   _____
Signature of Chief Nursing Officer   Date

ABSTRACT OF PROPOSED STUDY

1. CLINICAL RESOURCES:
   a. Location of unit(s) or type of unit(s) required.

   b. Types of activities required of nursing staff (briefly explain).

      1. Subject recruitment or identification:

      2. Data collection procedures:

      3. Research subject:

      4. Other:

   c. Types of activities requested of patients/significant others (briefly explain).

   d. Space requirements:

   e. Time of day/shift when data will be collected.

   f. Project time period (estimate beginning and end date of project).

_____   _____
Principal Investigator   Date

_____   _____
Advisor (for Graduate Student)   Date

ATTACH THE FOLLOWING: IRB approval, all data collection instruments, proposal approval (graduate student).

able the IRB to fulfill its purpose. These individuals, however, are not able to vote regarding the disposition of the proposed research.

The jurisdiction of an IRB is determined by the answering of two fundamental questions: "Is the activity research?" and "Does the activity involve human subjects?" For health care professionals, the first question may not be so easily answered because the distinction between research and therapy is not always readily apparent. Federal policy defines research as "a systematic investigation, including research development, testing, and evaluation, designed to develop or contribute to generalized knowledge" (National Institutes of Health, 1991, .102[d]). Furthermore, research itself is not inherently therapeutic in that the therapeutic benefit of experimental interventions are unknown and may prove to be ineffective (Office for Protection from Research Risks, 1993, p. 1–2). If the focus of the proposed activity is of currently accepted and standardized methods of care or if it addresses institutional or patient-specific care issues, then the activity is generally not considered research and consequently does not require IRB reporting and review. However, if there is any uncertainty as to whether the activity is research, the activity should be treated as research and reported to the IRB.

Once the activity has been deemed research, the investigator should ask whether the research activity involves human subjects, and, if so, whether the activity falls within the jurisdiction of the IRB. This question is more readily answered and must be answered "yes" if the activity consists of any systematic collection of data about human beings, including data obtained from surveys and observations, as well as that from any human tissues, for example, embryonic or cadaveric tissues.

There is one caveat. It is a common standard within the health care community that even though an activity may not be "research," if the activity is to be reported in a publication or presentation, the general practice is to consider the activity research and to report it to the IRB. In so doing, once the activity receives IRB approval, it is sanctioned, thereby assuring the public and health care community that the activity complies with commonly accepted ethical practices, with a consequent minimization of risks to all participating parties, that is, the human subjects, investigators, and institution.

Once it has been established that the activity falls within the jurisdiction of the IRB, that is, that the activity is one of research and that it involves human subjects, the level of IRB reporting and review must be identified. There are three levels of review determined on the basis of the degree of risk inherent in the proposed research. Risk is defined by federal policy as "the probability of harm or injury (physical, psychological, social, or economic) occurring as a result of participation in a research study. Both the probability and magnitude of risk can vary from minimal to significant" (Office for Protection from Research Risks, 1993, p. 3–1). The three levels of review are (1) exempt, (2) expedited, and (3) full. Each is described in greater detail later. It is important to determine which level of review is required because, typically, the extent of information required, forms to be completed, and time necessary for the review are determined by the type of review. Any questions about the level of review or the submission process generally can be discussed with the chair of the IRB. When a proposed research activity does not clearly fall into a distinct level of review, submission of materials for the next highest level of review is prudent and expeditious.

Any activity that is considered research must be reported to the IRB. Research activities that are exempt from review by the IRB are those that pose no risks to subjects, have no means by which a subject can be identified, and use human subjects who are capable of freely consenting to participate (Office for Protection from Research Risks, 1993). Examples of activities that are exempt from review, but for which reporting to the IRB is required, and an example of a form for the reporting of a research activity considered exempt from review can be found in the following boxes.

Copies of surveys, interview guides or questionnaires, and the exact introductory remarks and consent forms are to be submitted. Although not formally reviewed, an officer from the IRB assesses the materials to verify that the activity meets the stipulations for an exemption. This verification generally requires a few days, after which the investigator receives a document from the IRB indicating the exact criteria by which the activity does or does not fulfill

➤ Activities Exempt for Coverage Under 45 Code of Federal Regulations 46

Research in which the involvement of human subjects will be in one or more of the following categories is exempt from coverage under this Assurance:

1. Research conducted in established or commonly accepted educational settings, involving normal educational practices, such as
   a. research on regular and special education instructional strategies, or
   b. research on the effectiveness of or the comparison among instructional techniques, curricula, or classroom management methods
2. Research involving the use of educational tests (cognitive, diagnostic, aptitude, achievement), survey procedures, interview procedures, or observation of public behavior, unless
   a. information obtained is recorded in such a manner that human subjects' responses can be identified, directly or indirectly, through identifiers linked to the subjects; and
   b. any disclosure of the human subjects' responses outside the research could reasonably place the subjects at risk of criminal or civil liability, or be damaging to the subject's financial standing, employability, or reputation
3. Research involving the use of educational tests (cognitive, diagnostic, aptitude, achievement), survey procedures, interview procedures, or observation of public behavior that is not exempt under paragraph (2) above if
   a. the human subjects are elected to appointed public office or candidates for public office; or
   b. federal statutes require without exception that the confidentiality of the personally identifiable information will be maintained throughout the research and thereafter

4. Research, involving the collection or study of existing data, documents, records, pathological specimens, or diagnostic specimens, if these sources are publicly available or if the information is recorded by the investigator in such a manner that subjects cannot be identified, directly or through identifiers linked to the subjects
5. Research and demonstration projects that are conducted by or subject to the approval of department or agency heads and that are designed to study, evaluate, or otherwise examine
   a. public benefit or service programs
   b. procedures for obtaining benefits or services under those programs
   c. possible changes in or alternatives to those programs or procedures; or
   d. possible changes in methods or level of payment for benefits or services under those programs
6. Taste and food quality evaluation and consumer acceptance studies:
   a. if wholesome foods without additives are consumed, or
   b. if a food is consumed that contains a food ingredient at or below the level and for a use found to be safe, or agricultural chemical or environmental contaminant at or below the level found to be safe, by the Food and Drug Administration or approved by the Environmental Protection Agency of the Food Safety and Inspection Service of the U.S. Department of Agriculture

Adapted from National Institutes of Health. (1991). Protection of human subjects: Title 45, Code of Federal Regulations, part 46, revised June 18, 1991. Washington, DC: Office for Protection from Research Risks.

➤ Sample Form for Exempt Review of Research

Date Received _____

FORM X
(Submit with page one of form A)

CRITERIA BY WHICH RESEARCH DOES NOT REQUIRE REVIEW
(please type)

1. Short title: _____
                                      (limit to 60 spaces)

2. Principal investigator (PI): _____

3. Check one or more of 1–7 that indicate the criteria by which the study qualifies for exempt status under the Federal Regulations (common rule).

    _____ 1. Research of normal educational practices.
    _____ 2. Educational tests, surveys, interviews or observation of adults, except where damaging.
    _____ 3. Surveys or interviews of public officials.
    _____ 4. Existing data or specimens where they are otherwise available to PI.
    _____ 5. Evaluation of public benefit or service programs.
    _____ 6. Taste and food quality evaluation.
    _____ 7. Subjects will not be identified.

4. Brief description of study. Include sufficient detail to allow OPRR to determine if criteria are met. For questionnaire studies, you must attach a questionnaire and exact introductory remarks or consent form.

5. If psych students will be used, describe anonymity procedures and educational value to students.

6. Signature, PI   Date   7. Administrative check   Date

8. CoPI or Faculty sponsor   Date
    (For student)

the requirements for an exemption. If the initial assessment determines the activity does not fulfill the requirements for an exemption, the investigator may be asked for additional justification or to submit the appropriate materials for an expedited review.

There are three types of activities that may receive an expedited review.

1. Activities that pose no more than minimal risk to subjects for participation in the activity. Minimal risk is defined as "a risk where the probability and magnitude of harm or discomfort in the proposed research are not greater, in and of themselves, than those ordinarily encountered in daily life or during the performance of routine physical or psychological examinations or tests" (National Institutes of Health, 1991, .102[i]). If the risks are greater than minimal and if precautions, safeguards, or alternatives cannot be incorporated into the research activity to minimize the risks to such a level, then a full review is required.

2. Activities in which subjects are capable of providing consent to participate. If subjects are unable to freely choose whether to participate in the activity (for example, cognitively impaired individuals or comatose patients), particularly vulnerable subjects (for example, children and minors), prisoners, pregnant women, mentally disabled persons, or economically or educationally disadvantaged persons, a full review of the proposal by the IRB is required.

3. Activities requiring minor changes in previously approved research during the period for which approval is authorized (1 year or less) (National Institutes of Health, 1991, .110[b]).

Activities considered within the exempt category but that provide a means by which individual subjects can be identified must be reviewed at the expedited level because of the potential risk resulting from the loss of anonymity and confidentiality. Materials required for an expedited review generally consist of an abbreviated research protocol addressing the objectives, methods, subject selection criteria, theoretical or potential risks and benefits, precautions and safeguards, and a sample informed consent. Samples of forms for submitting a proposal for an expedited review can be found in the box. An expedited review typically requires a couple of weeks, although in extreme cases a quicker review can be arranged. The proposal is reviewed by two members of the research committee and the chair of the IRB.

As with all levels of review, the investigator receives a document from the IRB, indicating the exact criteria by which the activity fulfills the requirements for an expedited review. If the initial assessment determines that the activity does not fulfill the requirements, the investigator may be asked for additional justification or to submit the appropriate materials for a full review. Federal policy requires that all members of the IRB must be advised of all proposals that have been approved under the expedited review process (National Institutes of Health, 1991, .110[c]).

A full review of any proposed research activity involving human subjects must occur in all other situations—for example, those in which participation in the activity poses greater than minimal risk; those for which a subject, for whatever reason, cannot freely consent; or those involving vulnerable populations as subjects. Materials required for a full review are identical to those required for an expedited review; it is the review process that differs. A full review typically requires at least a month between the submission of materials and notification of the disposition of the proposal. The proposal is reviewed by at least three members of the IRB or the chair of the IRB. (A member cannot participate in the discussion and determination of disposition of a project in which that member is an investigator. In this instance, the investigator member must be absent from the discussion, and this absence must be reflected in the minutes of the meeting.) The review of the proposed research activity, which is to focus on the aspects listed in the box, must occur at a convened meeting at which a majority of members of the IRB are present. The impartial review conducted by the IRB typically focuses on (1) the mechanisms within the proposed research by which the subjects are safeguarded or protected from any undue risks of participation, and (2) on the process and content of informed consent, that is, the ethics of the research. However, scrutiny of the research methodology also falls within the purview of the IRB, because research

➤ Sample Forms for Research Requiring Either Expedited or Full Review

Date Received _____

FOR OFFICE USE ONLY
IRB NO. _____

FORM A

REQUEST FOR ETHICAL REVIEW OF AN EXPERIMENTAL PROJECT ON HUMAN SUBJECTS
(please type)

1. Short title: _____
   (limit to 60 spaces)

   a) Descriptive title of protocol _____
   _____

2. Principal investigator (PI):
   Name _____   Academic Title _____

   College _____   Dept/Unit _____

3. Campus mailing address/Telephone: Telephone numbers:
   Room No.   Bldg. Name & No.   M/C   Work   Emergency
   _____   _____   _____   _____   _____

4. Faculty member (all other investigators):   Telephone numbers:
   Name   Dept/Unit   Work   Emergency
   _____   _____   _____   _____
   _____   _____   _____   _____
   _____   _____   _____   _____

5. Locations at which research is to be conducted:

6. Funding Source (If Departmental funds, please state): _____
   Grant No. and/or Acct. No. (if available): _____

7. Anticipated duration of protocol: From ___ /___ /19___   To ___ /___ /19___

8. Will this study be conducted entirely within PI's department?   Y   N

9. Will this be a DRUG STUDY (not investigational)?   Y   N

10. Will this study involve any investigational new drugs or devices?   Y*   N
    *(If yes, complete and attach Form B)

11. Will this study involve any deception of human subjects?   Y*   N
    *(If yes, complete and attach Form C)

12. Will this study involve radioactive materials or exposure?   Y   N

13. Will this study involve blood or human immunodeficiency virus?   Y   N

14. Anticipated number of subjects:_____ . Will subjects be paid? Y   N
    Circle all that apply.

    Minors   Incompetents   Prisoners   Employees   Employees' children   Fetuses
    Students   Abortuses   Human tissues   Pregnant women   Other adults

➤ **Considerations During the Review of Research Proposals**

In the review of proposals, the members of the IRB are instructed to

1. Identify the risks associated with the research
2. Determine that these risks will be minimized (or managed) to the extent possible. Precautions, safeguards, and alternatives can be incorporated into a research activity to reduce the probability of harm or to limit its severity or duration.
3. Identify the probable benefits to be derived from the research. Both direct and indirect benefits to the subject (for example, the improvement in health status), as well as those to society (for example, the development of generalizable knowledge), are to be considered. Not to be considered within this calculation of benefits are cash payments to subjects for participation, or any subjective benefits (for example, altruistic or humanitarian contributions to science and humanity).
4. Determine that the risks are reasonable in relation to the risks and the importance of the knowledge to be gained. This determination is subjective, contextually bound, and primarily determined by prevailing community values and preferences—hence emphasizing the important contributions of the community member to the IRB functioning.

5. Ensure that potential subjects will be provided with an accurate and fair description of the risks, discomforts, and anticipated benefits of participation in the study.
6. Determine intervals of periodic review appropriate to the degree of risk, but not less than once a year. These periodic reviews are to determine that there has been no shift in the risk to benefit ratio, whether there have been any unanticipated risks to subjects, whether any information has been gained regarding risks and benefits, or whether new information has been gained from other studies that should be provided to subjects for their consent to remain informed and freely given.
7. Determine that the existing research procedures do in fact provide protection of privacy, maintain confidentiality, and protect the rights and welfare of the subjects.

Adapted from Office for Protection from Research Risks. (1993). *National Institutes of Health: Protecting human research subjects: Institutional Review Board Guidebook.* Washington, DC: U.S. Government Printing Office.

that is so poorly designed as to be invalid exposes the subjects, the investigator, and the institution to unnecessary risk. So, although a proposal may be deemed to be ethically sound, if it is methodologically unsound, the IRB must disapprove the application. For the proposed research to be approved, it must receive the approval of a majority of those members present at the meeting per the criteria listed in the box (National Institutes of Health, .108[b]).

A research proposal must receive approval from the IRB before the collection of data can be initiated. Once permission has been granted by the IRB, the researcher is obligated to conduct the study as proposed. If it becomes necessary to alter the study in any way, the researcher must report those alterations to the IRB for review before their implementation. The IRB also must be notified if any unforeseen problems arise during the conduct of the study. Although investigators are required to provide a progress report on at least an annual basis (see box), any changes in procedure, risks, or unforeseen problems should be reported to the IRB immediately.

The process of providing informed consent is not a distinct moment in time for simply obtaining the subject's signature on a form; it is an ongoing educational process between the investigator and subject, and it reflects the basic principle of respect for

➤ Criteria for Approval of Research Proposals

All of the following requirements must be met:

1. Risks to subjects are minimized.
2. Risks are reasonable relative to anticipated benefits.
3. Selection of subjects is equitable.
4. Informed consent is sought as required.
5. Informed consent is documented as appropriate and as required.
6. Adequate provisions for monitoring the safety of subjects during data collection are present.
7. Adequate provisions to protect privacy and maintain confidentiality of data exist.

➤ Aspects of an Annual Review of an Ongoing Project

1. Progress of the study, such as numbers and types of subjects enrolled
2. Changes in leadership responsibility or major personnel, such as principal investigator, project director, coinvestigators
3. Procedural changes affecting experimental conditions, risks, or methods for providing informed consent or its documentation

persons. Consequently, informed, voluntary participation of the subject should be verified with every interaction between the investigator, or a representative of the research team, and the subject. Because of the nature and complexity of some studies (for example, longitudinal multiphase studies), informed consent may be required for the various phases of the study.

Although some IRBs require the use of a standardized format for consent procedures, modifications are usually permitted as long as the process provides for full disclosure, adequate comprehension, and voluntary choice—elements easy to enumerate but not so easy to achieve (see box) (National Institutes of Health, 1991). Usually any element may be omitted that is not relevant to the study; however, a statement that the subject understands what will occur as a result of his or her participation in the study and that the subject freely agrees to participate must be included at the end of the form, followed with a place for the subject's and witness' signature and date (see box). When a parent or guardian signs for a subject, the subject's name should be clearly identified, as should the signatory's relationship to the subject. If the research is complex or poses a significant risk, the IRB may encourage the investigator to develop a "patient information sheet," which presents the information from the formal consent form in simple, unambiguous language that is void of all "legalese." In other instances, audiotaped verbal consents may be acceptable, for example, with interviews. With questionnaire or survey research, it is commonly assumed

➤ Essential Elements of Informed Consent

The following information must be provided to each subject, as stated in 45 CFR Part 46:

1. A statement that the study involves research, an explanation of the purposes of the research and the expected duration of the subject's participation, a description of the procedures to be followed, and identification of any procedures which are experimental;

2. A description of any reasonable foreseeable risks or discomforts to the subject;

3. A description of any benefits to the subject or to others which may reasonably be expected from the research;

4. A disclosure of appropriate alternative procedures or courses of treatment, if any, that might be advantageous to the subject;

5. A statement describing the extent, if any, to which confidentiality of records identifying the subject will be maintained;

6. For research involving more than minimal risk, and explanation as to whether any compensation and medical treatments are available if injury occurs and, if so, what they consist of or where further information may be obtained;

7. An explanation of whom to contact for answers to pertinent questions about the research and research subjects' rights, and whom to contact in the event of a research-related injury to the subject;

8. A statement that participation is voluntary, refusal to participate will involve no penalty or loss of benefits to which the subject is otherwise entitled, and the subject may discontinue participation at any time without loss of benefits to which the subject is otherwise entitled.

9. Additional elements of informed consent, when appropriate, one or more of the following elements of information may be provided to each subject:

   a. A statement that the particular treatment or procedure may involve risks to the subject (or to the embryo or fetus if the subject is or may become pregnant) which are currently unforeseeable;

   b. Anticipated circumstances under which the subject's participation may be terminated by the investigator without regard to the subject's consent;

   c. Any additional costs to the subject that may result from participation in the research;

   d. The consequences of a subject's decision to withdraw from the research and procedures for orderly termination of participation by the subject;

   e. A statement that significant new findings developed during the course of the research which may relate to the subject's willingness to continue participation will be provided to the subject; and

   f. The approximate number of subjects involved in the study.

Adapted from National Institutes of Health. (1991). Protection of human subjects: Title 45, Code of Federal Regulations, part 46, revised June 18, 1991. Washington, DC: Office for Protection from Research Risks.

that the return of a completed questionnaire implies consent. However, in any of these situations, the investigator is obligated to fully disclose the nature and extent of the subject's participation in such a way that the subject can understand and freely volunteer to participate. Guidelines for developing a consent form as well as sample consent forms can usually be obtained from the IRB.

Few circumstances allow for the waiver of consent. Situations in which this may

➤ Sample Consent Form

AGREEMENT TO CONSENT

The research project and the treatment procedures associated with it have been fully explained to me. All experimental procedures have been identified and no guarantee has been given about the possible results. I have had the opportunity to ask questions concerning any and all aspects of the project and any procedure involved. I am aware that I may withdraw my consent at any time and such withdrawal will not restrict my access to health care services normally available at the hospital. Confidentiality of records concerning my involvement in this project will be maintained in an appropriate manner. When required by law, the records of this research may be reviewed by applicable government agencies.

I understand that in the event of physical injury resulting from this research, the hospital will provide me with free emergency care, if such care is necessary. I also understand that if I wish, the hospital will provide me non-emergency care, but the hospital assumes no responsibility to pay for such care or to provide me with financial compensation.

I, the undersigned, hereby consent to participate as a subject in the above described research project conducted at the hospital. I have received a copy of this consent form for my records. I understand that if I have any questions concerning this research or my rights in connection with the research, I can contact the doctors named above or the Clinical Investigation Committee, at 123-456-7890.

After reading the entire consent form, if you have no further questions about giving consent, please sign where indicated.

Doctor: _____   _____
                                Signature of Subject

Witness: _____   Date: _____ Time: _____ AM PM
                                                            (circle)

---

be approved include the following: (1) the research involves no more than minimal risk to subjects, (2) the waiver or alteration will not adversely affect the rights and welfare of the subjects, (3) the research could not practically be carried out without the waiver or alteration, and (4) whenever appropriate, the subjects will be provided with additional pertinent information after they have participated in the study (National Institutes of Health, 1991, 116[d]).

In providing the information for consent, the investigator may want to consider using such devices as audiovisual aids, tests of the information provided, or consent advisors to verify comprehension by the potential subject (Office for Protection from Research Risks, 1993). Each oral presentation of the information for consent must be witnessed by a third person, who must sign both the consent form and, if used, a copy of the written summary of the presentation (also known as the patient information sheet).

Copies of each are given to the subject, and the investigator should retain the originals for at least 5 years.

GAINING ACCESS

Gaining access to subjects is subsequent to gaining entry to the clinical setting. Gaining entry involves formal support and approval for the study, whereas gaining access involves informal support and approval, as well as staff enthusiasm for the study. For a staff nurse in the clinical setting, gaining informal support and approval can result from discussions with peers, nurse managers, house staff, and attending physicians about the research idea and plan. Useful strategies for obtaining research support and approval from the informal structure of an organization include establishing credibility and attending to social amenities (Teplitz, 1993).

Establishing Credibility

An investigator can use many ways to establish credibility within the informal structure of an organization. First, the investigator can promote the benefits of the study (Oda, 1983). The nursing staff is interested not only in the potential contributions to knowledge but also in the more immediate contributions to patient care services. It is essential to emphasize how the information from the study will lead to the improvement in services provided to the target population. In addition, it is important for the nursing staff to know how this information will help in making their jobs better and easier.

Second, investigator credibility can be enhanced by visibility (Schatzman & Strauss, 1973). Clinical visibility conveys the idea that an investigator is personally interested in the progress of the study, the quality of the data generated, and the interaction between the study protocol and daily clinical operation. Clinical visibility also helps emphasize the clinical significance of the study and reduces personal barriers, such as perceived distance between clinical and research personnel (Stetler, 1983). The investigator's presence promotes interchange with the staff, indicating an interest in them beyond their contributions to the study.

Third, researchers can establish credibility by minimizing the intrusions and demands that the study protocol might make on the daily operation of the clinical site. A pilot study that evaluates the data collection procedure, questionnaires, and instruments can provide valuable information to this end (Oda, 1983). Conducting a pilot study also can (1) allow persons within the organization to provide feedback and advice, and, therefore, to experience a sense of involvement (Oda, 1983; Holm & Llewellyn, 1986, p. 258) and (2) demonstrate the investigator's consideration of the contribution of the organization to the study. Pilot studies are discussed in Chapter 25.

Attending to Social Amenities

Many of the aforementioned strategies also assist in attending to social amenities. It is prudent to emphasize the specific contributions of others to the implementation of the study. Common courtesies, keeping key figures informed of the progress of the study, acknowledging participation of staff, and maintaining professional conduct, although seemingly simple gestures, greatly assist in obtaining support and approval.

MAINTAINING SUPPORT

Because data collection can require months or years, it is essential that the support of a clinical setting for a study be maintained. With the current emphasis on developing research programs, it is vital that relationships for supporting future studies be sustained.

The importance of an investigator's fulfilling promises and commitments cannot be overemphasized. Failure to do so can result in mistrust and can lead to an abrupt and, perhaps, irreversible severance of the research partnership developed between the investigator and the clinical site. Breach of confidence, misuse of data, and lack of appreciation of the resources provided by the clinical setting by previous investigators have been given as reasons for complex and difficult research application procedures (Hodgman, 1981) and for refusals by certain organizations to serve as data collection sites (Oda, 1983). Wilson (1989) suggested that at the completion of a project, the investigator should acknowledge the support and resources from the clinical setting by having a celebration—an informal ceremony to report the findings and to treat the cessation of the research relationship as more of a "suspension" than a "termination."

Strategies for maintaining support are doubly important for staff members who conduct research. The aforementioned strategies not only serve to encourage support for research but also facilitate the investigator's ability to function as a practitioner.

SUMMARY

Gaining the support of a clinical setting for a study is an essential, preliminary step for conducting research. The process of gaining support is dynamic. It can consume large amounts of time and provide numerous opportunities for success or failure. The recommendations offered are intended to facilitate development of a partnership in pursuing knowledge that results in a positive research experience for the investigator and the clinical setting alike—the successful completion of the study.

REFERENCES

Abbott, N. K. (1981). Data collection: Gaining access to data. In S. D. Krampitz & N. Pavlovich (Eds.), *Readings for nursing research* (p. 98). St. Louis, Mosby.

Blichfeldt, M. P., Deane, D. M., & Lancaster, J. (1987). Facilitating research in critical care. *Dimensions of Critical Care Nursing, 6,* 284.

Flaskerud, J. H., & Janken, J. K. (1978). What are some successful strategies for negotiating field research in community agencies? *Nursing Research 27,* 375.

Hodgman, E. C. (1978). Student research in service agencies. *Nursing Outlook, 26,* 558.

Hodgman, E. C. (1981). Research policy for nursing services: Part I. *Journal of Nursing Administration, 11*(4), 30.

Holm, K., & Llewellyn, J. G. (1986). *Nursing research for nursing practice.* Philadelphia: W. B. Saunders.

Kirchhoff, K. T., & McGuire, D. B. (1985). The nursing review process in a clinical setting. *Journal of Professional Nursing, 1,* 311.

McHugh, N. G., & Johnson, J. E. (1980). Clinical nursing research: Beyond the method book. *Nursing Outlook, 28,* 352.

National Institutes of Health. (1991). Protection of human subjects: Title 45, Code of Federal Regulations, part 46, revised June 18, 1991. Washington, DC: Office of Protection from Research Risks.

Oberst, M. T. (1985). Integrating research and clinical practice roles. *Topics in Clinical Nursing, 7*(2), 45.

Oda, D. S. (1983). Social and political facilitation of research. *Advances in Nursing Science, 5*(2), 9.

Office for Protection from Research Risks. (1993). *National Institutes of Health: Protecting human research subjects: Institutional Review Board Guidebook.* Washington, DC: U.S. Government Printing Office.

Sayner, N. C. (1984). Research in the clinical setting: Potential barriers to implementation. *Journal of Neurosurgical Nursing, 16,* 279.

Schatzman, L., & Strauss, A. L. (1973). *Field research: Strategies for a natural sociology.* Englewood Cliffs, NJ: Prentice-Hall.

Smeltzer, C. H., & Hinshaw, A. S. (1988). Research: Clinical integration for excellent patient care. *Nurse Manager, 19,* 38.

Stetler, C. B. (1983). Nurses and research: Responsibility and involvement. *National Intravenous Therapy Association Journal, 6,* 207.

Teplitz, L. (1993). Gaining access to clinical sites and subjects for clinical research. *Progress in Cardiovascular Nursing, 8*(11), 24.

Williams, M. A. (1989). Research and the acute care setting (Editorial). *Research in Nursing & Health, 12*(1), iii.

Wilson, H. S. (1989). *Research in nursing.* (2nd ed.). Menlo Park, CA: Addison-Wesley.

Chapter 14

Seeking Funding for Clinical Research

Marguerite R. Kinney

Successful grantsmanship is an art that requires sound planning for the project, development of a well-written proposal, and selection of an appropriate funding source. Proposal development is discussed in Chapter 24. This chapter focuses on selection of a funding source and the proposal review procedures used by these sources.

SOURCES OF FUNDING

There are numerous potential sources of funding for clinical research projects. These sources include intramural, industry, associations, foundations, and government. Intramural funds typically are limited to small "seed" grants and are designed to support preliminary projects that will lead to funding from extramural sources. These funds may be restricted to investigators who are beginning a research career, or they may serve to bridge experienced investigators from one project to another. University-based health science centers typically offer these funds for their investigators, but clinicians in other settings should explore the availability of this type of funding. If no program exists, it may be possible to develop one using departmental funds or private contributions.

Companies in the health care industry are important sources of funding for clinical research. Projects supported by industry may be initiated either by the company or by the investigator. Clinical sites where new products are being introduced are of particular interest to pharmaceutical companies and equipment manufacturers. Discussions with company representatives may lead to the identification of questions of mutual interest that could be pursued through research. It is important that both advantages and disadvantages of partnering with corporations be considered. One issue requiring open and frank discussion is potential conflicts of interest, including the balance between freedom of information and the need for secrecy and patents; the question of control and direction of the research effort; the selection of investigators; and possible reporting biases or restrictions in reporting results (Keane, Larson, Naji, & Rom, 1986).

Professional and voluntary associations often have well-developed research award programs to support both targeted and untargeted research. Funds may be available from local chapters as well as from the national organization. Examples are provided in the box, but there are many others. In some cases, associations have joined efforts in research funding to maximize the resources available; for example, the American Association of Critical-Care Nurses (AACN), Sigma Theta Tau International, the Emergency Nurses Association, and the Emergency Medical Association.

> ## Potential Sources of Funding for Clinical Research

A selected list of potential sources of funding for clinical research projects with addresses follows:

- American Association of Critical-Care Nurses, 101 Columbia, Aliso Viejo, CA 92656; telephone: 1-800-899-2226
- American Cancer Society, 1599 Clifton Road, NE, Atlanta, GA 30329-4251; telephone: 404-329-7558
- American Diabetes Association, Scientific and Medical Division, 1660 Duke Street, Alexandria, VA 22314; telephone 703-549-1500, ext. 2376
- American Heart Association, Division of Research Administration, 7320 Greenville Avenue, Dallas, TX 75231; telephone: 214-706-1453
- American Lung Association, 1740 Broadway, New York, NY 10019-4374; telephone: 212-315-8793
- American Nurses' Foundation, Inc., 600 Maryland Avenue, SW, Suite 100W, Washington, DC 20024-2571; telephone: 202-554-4444
- Avon Products, Inc., 1345 Avenue of the Americas, New York, NY 10105-0196; 212-282-5515
- Cystic Fibrosis Foundation, 6931 Arlington Road, Bethesda, MD 20814; telephone: 1-800-FIGHT-CF or 301-951-4422; 800-344-4823
- Emergency Nurses Foundation, 216 Higgins Road, Park Ridge, IL 60068-5735; telephone: 708-698-9400 or 1-800-243-8362
- Fetzer Institute (mind and spirit as components of health and healing), 9292 West KL Avenue, Kalamazoo, MI 49009-9398; telephone: 616-375-2000
- William T. Grant Foundation (children, adolescents and youth), 515 Madison Avenue, New York, NY 10022-5403; telephone: 212-752-0071
- Harry Frank Guggenheim Foundation (violence, aggression and dominance), 527 Madison Avenue, New York, NY 10022-4301; telephone: 212-644-4907
- The JM Foundation (rehabilitation, prevention and wellness, health policy, alcohol/drug abuse), 60 East 42nd Street, Room 1651, New York, NY 10165; telephone: 212-687-7735
- Leukemia Society of America, Inc., 600 Third Avenue, New York, NY 10016; telephone: 212-856-9686
- March of Dimes Birth Defects Foundation, 1275 Mamaroneck Avenue, White Plains, NY 10605; telephone: 914-428-7100
- Ms. Foundation for Women (reproductive health, safety, rural women), 120 Wall Street, 33rd Floor, New York, NY 10005; telephone: 212-742-2300
- National Institute of Nursing Research, Building 45, Room 3AN12, Bethesda, MD 20892-6908; 301-594-6908
- National Multiple Sclerosis Society, Research Programs Department, 733 Third Avenue, New York, NY 10017-3288; telephone: 212-986-3240
- Oncology Nursing Society, 501 Holiday Drive, Pittsburgh, PA 15220-2749; telephone: 412-921-7373
- The Prudential Foundation (AIDS prevention education and services to people with AIDS; health care delivery focusing on quality and cost-containment; health policy), 751 Broad Street, 15th Floor, Newark, NJ 07102-3777; telephone: 973-802-7354
- The Retirement Research Foundation (improving the quality of life for older Americans), 8765 West Higgins Road, Suite 401, Chicago, IL 60631-4170; telephone: 773-714-8080
- Sigma Theta Tau International, 550 W. North Street, Indianapolis, IN 46202; telephone: 317-634-8171
- The Thrasher Research Fund (child health), 15 East South Temple Street, 3rd Floor, Salt Lake City, UT 84150; telephone: 801-240-4753
- Van Amerigen Foundation, Inc. (mental health issues, with an emphasis on the disadvantaged), 509 Madison Avenue, New York, NY 10022-5501; telephone: 212-758-6221

Foundations are non-profit organizations typically governed by a board of directors or trustees. The more than 35,000 grant-making foundations in the United States can be categorized into three basic types: corporate, independent, and community, each with its own rules for funding. Corporate foundations are particularly interested in funding projects that will benefit their employees and take place near their corporate offices. For example, a corporation with a large number of female employees may be interested in projects related to women's health. Community foundations obtain their funds from individuals, corporations, and bequests and are interested in projects targeted for a specific geographical location. Examples are the Retirement Research Foundation, which supports programs aimed at improving the quality of life for older Americans and targets the Chicago metropolitan area, and the Charles H. Hood Foundation, which supports child health projects in New England. The amount of funding available from corporate and community foundations is typically small, often ranging from $2000 to $5000, but larger sums are also available. Independent foundations vary considerably in research focus and the size of awards. The philanthropic purposes of the foundation guide the funding priorities, which may change over time. Foundations may fund projects of more than one kind. For example, The Robert Wood Johnson Foundation provides funding for projects that reflect an applicant's own interests, investigator-initiated projects developed in response to the request for proposals by the foundation in a specified program area, and projects that are a part of the national programs of the foundation. Some foundations limit funding to tax-exempt or public agencies whereas other foundations include individuals as grantees.

The U.S. government is a major source of funding for health care research. Much of this funding is awarded by the National Institutes of Health (NIH) through its various institutes, centers, and offices (see box). These awards are usually large and extend for several years. Other federal sources of funding include the Agency for Health Care Policy and Research (AHCPR), the National Science Foundation (NSF), and the Centers for Disease Control and Prevention (CDC). Competition has become intense as budgets have become more and more constrained.

➤ Institutes, Centers, and Divisions of NIH

- National Institute on Aging (NIA)
- National Institute on Alcohol Abuse and Alcoholism (NIAAA)
- National Institute of Allergy and Infectious Diseases (NIAID)
- National Institute of Arthritis and Musculoskeletal and Skin Diseases (NIAMS)
- National Cancer Institute (NCI)
- National Institute of Child Health and Human Development (NICHD)
- National Institute on Deafness and Other Communication Disorders (NIDCD)
- National Institute of Dental Research (NIDR)
- National Institute of Diabetes and Digestive and Kidney Diseases (NIDDK)
- National Institute on Drug Abuse (NIDA)
- National Institute of Environmental Health Sciences (NIEHS)
- National Eye Institute (NEI)
- National Institute of General Medical Sciences (NIGMS)
- National Heart, Lung, and Blood Institute (NHLBI)
- National Institute of Mental Health (NIMH)
- National Institute of Neurological Disorders and Stroke (NINDS)
- National Institute of Nursing Research (NINR)
- John E. Fogarty International Center for Advanced Study in the Human Sciences (FIC)
- National Human Genome Research Initiative (NHGRI)
- National Center for Research Resources (NCRR)
- National Library of Medicine (NLM)
- Office of AIDS Research
- Office of Alternative Medicine

Agencies within state and local government may also fund health-related research, particularly if the project is related to a recognized problem for the state or local area.

TYPES OF FUNDING

Funding for clinical research may take one of several forms: grants, cooperative agreements, fellowships, contracts, or gifts. Grants are awarded in response to an investigator-initiated proposal, which may or may not be in response to an agency request. Grants may also take several forms. For example, grants from the American Cancer Society include Research and Clinical Investigation Grants, Institutional Grants, and Grants for the Support of Personnel for Research. Cooperative agreements are similar to grants except that there is substantial programmatic involvement by the funding agency. In contrast to grants and cooperative agreements that support investigator-initiated research, contracts are a mechanism for supporting research proposed by a funding agency. A request for proposal or request for application is issued by an agency to publicize its interest in supporting a specific area of research that needs the stimulation of set-aside funds. In general, contracts are monitored more closely than grants, and budgets and allowable expenses are more constrained. Fellowships provide individual support for research training, and they also take several forms.

Fellowships to support research training are available from both public and private sources. For example, the American Lung Association offers financial support for nurses enrolled in a doctoral program whose research interest is in some area of lung health. The cornerstone of the research training program of the National Institute of Nursing Research (NINR) at NIH is the National Research Service Award (NRSA). Several mechanisms of support are available:

- Individual NRSA Predoctoral Fellowships (F31s), which support supervised research training leading to a doctoral degree. The fellowship provides a stipend and an allowance for tuition, research, and other expenses. The success rate across NIH for these awards in 1994 was close to 50%, considerably higher than for regular research grants.
- Individual NRSA Postdoctoral Fellowships (F32s), which support postdoctoral training with a stipend and an expense allowance. The success rate across NIH in 1994 was approximately 39%.
- Senior NRSA Fellowships (F33s), which provide stipends and expense allowances for experienced investigators who wish to make major changes in the direction of their research careers, broaden their scientific backgrounds, acquire new research capabilities, or enlarge their command of related research fields.
- Institutional NRSAs (T32s), which are training awards made to institutions offering predoctoral and postdoctoral research training in a specified area, such as women's health or interventional methods. Funds are available through the institution for trainee stipends, tuition and fees, and certain expenses.
- Minority Research Training Supplements, which are awarded to institutions with active institutional NRSAs to support research training for additional minority predoctoral or postdoctoral students.
- Mentored Patient-Oriented Research Career Development Award (K23), which supports the career development of investigators who have made a commitment to focusing their research endeavors on patient-oriented research.

The NINR has other mechanisms for providing a sponsored research experience be-

> ## ➤ Characteristics of Successful Mentored Research Awards

- A scientific focus of the proposed research that is timely and important
- Highly qualified candidates who are ready to undertake a research career award
- Suitable sponsors and sufficient resources and support from the university
- A feasible and adequate training plan
- An excellent research proposal
- Preliminary work in the research area conducted or cited
- Thorough description of instruments to be used in the proposed study
- Clearly described aims and methods
- Detailed data analysis plans

yond the NRSA program, although these awards are technically research grants and not training grants. They are the Mentored Research Scientist Development Awards (KO1) and Minority Research Supplements. The Mentored Research Scientist Development Award provides scientists with a period of sponsored research experience as a way to gain expertise in a research area new to the applicant or in an area that would demonstrably enhance the applicant's scientific career. It is expected that following this experience the investigator will be able to pursue an independent and productive research career. Characteristics of successful applications are listed in the box. The Minority Research Supplements are designed to supplement currently funded research grants to attract underrepresented minorities into careers in science. The awards are available to high school students, undergraduate students, graduate research assistants, postdoctoral trainees, and investigators.

Finally, gifts and donations may be a source of funding for specific projects. Many nursing departments are familiar with gifts and donations for purposes of staff development and education, but have not explored the availability of such funds for clinical research.

STRATEGIES FOR ENHANCING FUNDING POTENTIAL

The first step in seeking support for a project is to gather information about prospective funding sources. Federal sources are well publicized and information is readily available. The NIH Gopher Server is available via the Internet (gopher.nih.gov) and provides access to the *NIH Guide to Grants and Contracts* (also available in a printed form) and to CRISP (Computer Retrieval of Information on Scientific Projects), a database of information about all NIH-funded grants.

SPIN (Sponsored Programs Information Network) is a database of funding opportunities designed to assist in the identification of external support for research, education, and development projects. The database contains thousands of federal, nonfederal, and corporate opportunities. In addition, SPIN provides requests for proposals from the *Commerce Business Daily,* requests for

applications from the *NIH Guide for Grants and Contracts,* and the *Federal Register Weekly Reference Guide,* which lists agency announcements on the availability of funding, funding priorities, and regulations. The SPIN database is updated biweekly.

The Community of Science Web Server provides information about the National Science Foundation and NIH, and can be accessed via http://cos.gdb.org on the Internet. Readily available sources for nonfederal granting agencies include the public library, university health science center libraries, university grant offices, professional journals and newsletters, annual reports of foundations, and colleagues. Several directories of foundations are available in libraries and provide information such as funding interests, types of organizations funded, types of support awarded, and population groups of interest. (See Selected Resources at end of this chapter.)

The second step in seeking funding is to ask a set of questions about the prospective funding agency, about the project, and about the researcher's institution (see boxes). It is important that the researcher contact the program officer of the agency early in the proposal development process. This conversation allows the researcher to learn about any recent changes in the interests of the agency or its application procedures. Program officers also may be able to advise researchers about the direction that the proposal should take. They can also provide an annual report and other printed materials and a list of recently funded projects. These individuals often attend meetings of research societies where they may be spoken with in person.

Other strategies for enhancing funding potential are listed in the box titled Strategies for Enhancing Funding Potential. Research is a collaborative enterprise and investigators should seek out individuals and groups that can assist them in becoming more knowledgeable about funding opportunities and the application process.

PREPARING THE BUDGET

Reviewers examine the proposed budget to determine whether it is realistic and justified in relation to the aims and methods of the project. Thus, the researcher should approach preparation of the budget as a

➤ Questions to Ask About the Agency

- Do they have printed materials describing their organization, programs, research priorities, and grant policies? Is the information current?
- Does the research match their funding interests?
- Does the researcher qualify (eligibility, restrictions, and special stipulations)?
- Is the agency really interested in the project?
- Will the agency support all aspects of the project or just portions of the project?
- What parts of the project does the agency seem most enthused about?
- Are there any obligations for the future (payback clause)?
- What amounts of money does the agency grant?
- Is the amount of support enough to complete the project?
- How many awards does the agency support?
- Can the researcher obtain a list of past grantees and their projects?
- Is there a formal application kit? Is a preapplication or a letter of inquiry required?
- When is the application due? Does the date refer to date of postmark or date of arrival?
- Who will review the application? Is a site visit required?
- What is the time lag between application and approval? Between approval and funding?

Adapted from Reif-Lehrer, L. (1995). *Grant application writer's handbook.* Copyright 1995, Sudbury, MA: Jones and Bartlett Publishers. www.jbpub.com. Reprinted with permission.

restrictions on the use of funds are detailed. Small grants may exclude salaries and allow only supplies and minor equipment. Other funding sources may cover salaries only of technical personnel but not of professionals. The researcher should clearly understand the policies of the agency regarding indirect costs. *Direct costs,* such as salaries or necessary equipment, are applied directly to the study. *Indirect costs,* or overhead, include costs of operation that are not specific for any single project, such as administrative expenses and building or equipment maintenance.

Small grants may not provide all of the funding needed for a project. However, funds from more than one source may be pooled as long as the funds do not overlap and they are dispersed for the purpose requested.

Some granting agencies require a specific format for preparing the budget and may even provide a form for this purpose, whereas other agencies allow the investigator to create the format. If no format is specified, suggested major headings are per-

➤ Questions to Ask About the Project

- Does the researcher have a clear concept of what the project will require?
- Has the researcher defined what the project will accomplish?
- Has the researcher determined whether funding agencies are interested in your project?
- What methods will be used to achieve the goals?
- What personnel, equipment, supplies, and space are required for the project?
- How long will the project take?
- How much will the project cost? Has the researcher calculated a preliminary realistic budget?
- What is needed from the funding agency? Is institutional cost sharing required?

Adapted from Reif-Lehrer, L. (1995). *Grant application writer's handbook.* Copyright 1995, Sudbury, MA: Jones and Bartlett Publishers. www.jbpub.com. Reprinted with permission.

two-step process. The first step is to list the categories for which funds are being requested and the second is to provide a detailed and concise explanation for each category listed.

Funding agencies differ in the costs they allow; thus, the researcher should read carefully the application instructions where sonnel, equipment, supplies (consumable items), consultants (if necessary), travel (if planned), and other. If the project will cover more than 1 year, a budget for each year as well as an overall summary should be presented. Figure 14–1 provides a sample budget from a proposal titled *Facial Expressions of Pain During Chest Tube Removal* submitted for an intramural award, which could not exceed $20,000.

For personnel, each member of the project team is listed, indicating full-time or part-time status, percentage of time each will devote to the project, and fringe benefits (calculated at the same rate as for others at the research institution). For a multiyear project, yearly salary increases are calculated based on the average annual increases of the organization over a 5-year period.

Each piece of equipment to be purchased should be described in detail with the cost indicated. Supplies should be described in terms of amount needed to meet the aims of the project. Consultants should be listed, the specific contributions they will make to the project noted, and the number of days

➤ Questions to Ask About the Research Institution

- Is the researcher's institution willing to let him or her apply? Do they support the project? Are they willing to share costs?
- Does the researcher have to file an "intent to apply" with his or her institution?
- Is the institution willing to administer the grant?
- Is the institution willing to provide the necessary space and resources?
- Are there issues related to overhead, salary, copyright and patents, or equipment?
- Does the institution have on-file assurance of compliance with relevant regulations such as for treatment of human subjects and humane treatment of animals?

Adapted from Reif-Lehrer, L. (1995). *Grant application writer's handbook.* Copyright 1995, Sudbury, MA: Jones and Bartlett Publishers. www.jbpub.com. Reprinted with permission.

➤ Strategies for Enhancing Funding Potential

1. Attend grantsmanship courses that address proposal writing and potential funding sources.
2. Seek out a mentor for advice about writing and submitting a proposal.
3. Work with an experienced researcher to refine research skills.
4. Join a local research network to share ideas, learn about potential funding sources, and develop new contacts.
5. Join a research organization such as the ANA Council of Nurse Researchers or one of the regional research societies.
6. Serve on an institution research committee or professional organization to make contact with other researchers and to learn about funding sources.

Adapted from Burns, N., & Grove, S. K. (1987). *The practice of nursing research: Conduct, critique, and utilization.* Philadelphia: WB Saunders.

they will work on the project specified. If consultant travel is required, allowances should be consistent with the policies of the research institution. If travel by project staff is required, then the researcher should specify number of trips, purpose, and types of expense to be incurred (for example, airfare, hotel, meeting registration). A category called "other" can be used for expenses that do not fit the standard categories.

APPLICATION AND GRANT REVIEW PROCESS

The application and proposal review procedures depend on the funding source. Some sources request a succinct and descriptive letter providing essential details about the project. In some cases, projects may be funded on the basis of the letter, whereas in other cases, a full proposal may be requested. Other sources may request a "miniproposal" and then ask for a full proposal based on the initial review. The NIH uses the standard PHS-398 proposal format,

PERSONNEL

Name	Role on Project	Type Appt (months)	% Effort on Project	Base Salary	Salary Requested	Fringe Benefits	Totals
Marguerite R. Kinney	Principal investigator	12	.20		0	0	0
TBA	Research assistant	12	.50	20,000	10,000	920	10,920

CONSULTANT COSTS

2 coders for Facial Action Coding System	4500

EQUIPMENT

1 Sony camcorder	2500

SUPPLIES

Videotapes	64.50	
Videotape conversion	108.40	
Batteries	191.36	
Mailing folders	30.00	
Postage	58.00	
Duplication	30.00	482.26

TRAVEL	0
OTHER EXPENSES	0
TOTAL DIRECT COSTS FOR BUDGET PERIOD	18,402.26

BUDGET JUSTIFICATION

Personnel

Principal Investigator — No salary requested (need to provide letter from the institution indicating that the PI's time is being donated by the institution). The PI will assume responsibility for the conduct of the study including supervision of the RA, data collection, data analysis, and writing the research report.

Research Assistant — The RA will be responsible for recruiting subjects, obtaining informed consent, assisting the PI in data collection, and cleaning and entering data.

Consultants — The coding of the facial action units requires certification in the use of the Facial Action Coding System. Two observers are necessary for purposes of reliability. Observers charge 15.00/hour for coding and it is estimated that one hour of coding will be required for each subject. Thus, 15.00/hour × 150 subjects × 2 coders = 4500.00.

Equipment — 1 Sony Handycam camcorder CCD-TR 700 = 2500.00.

Supplies

Videotapes — 8 mm videotapes: 120 minutes/tape = 30 subjects/tape = 5 tapes @ 12.90 = 64.50

Conversion — 8 mm videotapes converted to VHS @ 10.84/tape = 5 × 10.84 = 54.20 × 2 coders = 108.40

Batteries — 2 lithium-powered batteries @ 95.68 = 191.36

Mailing folders — 5 folders @ 3.00 × 2 coders = 30.00

Postage — 2-day mail @ 2.90 × 5 tapes × 2 coders = 29.00

Return postage — 2-day mail @ 2.90 × 5 tapes × 2 coders = 29.00

Duplication — Demographic form × 150 × .10 = 15.00
Numeric Rating Scale × 150 × .10 = 15.00

Figure 14–1
Sample budget.

which can be obtained from a university grants and contracts office or from NIH. (See Selected Resources at end of this chapter.)

If a funding agency specifies the content of a letter of inquiry, instructions should be followed carefully. If no specific instructions are provided, the following should be considered:

- Focus on the opportunity that the project presents to the agency, not on how their funding will fill the researcher's needs.
- Be brief. Summarize the project in one page.
- Address the letter to the person responsible for funding by name.
- Be sure that the mandate of the agency is addressed.
- Explain clearly and succinctly what is proposed and what is hoped to be accomplished (or enclose a separate summary of the project).
- Discuss the suitability of the project for the mandate of the agency.
- Discuss the amount of funding required.
- Include a current biosketch.
- If appropriate, request an appointment with the program officer.
- Be persuasive but not overbearing (Reif-Lehrer, 1995, p. 315).

➣ Common Reasons for Disapproval of Funding Requests

1. Lack of new or original ideas
2. Diffuse, superficial, or unfocused research plan
3. Lack of knowledge of published relevant work
4. Lack of experience with the methodology
5. Uncertainty concerning future directions
6. Questionable reasoning in experimental approach
7. Absence of an acceptable scientific rationale
8. Unrealistic scope of the study
9. Lack of sufficient experimental detail
10. Uncritical approach to the study

Review procedures at private funding agencies vary and may be less formal than at government agencies, and it may be difficult to obtain information about their review procedures. Applicants may be asked to present their proposal in person or a site visit may be made by the agency. Reviewers may be outside consultants with the second level of review provided by an in-house staff committee. A board of directors may make the final decision based on the recommendation of the reviewers.

Proposals sent to the NIH receive two levels of review. The first level of review is by a study section, which evaluates the scientific merit of the proposal. Rosters of study section members are available online and in print. Applications not likely to be funded in the current funding climate may be designated as "noncompetitive" and are not assigned a priority score. Scored applications receive a numerical rating from each member of the study section as follows:

Numerical Rating	Corresponding Merit Descriptor
1.0–1.5	Outstanding
1.5–2.0	Excellent
2.0–2.5	Very Good
2.5–3.5	Good
3.5–5.0	Acceptable

The numerical scores are averaged and multiplied by 100 to provide a rating, or priority score, for the proposal. Finally, percentile ranks are calculated to indicate the percent of reviewed applications that have scores equal to or better than a given proposal. Percentile ranks are calculated for particular study sections during a 1-year period and are used for making funding decisions.

Judgments about scientific merit are based on the strengths and weaknesses of the research plan as well as on general strengths and weaknesses (see box). Typically highly rated proposals have a broad range of strengths in various categories and weaknesses are found in few of the categories. Conversely, proposals not rated highly are judged to have a narrow range of strengths and the weaknesses span a wide range of categories. A large number of weaknesses are often identified in the categories of design, sample, techniques, and data analysis. Thus, successful proposals are those addressing an important problem that is solvable using the proposed techniques. In addition, the proposal presents a clear, comprehensive, balanced, and well-synthesized literature review and describes adequate resources to complete the project (Fuller, Hasselmeyer, Hunter, Abdellah, & Hinshaw, 1991).

The second level of review is done by the National Advisory Council for the institute or center. Recommendations for funding are made based on the summary statements and percentile ranking from the study section and relevance to the program goals of the institute or center. Thus, NIH awards are based on scientific merit and program relevance.

Dave Bauer (1996), the author of a number of texts on grant seeking, suggests that there are six "deadly sins" that researchers often commit when seeking funding for their projects. Sins to be avoided include

1. Failing to contact the program officer early in the development of the proposal.
2. Not asking to be a peer reviewer for the program in which you (the researcher) are interested.
3. Overstating the goals. Resist the temptation to include too much in the project.
4. Inadvertently discrediting other researchers with a tone in the literature review that casts previous researchers as having missed the mark. Those researchers or their colleagues or former students may be serving on the review panel.
5. Not holding a proper mock review in which individuals not familiar with the proposal mimic the real review process as closely as possible. Objective opinions and constructive criticism will improve the submitted proposal considerably.
6. Submitting the proposal at the last minute, which may be the deadliest sin of all.

If a proposal is not funded, it may be appropriate to revise and improve the proposal and resubmit it in the next application cycle. The summary statement is very helpful in identifying areas of strengths and weaknesses. New investigators may find it helpful to seek consultation from an experienced researcher in planning for the resubmission to be sure that the revised application is responsive to the original critique. Funding sources may have explicit requirements for resubmitted applications, and the investigator must be knowledgeable about them. An important step in planning for resubmission is to seek advice from the program officer of the agency. The revised application should

- Contain substantive improvements
- Be responsive to all questions and criticisms in the summary statement
- Incorporate any pertinent work done since the original submission
- Make clear the changes that have been made

SUMMARY

Seeking funding for clinical research requires that the researcher carefully plans to learn about potential funding sources, contacts program officers early to discuss ideas, and writes a proposal that funding agencies will want to invest their resources in. The budget is an important component of the proposal and should be realistic and justified. Becoming part of a network of clinical researchers has many advantages and should not be ignored. It is a wonderful feeling to receive an award notice and realize that someone is willing to invest in your project. That feeling makes the effort worthwhile.

REFERENCES

Bauer, D. (1996). Six deadly sins cause researchers to get grief instead of grants. *UAB Reporter*, May 26, p. 6.

Burns, N., Grove, S. K. (1987). *The practice of nursing research: Conduct, critique and utilization* (pp. 385–387). Philadelphia, W. B. Saunders.

Fuller, E. O., Hasselmeyer, E. G., Hunter, J. C., Abdellah, F. G., Hinshaw, A. S. (1991). Summary statements of the NIH nursing research grant applications. *Nursing Research, 40,* 346–351.

Keane, A., Larson, E., Naji, P., Rom, M. (1986). Industry and nursing research: A compatible couple? *Nursing Economics, 4,* 128–130.

Reif-Lehrer, L. (1995). *Grant application writer's handbook* (p. 315). Boston: Jones and Bartlett.

SELECTED RESOURCES

(1997). *Annual register of grant support: A directory of funding sources* (31st ed.). New Providence, NJ: RR Bowker.

(1994). *Corporate foundation profiles* (8th ed.). New York: The Foundation Center.

Baumgartner, J. E. (1995). *National directory of grantmaking public charities*. New York: The Foundation Center.

Guide to Proposal Writing: An excellent resource providing advice on how to create a funding request; how to research, contact, and cultivate potential funders; and how to fine-tune each part for different proposals is available for $34.95 plus $4.50 shipping from the Foundation Center, 79 Fifth Avenue, New York, NY 10003-3076; 1-800-424-9836 or 212-620-4230; FAX: 212-807-3677. Includes excerpts from actual grant proposals.

Margolin, J. (Ed.). (1994). *Foundation fundamentals: A guide for grantseekers* (5th ed.). New York: The Foundation Center.

MacLean, R. (Ed.). (1997). *Foundation grants index* (26th ed.). New York: The Foundation Center.

Reif-Lehrer, L. (1995). *Grant application writer's handbook*. Boston: Jones and Bartlett.

Renz, L. (Ed.). (1994). *Foundation giving: Yearbook of facts and figures on private, corporate and community foundations*. New York: The Foundation Center.

Rich, E. H. (1998). *The Foundation directory*. New York: The Foundation Center.

Ries, J. B., Leukefeld, C. G. (1995). Applying for research funding: Getting started and getting funded. Thousand Oaks, CA: Sage.

Schumacher, D. (1992). *Get funded! A practical guide for scholars seeking research support from business*. Thousand Oaks, CA: Sage.

To obtain PHS-398 Application Forms:
Center for Scientific Review
National Institutes of Health
6701 Rockledge Drive, Room 1040, MSC 7710
Bethesda, MD 20892-7710
(301) 435-0714.

Collaboration

Kathleen S. Stone

Collaborative research is the process of working with others in the pursuit of scientific discovery. The primary advantage of collaboration is the multidimensional research that results from melding the expertise of various persons (Matthews, 1985). Collaborative research is ideally suited to addressing complex patient care problems. The focus of this chapter is on the need for collaboration, forms of collaboration, characteristics of successful collaborators, advantages of collaboration, and obstacles to collaboration.

NEED FOR COLLABORATION

The application of clinical research findings to patient care has the potential of enhancing quality nursing care and predicting patient care outcomes. Evidence-based practice creates an increased demand for research to evaluate and test practice (McWilliam, Desai, & Greig, 1997). However, there is a paucity of clinical research to guide clinical practice. One method of increasing the research base for clinical practice is collaborative nursing research. Collaborative nursing research among staff nurses, clinical nurse specialists, and doctorally prepared nurse researchers holds the greatest promise for the generation of research findings that can be directly applied to clinical practice. Collaboration maximizes the use of time available within clinical practice (Govoni & Pierce, 1997). Staff nurses are in the ideal position to identify the important clinical problems that arise in practice. The collaborating clinical nurse specialist and the nurse researcher can assist in the development of the research project by sharing their knowledge and expertise of the research process. Together, these professionals can make a difference in clinical practice by melding their talents through research (Govoni & Pierce, 1997).

FORMS OF COLLABORATION

There are different forms of collaborative research, which include (1) intranursing and interdisciplinary and (2) intrainstitutional and interinstitutional. Intranursing collaborative research brings together nurses with different areas of expertise to examine a particular research question. For example, an intranursing collaborative group to examine a patient care problem might consist of a nurse academician with a doctoral degree, a clinical nurse specialist with a master's degree, and several clinicians. To address a complex research question, an intranursing collaborative group might also include nurses with basic preparation in nursing but whose advanced doctoral preparation includes physiology, exercise physiology, psychology, sociology, or anthropology. An interdisciplinary collaborative research group includes researchers from disciplines other than nursing, for example, medicine, respiratory therapy, pharmacology, or biomedical engineering.

Collaborative research accomplished by researchers in the same institution is called intrainstitutional. Interinstitutional research involves researchers from different institutions. Multicenter clinical trials are an example of interinstitutional collaborative research. Whatever the configuration of the collaborative research group, the research question dictates the necessary participants.

CHARACTERISTICS OF SUCCESSFUL COLLABORATORS

Working with persons from the same or different disciplines can be challenging. A key ingredient for successful collaboration is the unique contribution of the individual participants. It is vital, therefore, that participants possess the following characteristics:

- The ability to accept new ideas and perspectives. Because each participant has a unique perspective, this attribute must be recognized and appreciated for the multidimensional aspect it lends to the research.
- Openness and tolerance of review, critique, and challenges to beliefs and thoughts, particularly during the development of the research project. The excitement and challenge of collaborative research is the discovery of new approaches to the research problem. Collaborative efforts require open-mindedness.

- Willingness to negotiate and compromise. Because the collaborative group must reach a consensus in the decision-making process, it is vital that participants be willing to negotiate and compromise to facilitate the melding of research expertise.
- Ability to function independently and interdependently.
- Conscientiousness in completing individual assignments and willingness to communicate problems and accomplishments to the group (Iwasiw & Olson, 1984).
- Sense of ethics. To have a cohesive collaborative group, it is critical that there be a sense of trust in the sharing of ideas, results of previous work, and current findings.

ADVANTAGES OF COLLABORATION

Although the primary advantage of collaborative research is the melding of expertise to address complex patient care problems, there are a number of additional advantages. Persons with different educational levels and backgrounds come together and grow, learn, and receive mentorship (Hanson, 1988). Working together to develop the project and to mutually solve a problem can assist in the development or reestablishment of working relationships that go well beyond the research study (Govoni & Pierce, 1997). Successful collaborative research endeavors hold the potential for continued or future collaboration.

As stated earlier, the primary advantage to collaborative work groups with members from all levels—academicians with doctoral degrees, clinical nurse specialists, and staff nurses—is the development of clinically relevant research that directly enhances patient care. Staff nurses are particularly adept at identifying research questions and methodological issues that address the clinical applicability of research.

Working with persons from the same or a different discipline can facilitate entrance into data collection sites (Matthews, 1985). For example, academicians frequently have difficulty gaining entry into acute and chronic care facilities. When members of the collaborative research group, namely the clinical nurse specialist or the staff nurse, are already employed by the institution, entry into the system can be facilitated. Frequently, interdisciplinary members of the group (for example, an exercise physiologist or psychologist) have difficulty gaining entry into nontraditional areas and can be aided by the nurse member of the research group. Members of the collaborative research team can be helpful in obtaining institutional and human subject approval for a study conducted at their institution. Access to subjects and subject recruitment can be enhanced by a collaborative effort. Patients and significant others are more likely to consent to participate in a research study if they are approached by the staff nurse with whom they are familiar and with whom they are comfortable.

Another advantage of collaboration is the "pooling" of resources, which include subjects, finances, equipment, access to statistical consultation, and data entry and analysis. Frequently, staff nurses have limited access to research resources. Another major advantage of collaborative research is the larger sample size, which enhances the universality of the findings. Interinstitutional and multicenter clinical trials augment the collaborative research effort by replicating studies to improve the generalizability of the results.

OBSTACLES TO COLLABORATION

Although collaboration is beneficial, potential obstacles need to be addressed. These include lack of motivation and time, territoriality, problems with communication, unequal work distribution, and inconsistency in data collection.

Lack of Motivation and Time

In the real world of nursing, the ability to question is virtually lost among scheduling, lack of sleep, and the continual demands of meeting patient care needs (Govoni & Pierce, 1997). Expert staff nurses have a high degree of "know how" but have often lost the opportunity to ask the "know why?" Collaboration with clinical nurse specialists and nurse researchers offers the opportunity to explore the "know why?" of clinical problems. Career development can be a motivating factor for nursing staff who participate in clinical research. Participation in research may be considered as a form of staff development (McWilliam et al., 1997).

Clinical ladders that incorporate participation in research can enhance motivation, particularly if it is associated with financial incentives. Management of time constraints and scheduling are issues critical to the success of the collaborative research project. It is imperative to work with nurse managers to schedule staff to facilitate the research process. Peers on the units where staff nurses are involved in research can be supportive or destructive to the collaborative process (Govoni & Pierce, 1997).

Territoriality

Whenever a sole participant in a research project wants credit for an idea, study, or a publication, the term *territoriality* is applied. Prior written agreement and guidelines can help in avoiding this difficulty. Consensus can be difficult to attain when working with divergent personalities and perspectives. Mutuality requires a high level of reciprocity with a balanced exchange among individuals (Oda, O'Grady, & Strauss, 1994). As discussed earlier, a successful collaborator is that person who is willing to negotiate and compromise. Often, the group leader must facilitate consensus by identifying areas of commonality and then must negotiate with the participants to reach a mutually satisfactory resolution.

Problems with Communication

One way to overcome problems with communication is to identify, at the outset, the appropriate methods to be used (meetings, telephone calls, written correspondence, reports), as well as paths of communication, and to assign individual responsibilities. For example, the person who will call the meetings should be identified and the meeting place should be established. Frequent meetings facilitate communication among participants. If the collaboration is between an academic and a service setting, then intercommunication must be maintained within each setting; this becomes the responsibility of each of the appropriate participants. The academic participant must communicate regularly with the department chairperson, associate dean, and dean in the academic setting. The staff nurse and clinical nurse specialists are responsible for maintaining communication with the nurse manager, division director, and director of nursing services so that everyone is informed of the research progress and is supportive. Opportunities for hospital administrators and academic administrators to get together are also desirable to help facilitate communication and to solve problems (Ingersoll et al., 1995). In interinstitutional collaborative research, the research budget must include financial support for meetings, telephone calls, conference calls, and correspondence (Bergstrom et al., 1984).

Unequal Work Distribution

Unequal work distribution is a significant deterrent to successful collaboration. Individual assignments should be equitable and mutually agreed on by the collaborators. The work can be divided according to the research expertise of the collaborators or by the sections of the proposal (for example, literature review, methods, and data analysis). Once the work assignments have been made, the next obstacle is meeting the deadlines for assigned work. From a staff nurse perspective, asking a question and finding an answer in this high technology era is usually fairly easy and quick. The length of time to develop a project, obtain approval, collect the data, analyze the data, prepare the manuscript, and submit for publication is variable and completely unknown to the novice staff nurse (Govoni & Pierce, 1997). Hence, a realistic timetable should be developed, keeping in mind the various commitments of the participants. The leader is responsible for reminding the participants of their commitments, either in verbal or in written form. In collaborative groups consisting of academicians and clinicians, the issue of data collection should be discussed and roles should be determined. All too often staff nurses carry the burden of data collection, and this is not the expectation of collaborative research.

Inconsistency in Data Collection

In collaborative research, maintaining consistency in data collection can be difficult. Reliability and validity of the data are major concerns. To overcome any obstacles, careful planning is required. The research protocol should be a detailed, step-by-step, written document easily understood by all participants. The data collection instruments should be standardized with documented reliability and validity. In multisite collaborative research, it is useful for data collectors to learn how to use biomedical equipment or data collection instruments at a central site. In addition to on-site training, videotaped training films and pictures showing how to set up equipment for data collection are recommended (Bergstrom et al., 1984). Visits to data collection sites to ensure consistency in data collection and to establish interrater reliability should be arranged for and planned for in the budget. Meetings are essential for collaborators to review data, select data collection points, and discuss data analysis methods.

STEPS IN THE COLLABORATIVE PROCESS

Identifying Research Collaborators

Iwasiw and Olson (1984) noted that the success of a collaborative research project hinges on the relationships among the collaborators, with selection of researchers being the critical first step. To identify potential collaborators, consideration should be given to persons with similar research interests within and outside the institution. Hospitals affiliated with or near either a school or a college of nursing share a rich resource—a pool of research partners to facilitate the development of collaboration between clinicians and academic researchers. Potential collaborators can be identified through nurse researcher directories published by organizations such as The American Nurses' Association, Sigma Theta Tau, and Journal of Nursing Administration. These publications list nurses with doctoral degrees by geographical area, type of doctoral degree, and area of research interest and expertise (Larson, Wells, & McHugh, 1985). Another way of identifying possible collaborators is by reviewing the literature to find the names of persons conducting research in specific fields.

To determine compatibility, the potential collaborators should be brought together for several meetings to discuss their backgrounds, interests, goals and objectives, philosophies, and past experiences in collaborative research. It should be emphasized at the initial meetings that there is no pressure to participate in the research. The size of the research team can be critical to the development of cohesion and to promote effective communication. Usually six to eight core research team members are ideal to ensure project completion (Govoni & Pierce, 1997).

The following are questions to ask when determining compatibility of research collaborators (Iwasiw and Olson, 1984; Williams, 1987):

- What are the major goals of the research project?
- What are each collaborator's goals and are they compatible with the project?
- Are the individual research philosophies of the participants similar?
- Is there a strong mutual commitment to the research objectives?
- Are work habits and time schedules compatible?
- Do the participants communicate well?
- Can differences among the participants be tolerated?
- Is there a sense of trust among group members?

Defining Roles of the Collaborators

A director for research in an academic or service setting sometimes acts as facilitator for a collaborative research group. This person can assist by

- Bringing collaborators together
- Setting meeting dates
- Serving as liaison with institutional administrations
- Communicating with collaborators
- Providing access to resources (research literature, equipment, space, computers, typing, and data entry and analysis)

When one person manages these tasks, participants are free to concentrate on the project.

After the exploratory meetings have been held and participants have been confirmed, it is important that a leader be selected by the group. Generally, the person who initiated the research idea emerges as group leader and facilitator of the group process (Hunt et al., 1983). However, the group leader might or might not be the principal

investigator (PI) for the proposed research project. Requirements of the research project determine who will be the PI. If the project requires extramural funding, there is greater likelihood of its being funded if the PI has a doctorate, has previous research experience, and has refereed publications in the area of interest, or at least in a related area. Collaborators can serve as coinvestigators or research associates on the grant, but the PI is ultimately responsible for the development of the objectives, method, scientific merit, and administration of the research. Although the titles "principal investigator" and "coinvestigator" are designated for a grant submission, true collaboration is nonhierarchical, with all collaborators sharing responsibilities (see box) (Hoare, 1985).

Developing Operating Guidelines

Written operating guidelines developed by the collaborative group should address the responsibilities of the group facilitator or the PI. In addition, responsibilities of individual investigators should be determined early in the collaborative process. If the project is funded, the collaborative group should discuss and establish written guidelines that address the management of intramural and extramural monies from nonfederal, private industry, and federal sources.

It is imperative to the success of the collaborative group that the written guidelines detail the overall plan for dissemination of study results. The group needs to consider coauthorship of articles and participation in paper and poster presentations at the local, regional, national, and international levels. These guidelines must be developed and agreed on before the research effort. Ambiguity can lead to uncomfortable personal and professional relationships and to the undoing of collaboration (Stevens, 1986). Several writers (Spiegel and Keith-Spiegel, 1970; Werley, Murphy, Gosch, Gottesmann, & Newcomb, 1981; Burman, 1982; Huth, 1982; Waltz, Nelson, & Chambers, 1985; Brooten, 1986; Stevens, 1986; Hanson, 1988) have addressed the issue of authorship and, whereas all agreed that guidelines had to be developed regarding coauthorship, there still remains a lack of overall agreement regarding norms. The American Psychological Association (APA)

Responsibilities of the Group Facilitator or Principal Investigator and Individual Investigators

The group facilitator coordinates and manages

- Meetings
- Conference calls
- Communication
- Decision making
- Assignment of responsibilities
- Grant preparation
- Grant budget
- Data collection
- Data analysis of collated group data
- Preparation of interim and final reports

Individual investigators assume responsibilities for

- Development of the proposals and submission for human subject approval
- Data collection and analysis and format for pooled data
- Interim reports

publication manual states that "Authorship is reserved for persons who receive primary credit and hold primary responsibility for a published work. Authorship encompasses, therefore, not only those who do the actual writing but also those who have made substantial scientific contributions to a study" (American Psychological Association, 1994, p. 294). The APA states that the name of the principal contributor should appear first, with subsequent names in order of descending contribution. Hanson (1988) indicated that some writing teams decide to alphabetize authors by last name, giving equal credit to all through a footnote. (Other groups rotate names so that everyone has the opportunity to be cited as first author when several publications are forthcoming.) Burman (1982) stated that the last name in a list is construed by convention as the senior supervising author. Whatever the group decision, prior discussion about authorship and written agreement in advance are critical to successful collaboration. Refer

to Chapter 27 for more information on authorship.

Developing the Research Plan

After written guidelines are established, the group must develop a research plan, which includes the following: (1) research objectives, (2) estimation of cost and resources, (3) division of labor, and (4) a timetable.

RESEARCH OBJECTIVES

The first step in the research process is to discuss research objectives and arrive at a consensus. Clear, well-defined, and focused objectives should guide the collaborative effort to prevent later misunderstandings.

ESTIMATION OF COST AND RESOURCES

In the era of limited health care resources, it is imperative that the collaborators estimate accurately the cost-benefit ratio of the proposed project. Administrators are interested in the time, labor, and supply costs that will be involved in the project. If the project has the potential of determining an outcome that will have a future cost savings, this needs to be estimated to enhance administrative approval and support. As discussed earlier, a pooling of resources is one major advantage of collaborative research. An inventory of resources should include secretarial support, computer access, bibliographic software, literature search capability, duplication service, access to research equipment, statistical consultation, data entry and analysis, and financial support. A resources inventory helps to determine the feasibility of the project and the need to develop proposals for obtaining intramural and extramural funding (Matthews, 1985).

DIVISION OF LABOR

Some collaborative groups divide projects along the lines of members' knowledge, interests, and expertise. Others divide the work to reflect the sections of the research proposal—literature review, methods, and data analysis (Hoare & Earenfight, 1986). Regardless of the method of division, it is important to give sufficient time for a thorough discussion of the literature and for brainstorming sessions to identify new approaches (Matthews, 1985). The advantage of collaborative research is in the multidimensional approach, and time is needed to bring a new perspective into focus (Pender, Sechrist, Frank-Stromborg, & Walker, 1987). In some collaborative groups, discussions are tape-recorded and transcribed; then one member of the group writes a proposal based on the discussions. A draft of the proposal is then circulated for review (Pender et al., 1987). Occasionally it is necessary to develop separate proposals for different funding agencies. Different members of the collaborative group can write these proposals. Refer to Chapter 24 for details on proposal writing.

TIMETABLE

A realistic timetable should be developed to reflect the stages and appropriate deadlines for the research project. The timeline should account for drafts of sections of the proposal, pilot studies, editing, packaging of the proposal, completion of human subject forms, start-up date, data collection, analysis, and dissemination through presentations and publications. The timeline must be realistic so that expectations can be met. In clinically focused studies, it is important that sufficient time be allocated for pilot studies to refine the methods and to assess project feasibility. Because of the inherent difficulties in recruiting human subjects for clinical studies, the timeline must also provide adequate time for data collection. It is difficult for a collaborative group to remain motivated if time estimates are inappropriate.

Conducting Collaborative Research

Although overall coordination of the study is the responsibility of the PI, responsibility for implementing the collaborative research is shared equally by all collaborators (Hoare, 1985). As discussed earlier, a detailed written protocol, centralized training in data collection procedures, videotaped training films, and visits to data collection sites can facilitate implementation. Whereas these recommendations are frequently suggested for interinstitutional research, they also have applicability for clinical research conducted on different shifts or on different units of a single institution. During the conduct of research, communication among collaborators is essential to facilitate problem solving and decision making. Such collaboration ensures consistency in data collection, which affects the reliability and validity of the results. Because each collaborator is equally vested in the study design, it is the responsibility of all collaborators to maintain the integrity of the study. Although the PI has a major responsibility in the legalistic sense, in true collaboration each collaborator is equally vested. In a federal grant, a PI must be named to be legally responsible for the money expenditures and the integrity of the research.

Analysis of Collaborative Data

Group meetings are required to evaluate the data and to select common data points for analysis. Although the proposal delineates the method of analysis, it is not uncommon to make adjustments once the data have been collected. Clinically focused collaborative research studies frequently have gaps in data points because of the nature of the study. The group, therefore, needs to agree on how this problem will be resolved. Multisite and multiunit collaborative research must answer two questions:

1. How will the data from different sites be collated?
2. Are data affected by site location?

Because members of collaborative research teams are frequently mobile and in different locations, one person (usually the PI) is responsible for the safekeeping of the raw data and the computerized data (Hanson, 1988).

Disseminating Research Findings

Written operating guidelines serve as a framework for dissemination of research findings. Not every member of the group, however, will make the necessary effort to complete the process (that is, presentations and publications). At the end of the study, an objective assessment of each member's contribution should be made because this could influence authorship (Stevens, 1986). Collaborators should give as many other collaborators as possible the opportunity to present findings at the local, regional, or national levels. Which collaborator will present what and where should be weighed and discussed. The novice researcher should be given a nonthreatening, enjoyable experience that meets academic career requirements. It is not uncommon for researchers to write several articles for different journals based on one study (Hanson, 1988). When the collaborators are academicians and clinicians, it is appropriate that manuscripts be prepared for research and clinical practice journals alike. In the case of multidisciplinary research, discipline-specific journals should be considered. The collaborative group leader should facilitate the publication process, because the final step in any research process is the dissemination of research findings.

SUMMARY

There are different forms of collaborative efforts—intranursing and interdisciplinary, as well as intrainstitutional and interinstitutional. Research questions can be used to determine participants and types of collaboration needed to facilitate research studies.

Collaborative efforts generate tremendous benefits including (1) the ability to address complex patient care problems, (2) the generation of clinically relevant research, (3) entry into acute and chronic care facilities, and (4) acquisition of a larger sample size from which the generalizability of results improves patient care. Participants in collaborative projects also have the opportunity for professional growth through mentorship.

To accrue the benefits of collaboration it is necessary to overcome obstacles—lack of motivation and time, territoriality, problems with communication, unequal work distribution, and inconsistencies in data collection. Two ways to overcome obstacles are (1) to search out participants who possess the attributes of successful collaborators and (2) to establish operating guidelines. Characteristics of successful collaborators include the ability to (1) accept new ideas, (2) be open to review and critique when ideas are challenged, and (3) be able to negotiate and compromise to facilitate the melding of research expertise. Successful collaborators also complete assignments, communicate problems and accomplishments to the group, work independently as well as interdependently, and are ethical.

REFERENCES

American Psychological Association. (1994). *Publication manual of the American Psychological Association* (4th ed., p. 294). Washington, DC: Author.

Bergstrom, N., Hansen, B. C., Grant M., Hanson, R., Kubo, W., Padilla, G., & Wong, H. L. (1984). Collaborative nursing research: Anatomy of a successful consortium. *Nursing Research, 33,* 20–25.

Brooten, D. A. (1986). Who's on first [Guest Editorial]. *Nursing Research,* 35, 259.

Burman, K. D. (1982). "Hanging from the masthead": Reflections on authorship. *Annals of Internal Medicine, 97,* 602–605.

Govoni, A. L., & Pierce, L. L. (1997). Collaborative research among clinical nurse specialists and staff nurses. The *Journal of Continuing Education in Nursing, 28*(4), 181–187.

Hanson, S. M. H. (1988). Collaborative research and authorship credit: Beginning guidelines. *Nursing Research, 37,* 49–52.

Hoare, K. (1985). Research collaboration or participation: What's the difference? *Perioperative Nursing Quarterly, 1*(4), 7–9.

Hoare, K., & Earenfight, J. (1986). Unit-based research in a service setting. *Journal of Nursing Administration, 16*(4), 35–39.

Hunt, V., Stark, J. L., Fisher, F., Hegedus, K., Joy, L., & Woldum, K. (1983). Networking: A managerial strategy for research development in a service setting. *Journal of Nursing Administration, 13*(7,8), 27–32.

Huth, E. J. (1982). Authorship from the reader's side [Editorial]. *Annals of Internal Medicine, 97,* 613–614.

Ingersoll, G. L., Brooks, A. M., Fischer, M. S., Hoffere, D. A., Lodge, R. H., Wigsten, K. S., Costello, D., Hartung, D. A., Kiernan, M. E., Parrinello, K. M., & Schultz, A. W. (1995). Professional practice model research collaboration: Issues in longitudinal, multisite designs. *Journal of Nursing Administration, 25*(1), 39–46.

Iwasiw, C. L., & Olson, J. K. (1984). Collaboration; A research strategy that works. *Canadian Nurse, 80*(2), 39–41.

Larson, E., Wells, M. P., & McHugh, N. (1985). Perioperative nursing research. Collaboration between clinical nurse and researcher. *AORN Journal, 41,* 868–973.

Matthews, I. P. (1985). Collaboration in applied research. *Radiography, 51,* 231–232.

McWilliam, C. L., Desai, K., & Greig, B. (1997). Bridging town and gown: Building research partnerships between community-based professional providers and academia. *Journal of Professional Nursing, 13*(5), 307–315.

Oda, D. S., O'Grady, R. S., & Strauss, J. A. (1994). Collaboration in investigator initiated public health nursing research: University and agency considerations. *Public Health Nursing, 11*(5), 285–290.

Pender, N. J., Sechrist, K. R., Frank-Stromborg, M., & Walker, S. N. (1987). Collaboration in developing a research program grant. *Image: Journal of Nursing Scholarship, 19*(2), 75–77.

Spiegel, D., & Keith-Spiegel, P. (1970). Assignment of

publication credits: Ethics and practices of psychologists. *The American Psychologist, 25,* 738–747.

Stevens, K. R. (1986). Authorship: Yours, mine, or ours? *Image: Journal of Nursing Scholarship, 18,* 151–154.

Waltz, C. F., Nelson, B., & Chambers, S. B. (1985). Assigning publication credits. *Nursing Outlook, 33,* 233–238.

Werley, H. H., Murphy, P. A., Gosch, S. M., Gottesmann, H., & Newcomb, B. J. (1981). Research publication credit assignment: Nurses' views. *Research in Nursing and Health, 4,* 261–279.

Williams, C. A. (1987). Collaborative research: A commentary. *Journal of Professional Nursing, 3,* 82-124–125.

SUGGESTED READINGS

Breu, C., & Dracup, K. (1976). Implementing nursing research in a critical care setting. *Journal of Nursing Administration, 6*(10), 14–17.

Cronenwett, L. R. (1987). Clinical research by master's students. *Journal of Nursing Administration, 17*(1), 6–7.

Egan, E. C., McElmurry, B. J., & Jameson, H. M. (1981). Practice-based research: Assessing your department's readiness. *Journal of Nursing Administration, 11*(10), 26–32.

Engstrom, J. L. (1984). University, agency, and collaborative models for nursing research: An overview. *Image: Journal of Nursing Scholarship, 16,* 76–80.

Felton, G., & McLaughlin, F. E. (1976). The collaborative process in generating a nursing research study. *Nursing Research, 25,* 115–120.

Haller, K. B. (1986). Research in clinical settings. *MCN: The American Journal of Maternal/Child Nursing, 11*(4), 290.

Lasoff, E. M. (1986). Improving nurses' cooperation with clinical research. *Journal of Nursing Administration, 16*(9), 6–7.

Lindeman, C. A. (1973). Nursing research: A visible, viable component of nursing practice. *Journal of Nursing Administration, 3*(2), 18–21.

McArt, E. W. (1987). Research facilitation in academic and practice settings. *Journal of Professional Nursing, 3,* 84–91.

McClure, M. L. (1981). Promoting practice-based research: A critical need. *Journal of Nursing Administration, 11*(11,12), 66–70.

Padilla, G. V. (1979). Incorporating research in a service setting. *Journal of Nursing Administration, 9*(1), 44–49.

Singleton, E. K., Edmunds, M. W., Rapson, M., & Steele, S. (1982). An experience in collaborative research. *Nursing Outlook, 30,* 395–401.

Werley, H. H. (1972). This I believe . . . about clinical nursing research. *Nursing Outlook, 20,* 718–722.

Whitney, F. W., & Roncoli, M. (1986). Turning clinical problems into research. *Heart & Lung, 15,* 57–59.

Chapter 16

Progressing from an Idea to a Research Question

Magdalena A. Mateo and Cheryl Newton

Ideas for research problems emerge from clinical practice, continuous improvement trends, literature, priorities set by professional organizations, and discussions and presentations at professional conferences. This chapter includes information on how to identify a researchable problem, how to formulate the problem, how to pose the research question, and how to develop the hypothesis.

IDENTIFYING A RESEARCHABLE PROBLEM

Sources of Research Topics

Although nurses face a multitude of patient care problems, researchable problems are sometimes difficult to identify either because situations are obvious or because nurses become accustomed to the problem or patient situation. Nurses working in practice settings do not always consider doing research simply because they think they are already too busy providing care to patients (Diers, 1971). In addition, there is an inherent belief that practicing nurses are "doers," whereas researchers are "thinkers." Theoretical conceptions of the research process traditionally have been designated for graduate and doctoral study (Parker & Labadie, 1983). There is, therefore, a need for practicing nurses to develop their skills in identifying researchable problems relevant to practice.

Some clinical problems are obvious; others are difficult to recognize because the ideas seem vague. Artinian and Anderson (1980) identified approaches that can be used to facilitate the identification of problems in familiar settings (see box).

➤ How to Identify Problems in Familiar Settings

1. Assume the perspective of an outsider by going to a familiar setting or situation at an unusual time. Listen to what is said by patients and to whom and then ask questions.
2. Keep a daily record of what occurs (date, time, place, persons, actions, quotes) and record observations as soon as possible after leaving the setting.
3. Develop a new awareness of the patient setting by trying to identify patterns and trends from the recorded observations. The identification of patterns and trends directs the focus onto new observations that can identify repetitive trends or issues.
4. Review the literature for articles about patient care situations comparable to those identified and try to apply interpretations to the preliminary analysis of the collected data (date, time, place, persons, actions, quotes).
5. Discuss the data with uninvolved colleagues or researchers to get other perspectives on the events.

From Artinian, B. M., & Anderson, N. (1980). Guidelines for the identification of researchable problems. *Journal of Nursing Education, 19*(4), 54–58.

CLINICAL PRACTICE

Researchable problems sometimes result from a complaint or a feeling that something is "not quite right" (Diers, 1979). For example, why do patients using epidural catheters for pain relief require so much nursing time? Patients using epidural analgesia should require less nursing time. Why are vital signs ordered two times per shift on all patients even if vital signs have been stable and within normal values for the past 3 days?

Ideas for research can be triggered by personal experiences (Adebo, 1974). The nurse may be able to compare the actual situation to the ideal and then examine the existing discrepancy by imagining what the ideal situation should be. Similarly, the nurse's ability to discriminate researchable problems can be enhanced by evaluating past experiences, by keeping abreast of practice changes and recommendations from research reported at conferences and in the literature, and by being alert to the possibility of making changes in practice (Eells, 1981). For example, a nurse might notice a difference in the length of time needed for wounds to heal between two groups of patients. Or perhaps two nurses might perform a routine procedure differently, yet each may believe that his or her way is best. Networking with colleagues is helpful in identifying trends in practice.

Patterns and trends in clinical and fiscal arenas can be excellent sources for research questions. Although it may be easier to focus on problematic areas because they are more obvious, one may want to explore areas that have positive outcomes, such as a decreased length of stay in the cardiothoracic patient population.

CONTINUOUS IMPROVEMENT

Continuous improvement issues are reliable sources of research problems because they often target a defined population experiencing a common problem. The initial investigation of the issue serves to evaluate whether further study is needed. Results of continuous improvement projects can also be used as background information for a proposed study; for example, the occurrence of sentinel events or frequency of events over a period of time could give an idea about availability of sufficient data.

LITERATURE

Research and nonresearch literature are good sources for research projects, especially when sections on recommendations and implications for practice are included. Because reports of completed research studies include recommendations for further research, these are viable sources of topics. Sometimes studies need to be replicated or explanations for the recurrence of a phenomenon must be reinvestigated. Whether interventions used in certain populations produce the same outcomes when applied to other groups always presents a viable study issue. There are also articles that focus on research priorities. Cronin and Owsley (1993) used the Delphi technique to identify nursing research priorities. Nursing administrators, nursing educators, clinical nurse specialists, clinicians, and staff nurses from various patient care areas were asked to identify topics for research. They categorized topics into nursing intervention (pain management), care delivery (effects of critical paths), and patient education (family support during crisis).

The literature is useful when researchers refine the parameters of the study (Grant & Davis, 1995). The literature could also be used to support the importance of a research problem to practice, identification of potential frameworks to guide a study, and determination of the type of design and methods appropriate for the study.

PROFESSIONAL ORGANIZATIONS

Priorities set by professional organizations reflect not only changing health care needs but also evolving issues encountered by the organizations themselves (Notter & Hott, 1988). A review of the priorities of an organization can be helpful in identifying important areas of investigation.

Publications identifying priorities for nursing research as a result of trends in health care are useful. Forte, Ritz, and Balestracci (1997) reported opportunities for research following the merging of a health care system. They used the Delphi technique to identify priorities from the inpatient and ambulatory setting perspectives. This was followed by asking research participants to rank topics based on the combined inpatient and ambulatory setting lists. The focus of the three top research topics identified were related to nursing interventions and outcomes, pain, and care delivery for ambulatory care.

CONFERENCES

Professional conferences provide another source for research ideas. Paper and poster presentations offer a forum for discussing study findings and their applications to practice, thereby generating new ideas or directions for further research. Through discussion of studies or presentations with peers, common interests in issues emerge, paving the way for the possibility of collaboration.

Considerations in Problem Selection

Fuller (1982) reported that good clinical studies include the following: (1) frequent and evident occurrence of the problem in a distinct patient population, (2) a feeling that the current way of dealing with the problem is unsatisfactory, and (3) a way of reliably measuring any aspect of the problem. The nurse researcher should examine all research possibilities closely through set criteria (Diers, 1971; Adebo, 1974; Beckingham, 1974; Artinian & Anderson, 1980; Gordon, 1980; Fuller, 1982; Lindeman & Schantz, 1982; Fleming, 1984; Valiga & Mermel, 1985; Whitney & Roncoli, 1986; Rogers, 1987). The problem to be studied should be based on this examination. Four questions relevant to this analysis follow.

First, can the problem be answered by collecting observable data that explain the phenomena or the magnitude of any discrepancy? Whether observable data can be collected is determined by identifying the types of data to be collected. For example, if the question is "What are the effects of epidural analgesia on surgical patients?" the data collected might include the incidence of urinary retention and vital signs. Because these data are observable, the nurse could consider this question as a research possibility. On the other hand, if the question is "What is patient care?" further exploration of what the nurse really wants to find out is required because the question is asked in such a way that it cannot be answered by collecting observable data.

Second, will the proposed solution to the problem result in the delivery of better patient care? It is important to anticipate probable results so that the significance of the study to patient care can be ascertained. For example, if the purpose of a study is to assess the need to obtain routine vital signs every 4 hours for 5 days regardless of the patient's condition, then the need to obtain the patient's vital signs should be examined. The study result might prove that there is no need to continue the practice, because changes in vital signs are not clinically significant. Better patient care might result because time used in obtaining vital signs is then directed toward other aspects of patient care, and patients are no longer awakened during the night.

Third, are resources available? Human, financial, and environmental resources need to be available. *Human* resources include the following: (1) availability of a consultant to assist in designing the study, analyzing data, and identifying or developing data instrument tools for measuring changes in the variables under study (physiological or psychological), (2) availability of subjects within the specified time frame, and (3) availability of the nurse's time to plan and implement the study and to disseminate findings. *Financial* resources relate to expenses for purchasing equipment, obtaining tests, duplicating materials, collecting data—including travel if needed—and analyzing data. *Environmental* resources are related to the study setting, including physical facilities and administrative and staff support.

Fourth, is the problem an ethical one? Sometimes the collective good of society and the individual good of a participant pose a conflict of clinical and social interests (Jameton & Fowler, 1989). It is important to determine whether participation in the study will result in unpleasant effects for the subjects. Of equal importance is assessment of the risk-versus-benefit ratio, which means answering the question, "Will participation in the study result in some benefit for the subjects or society?" The identification of the risks and benefits in a study is essential for determining whether the proposed study is ethical.

Other important considerations when determining the focus of a study are the researcher's interest in the topic and the length of time required to conduct a study. The interest in a topic is vital to sustain one's motivation, especially when problems in the study implementation arise. The length of time in which a study is to be completed is vital to ensure that organizational resources are available throughout the duration of a project.

FORMULATION OF A PROBLEM

Brainstorming

Although most nurses are faced with similar practice situations, observations and reactions to a specific situation are based on previous experience. For this reason, brainstorming is helpful for narrowing the focus and determining the importance of the study and its researchability. Before formulating the problem, variables under examination should be named, discrepancies should be clearly delineated, and questions to be answered should be identified (Diers, 1971). For example, it is observed that caring for a patient on epidural analgesia seems to require considerable nursing time; this "hunch" can be validated by asking other staff if they agree. A meeting can be held to brainstorm this subject and elicit reasons to explain why more staff time is used and for what types of patients and activities. This brainstorming session might result in a survey to determine answers to these questions.

Variables

IDENTIFYING VARIABLES

A variable is something that changes or differs within the population under study; it is an operational concept (Polit & Hungler, 1995). Variables can be dichotomous, independent, dependent, intervening, or extraneous.

Dichotomous variables take on only two values (for example, skier/nonskier, drinker/nondrinker, smoker/nonsmoker). An *independent variable* stands alone and can be manipulated or not. If it is manipulated in the study, it is called treatment or intervention; if it is not manipulated, it is called an attribute. A *dependent variable* is the outcome, response, or effect that the researcher is interested in understanding or predicting. For example, in a study exploring differences in tolerance to chemotherapy between women with breast cancer who do aerobic exercise three to four times a week and those who do not exercise, the *independent variable* is aerobic exercise, and the *dependent variable* is the person's tolerance to chemotherapy. The independent variable has two levels, exercise and nonexercise, but is only one independent variable. If there were three levels of exercise and no exercise group, there would still be one independent variable but with four levels.

Intervening or *extraneous variables* are factors that affect (or are related to) the independent and dependent variables and therefore need to be controlled or measured.

The most common extraneous variables are related to the demographic characteristics of subjects. These characteristics include age, sex, socioeconomic background, and educational level. Other examples of extraneous variables relate to a variety of environmental and contextual factors that affect the results of the study. These factors include room temperature, time of day data are collected, type of disease, medications, length of time needed to carry out a task, or presence of family members during an interview. One way to control extraneous variables is to include subjects who are as alike as possible. For example, if the purpose of a study is to find what effect aerobic exercise has on tolerance to chemotherapy, the nurse should use subjects with similar characteristics (for example, females within a specified age range who have been diagnosed with breast cancer, are receiving the same medical treatment, and are physically able to do aerobic exercise).

DEFINING VARIABLES

Once the variables are identified, the next step is to translate the concept so that the researcher can measure the characteristics (dependent variable) and the treatment (independent variable) (Polit & Hungler, 1995). It is important to define a variable according to the way it is used in the study because, based on context, concepts differ. For example, there are different ways of measuring individual smoking behaviors. Smoking behavior can be measured by the number of cigarettes smoked in a day or by the type of cigarettes smoked based on nicotine content. The operational definition (measurement) of the variable (smoking behavior) might specify that smoking behavior is the individual consumption of a brand of cigarettes and the number of cigarettes smoked from 7 AM to 7 PM. A brief description of the treatment and how it is administered illustrates how a variable can be manipulated. For example, if a smoking cessation program is being instituted, the teaching mode should be specified.

Statement of the Problem

The research problem serves as a guide for determining the study method. Major variables being examined, the relation between variables, the nature of the population, and the research design should be included in the problem statement. A research problem can be expressed as a declarative statement or as a question. An example of a declarative statement follows: "The purpose of this research is to examine the relationship between epidural analgesia and urinary retention in peripheral vascular surgical patients." An example of a question follows: "What is the relationship between the use of epidural analgesia and urinary retention in peripheral vascular surgical patients?" As these examples indicate, the question format is simpler and more direct than the declarative statement (Polit & Hungler, 1995).

THE RESEARCH QUESTION

The research question summarizes the past in the present and at the same time heralds the future (Ellis, 1973). It determines the research method for answering the problem. Formulating the proper research question can be difficult because design, statistics, and groups and events are implied. It is important to keep in mind, however, that the research question can be revised or updated during the proposal development stage as more information about the topic is obtained. The purpose of *descriptive design* research questions is to describe, explore, and determine incidence. *Experimentally designed* questions are used to assess relationships between two or more variables or to test for differences (see box).

Good research questions meet three basic criteria (Lindeman & Schantz, 1982): (1) the question can be answered by collecting observable data, (2) the question includes the relationship between two or more variables, and (3) the question is logical and consistent with what is already known about the topic, suggesting that future knowledge can be acquired.

Sutherland, Meslin, Cunha, and Till (1993) identified criteria that 40 clinical investigators and laboratory scientists thought were important and useful in evaluating the merit of research questions. The three most frequently identified were potential impact, justification (preclinical testing), and feasibility. Other criteria less often mentioned were innovation (originality), aesthetics (clarity of idea), and politics (funding).

➤ Examples of Research Questions

Descriptive

1. What factors are associated with accidental extubation in critically ill patients?
2. Is there a relationship between circadian rhythms and body temperature?

Experimental

1. Do anorexia nervosa patients who use relaxation exercises before meals (independent variable) maintain weight (dependent variable) better than those who use no relaxation exercises before meals?
2. Does seclusion room use decrease (dependent variable) when adolescent psychiatric patients who, following confinement, engage in a 1-hour interaction with the nurse (independent variable) compared to patients who do not interact after confinement?

Artinian, B. M., & Anderson, N. (1980). Guidelines for the identification of researchable problems. *Journal of Nursing Education, 19*(4), 54–58.

To use a previously stated example, "What is the difference in tolerance to chemotherapy between women with breast cancer who *do* aerobic exercise three to four times a week and those who *do not* exercise?" This question proposes to examine the difference in chemotherapy tolerance between women with breast cancer who do aerobic exercise and those who do not. This question not only includes the relationship between variables (tolerance to chemotherapy and aerobic exercise) but also gives an indication of the design that will be used (a comparison of two groups of women with breast cancer).

THE HYPOTHESIS

The hypothesis is a statement of the predicted relationship between two or more variables. It flows from the problem statement, literature review, and theoretical framework. Hypotheses are testable. This means that variables can be measured, implications for testing the stated relationships are clear, only one prediction is made, and only criteria that accept or reject the hypothesis are specified. Hypotheses are justifiable. This means that hypotheses should be consistent with existing theory, with the knowledge and experience of the researcher, and with logical reasoning.

As illustrated in the following example, the research question reveals related variables or phenomena. The hypothesis is the tentative answer to the problem.

Research Question: Is there a difference in the tolerance to chemotherapy between women with breast cancer who do aerobics three to four times a week and those who do not exercise?
Hypothesis: There is no difference in the tolerance to chemotherapy between women with breast cancer who do aerobics three to four times a week and those who do not exercise.

There are several types of hypotheses. A brief explanation and examples are presented.

Inductive Versus Deductive Hypothesis

An inductive hypothesis is a generalization based on observed relationships (Polit & Hungler, 1995). Nurses observe patients' responses to treatment every day; therefore, deriving a hypothesis based on outcomes and trends observed in practice can be done easily. For example, a nurse might notice that patients who attend fall prevention educational programs with their families experience fewer falls during hospital stays than those who attend these educational programs by themselves. An inductive hypothesis that can be derived is "Patients who attend fall prevention educational programs with their families experience fewer falls during hospital stays than patients who attend these educational programs by themselves."

A deductive hypothesis is formulated by applying laws and theories to a situation. Assuming that the theory is correct, the nurse derives the hypothesis to strengthen the theory by assuming that certain outcomes can be expected. In the earlier example about attendance at fall prevention educational programs, it can be assumed that "Being alone in a different environment produces stress in a patient. Stress inhibits learning." If this is correct, a nurse can deduce that patients who are hospitalized for the first time will benefit more from an educational program on falls if they attend with their families than if they attend by themselves.

Simple Versus Complex Hypothesis

A *simple hypothesis* predicts the relationship between one independent variable and one dependent variable, whereas a *complex hypothesis* predicts the relationship between two or more independent variables and two or more dependent variables (Polit & Hungler, 1995). An example of a simple hypothesis follows: "Women with breast cancer who swim three times a week experience less nausea from chemotherapy than women with breast cancer who do not swim regularly." An example of a complex hypothesis follows: "Women with breast cancer who swim and do aerobic exercises three times a week report the occurrence of less nausea and a lesser degree of depression than women with breast cancer who do not swim but do aerobic exercises regularly."

In the examples, the simple hypothesis includes one independent variable (swimming three times a week) and one dependent variable (nausea). The complex hypothesis includes two independent variables (swimming and aerobic exercises three times a week) and two dependent variables (nausea and degree of depression).

Directional Versus Nondirectional Hypothesis

A *directional hypothesis* is one that specifies the nature of the relationship between two or more variables. An example of a directional hypothesis follows: "Nurses who participate in determining their work schedules use less sick time than those who do not participate in determining their work schedules."

A *nondirectional hypothesis* is one that does not predict the exact nature of the relationship between variables. The researcher usually uses a nondirectional hypothesis when there is no clear indication of the relationship between variables. An example of a nondirectional hypothesis follows: "There is a relationship between work schedules and work satisfaction among nurses working in a hospital."

Research Versus Statistical Hypothesis

A research hypothesis is a statement of the expected relationship between variables. The researcher's prediction is based on theory, previous research findings, or clinical experience (Burns & Grove, 1997). An example of a research hypothesis follows: "There is a relationship between job satisfaction and retention of nurses."

A statistical hypothesis (also called a null hypothesis) is a statement that shows *no* relationship between the independent and dependent variables. The researcher assumes that the statement is true unless results of a statistical test of significance indicate otherwise. An example of a null hypothesis is "There is no relationship between immobility and development of pressure sores in paralyzed patients who are bedridden."

SUMMARY

Nurses have an important and unique role in generating clinically relevant research. Research meaningful to practice must reflect issues encountered in the practice setting. Steps essential to the investigation of problems confronting nurses—from sources of topics to the formulation of researchable questions and testable hypotheses—were presented in this chapter. Figure 16–1 illustrates the progression from an idea to a formulated research question.

Personal experiences, staff and patient complaints, continuous improvement issues, literature, organizational priorities, and conferences provide materials for researchable problems. Before determining the focus of a study, it is wise to remember that the requisites for legitimate clinical studies include the following: (1) occurrence of the phenomena in specific patient groups, (2) a need to change the way of dealing with the problem, and (3) a reliable measure that can be used to evaluate outcomes. Brainstorming

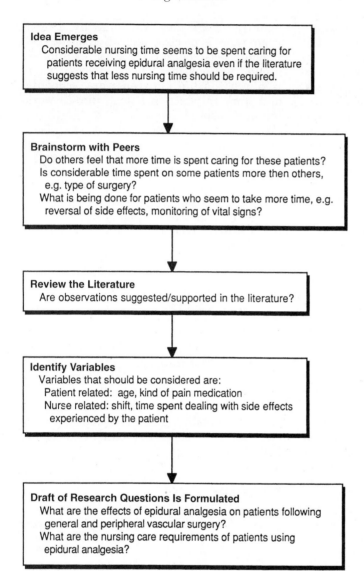

Figure 16–1
From an idea to the research question: a model.

ideas with peers and reviewing the literature are valuable tools for progressing from an idea to formulating the research problem. These steps elucidate the focus of the study, the variables to be examined, and the methods for evaluation.

REFERENCES

Adebo, E. O. (1974). Identifying problems for nursing research. *International Nursing Review, 21*, 53–59.

Artinian, B. M., & Anderson, N. (1980). Guidelines for the identification of researchable problems. *Journal of Nursing Education, 19*(4), 54–58.

Beckingham, A. C. (1974). Identifying problems for nursing research. *International Nursing Review, 21*, 49–52.

Burns, N., & Grove, S. K. (1997). *The practice of nursing research: Conduct, critique and utilization* (3rd ed.). Philadelphia: W. B. Saunders.

Cronin, S., & Owsley, V. B. (1993). Identifying nursing research priorities in an acute care hospital. *Journal of Nursing Administration, 23*(11), 58–62.

Diers, D. (1971). Finding clinical problems for study. *Journal of Nursing Administration, 1*(6), 15–18.

Diers, D. (1979). *Research in nursing practice.* New York: J. B. Lippincott.

Eells, M. A. W. (1981). The research problem. In S. D. Krampitz & N. Pavlovich (Eds.), *Readings for nursing research* (pp. 3–10). St. Louis: Mosby.

Ellis, R. (1973). Asking the Research Question. *Issues in research: Social, professional, and methodological.* Program meeting of the American Nurses' Association Council of Nurse Researchers, 31–35.

Fleming, J. W. (1984). Selecting a clinical nursing problem for research. *Image: The Journal of Nursing Scholarship, 16*, 62–64.

Forte, P. S., Ritz, L. J., & Balestracci, D. (1997). Identifying nursing research priorities in a newly merged healthcare system. *Journal of Nursing Administration, 27*(6), 51–55.

Fuller, E. O. (1982). Selecting a clinical nursing problem for research. *Image: The Journal of Nursing Scholarship, 14,* 60–61.

Gordon, M. (1980). Determining study topics. *Nursing Research, 29,* 83–87.

Grant, J. S., & Davis, L. L. (1995). Using the literature to design a study in the rehabilitation setting: An example with stroke patients. *Rehabilitation Nursing, 20*(3), 144–148, 154.

Jameton, A., & Fowler, M. D. M. (1989). Ethical inquiry and the concept of research. *Advances in Nursing Science, 11*(3), 11–24.

Lindeman, C. A., & Schantz, D. (1982). The research question. *Journal of Nursing Administration, 12*(1), 6–10.

Notter, L. E., & Hott, J. R. (1988). *Essentials of nursing research* (4th ed.). New York: Springer-Verlag.

Parker, M. L., & Labadie, G. C. (1983). Demystifying research mystique. *Nursing & Health Care, 4,* 383–386.

Polit, D. F., & Hungler, B. P. (1995). *Nursing research principles and methods* (5th ed.). Philadelphia: J. B. Lippincott.

Rogers, B. (1987). Is the research project feasible? *Occupational Health Nursing, 35,* 327–328.

Sutherland, H. J., Meslin, E. M., Cunha, D. A., & Till, J. E. (1993). Judging clinical research questions: What criteria are used? *Social Science Medicine, 37*(12), 1427–1430.

Valiga, T. M., & Mermel, V. M. (1985). Formulating the researchable question. *Topics in Clinical Nursing, 7*(2), 1–14.

Whitney, F. W., & Roncoli, M. (1986). Turning clinical problems into research. *Heart & Lung, 15,* 57–59.

Looking in the Literature

Mary G. Schira

A review of the literature is essential early in the research process. For many nurses, the literature review is probably the most familiar part of the research process. Nurses frequently read journal articles as a continuing education strategy to stay current in nursing practice. Developing a few additional critical thinking skills helps nurses review the literature from a research perspective.

To do the literature review, the beginning researcher must know how to locate pertinent references, organize the literature that has been read, and critically evaluate the research literature (Schira & Pass, 1991). The tangible outcome of the literature review is a concise written summary in the research proposal or report. The intangible outcome is the researcher's increased confidence in the subject area. This chapter addresses how to complete a literature re-

view and provides guidelines for evaluating the research literature.

LOCATING THE LITERATURE

Purpose

A literature review is usually done after the research problem or questions have been formulated (Schira, 1992). There are four primary purposes for doing a literature review (see box). First, the literature provides an in-depth understanding of what is known and not known about the topic, allowing the researcher to fit the proposed study into the context of existing knowledge. Through the literature review, the researcher identifies research that supports the proposed study, previous work that does not support the

➤ Purposes of the Literature Review

1. Provide in-depth understanding of the topic.
2. Identify whether the study has already been conducted.
3. Generate additional ideas, methods, or instruments.
4. Provide a conceptual framework within which the study fits.

study, and the ways in which the proposed study differs from preceding research. Second, an extensive review of the literature reveals whether a similar study has been conducted. Finding the proposed study in the literature is not reason for the researcher to give up on the study. Rather, the researcher needs to determine differences and similarities between the previous and proposed study and decide whether replication is needed. Third, the review often strengthens the proposed study by generating new ideas or problems not previously considered, identifying data collection instruments or methods that can be used or adapted, and posing additional research questions or hypotheses. Fourth, a literature review provides conceptual frameworks that were used in previous studies that might assist the researcher in the current project.

Although a somewhat familiar activity, the literature review can seem overwhelming. Before doing the literature search, the researcher needs to locate a library or identify computer online services with appropriate resource materials. There are many resources available to assist the researcher in obtaining the necessary literature. If a library is to be used, access to a university or a well-equipped hospital library is needed. Community or public libraries usually do not have the indexes or the capabilities to do the necessary computer searches for a literature review in the health care field. In addition to a well-equipped library, a reference librarian aware of potential resources and skilled in searching out appropriate references is invaluable to the researcher.

In the absence of an appropriate library,

computer online services can be accessed to search the literature. In the case of online or Internet searches, the researcher needs to have or develop a few basic computer skills. Another valuable resource in obtaining the literature is the Center for Nursing Scholarship located in Indianapolis, IN. The center contains a comprehensive collection of national and international nursing materials and publishes *The Online Journal of Knowledge Synthesis for Nursing*. This online journal contains research and research summary articles and can be electronically searched by subject, title, author, key word, date, phrase, or combination of words. The online journal also allows the user to link to external databases that are on the library reference systems. The center is funded by donations from Sigma Theta Tau International Honor Society members and chapters, and the health care community at large, and is available to both members of the society and nonmembers. The journal can be accessed through online services (stti@stti.iupui.edu) or the center can be visited in Indianapolis.

Sources

Sources of literature include printed indexes, computerized databases, references, review articles, and content experts.

PRINTED INDEXES

Indexes are most frequently found in a library and are used to find journal references. Most indexes follow a basic, standard format that includes author, title of the article, journal name, date of publication, volume and issue number, and the pages of the article (Fig. 17–1). Indexes frequently abbreviate journal titles; the full title can be found at the front of the index. Articles can usually be located by subject area or by author (see box).

The Cumulative Index to Nursing and Allied Health Literature (CINAHL) includes entries from nursing, allied health, and biomedical journals, and some popular journals (such as *Time* and *Newsweek*). Only journals printed in English are listed. Helpful features of CINAHL include identification of articles that are research reports and a note regarding the number of references included at the end of the article. CINAHL

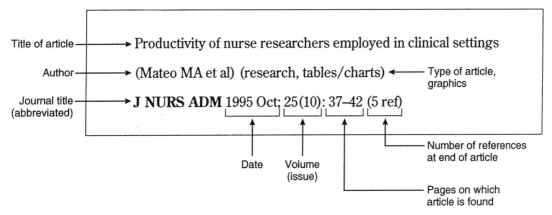

Figure 17–1
Publication information.

also includes an author index so that publications from known experts in the field can be located. This database is accessible online for a fee.

The International Nursing Index (INI) contains nursing and non-nursing journals with articles printed in English and in other languages. The INI also indexes publications from the National League of Nursing, The American Nurses' Association, and nursing associations throughout the world. Publications from nursing organizations may be helpful in providing policy statements regarding the topic of interest or statistical information to support the proposed study.

> ## Printed Indexes

1. Articles are grouped according to subject area and are frequently cross referenced. For example, an article on compliance in taking antihypertensive medicines could be found under both hypertension and compliance subject headings.
2. Each entry in the subject area usually includes the title, author, journal name, year, and volume and issue number, as well as page numbers on which the article appears.
3. Abbreviations used in the index, as well as the meaning of each part of the citation, are referenced at the beginning of the index.

Index Medicus is produced by the National Library of Medicine and is the most comprehensive listing of biomedical journal articles available. Index Medicus contains citations of articles printed in English and other languages. The majority of the citations are not from nursing journals, although several major nursing journals are included. The non-nursing literature may be helpful in identifying how other disciplines view the topic of interest from a theory and research perspective.

The Science Citation Index (SCI) focuses on journal articles in the scientific literature. Each journal is completely indexed, including cited references. The SCI contains a subject index, a corporate index, a source index, and a citation index. The latter comprises the major portion of this source and lists under each author's name all articles referencing the specific work. The SCI may be especially helpful in locating basic research that has been conducted on the topic of interest or to find work quoting an author that is key to the researcher's study.

Dissertation Abstracts International is a compilation of abstracts of doctoral dissertations submitted by more than 450 academic institutions. Compiled monthly, it frequently references research that has not yet been published as a journal article. Both nursing and non-nursing research can be located to help the researcher be as current as possible in the topic of interest. Like most printed indexes, Dissertation Abstracts International and SCI are available online for a fee or by searching a library database on computer.

Individual journal indexes can also be

useful. Some journals, such as *Nursing Research* and the *American Nephrology Nurses' Association (ANNA) Journal* publish a yearly index of articles included in the journal from the preceding year. The journal may also provide an index of authors that contributed to the journal the preceding year. Individual journal indexes can be especially helpful in locating specialty-specific literature (as in the *ANNA Journal*). Most journal indexes are published in the final volume of the year.

COMPUTERIZED DATABASES

Computerized databases are increasingly popular and necessary as the volume of published material continues to grow. Computer searches are more advantageous than hand searches of indexes because they take less time and allow concepts to be linked (Sinclair, 1987). Searching by computer can be accomplished using a library-based computer system or a personal computer and online resources in the home or workplace. The computer search yields a list of articles with complete bibliographical citations. For many of the articles, an abstract is also available on request (Nicoll, 1993). The computer allows the researcher to choose only the references of interest from those presented and to obtain a printed list of the articles chosen for review (see box).

Several databases apply specifically to nursing and health care. When doing a computer search, the researcher identifies the database for the search. Two of the most common databases used by nurses are CINAHL and MEDLARS (Medical Literature Analysis and Retrieval System). The CINAHL computer database contains the same information as the printed index, and includes citations from nursing, allied health, and biomedical journals published since 1983. MEDLARS is the most comprehensive online resource for medical literature and includes national and international journal article references. MEDLINE is probably the best known of the MEDLARS databases; it includes journals indexed in the International Nursing Index and Index Medicus since 1966. However, MEDLARS contains numerous other databases of interest to nurses, including CANCERLIT, BIOETHICSLINE, and AIDSLINE. One of the advantages of the MEDLARS database is that an abstract of the article is available; the CINAHL database does not include abstracts. However, the list of search terms in MEDLARS does not include a large number of nursing terms, which may make initial retrieval of information from the MEDLARS database more difficult than searching the CINAHL database.

Two other readily accessible computer databases available in most libraries are the Educational Resources Information Center (ERIC) and the Mechanized Information Center (MIC). ERIC contains an index of selected educational literature citing research-based and non–research-based journal articles and papers from presentations, which could be useful to the nurse researcher.

The MIC identifies the information available in U.S. government publications. In addition to bibliographical citations, abstracts or summaries are available in some of the reference areas. The information in the MIC may also be helpful in providing statistics related to disease prevalence or demographic characteristics that could be used in supporting the significance of the proposed research study.

Table 17–1 summarizes the printed indexes and computerized databases frequently used by nurses.

A computerized search can be done by a librarian or by the researcher, depending on the resources of the library and the researcher. Whether the search is done by a

➤ Doing a Computer Search: Benefits

A computer search

1. Is less time consuming.
2. Contains more current resources.
3. Allows retrieval from one source rather than from several printed indexes.
4. Permits concepts to be linked together. For example, if the goal is to find literature on anorexia and cancer, the terms can be combined in the search, and only relevant material will be selected from these two large subject headings.

Table 17–1

The Literature Review: Summary of Sources

SOURCES OF LITERATURE	TYPE OF REFERENCE	COMMENTS
Printed Indexes		
International Nursing Index	Nursing Nursing organizations Non-nursing	English and other languages
Cumulative Index to Nursing and Allied Health	Nursing Allied health Biomedical (selected) Popular (selected)	Primarily journal articles English language only
Index Medicus	Biomedical, medical Nursing (selected)	English and other languages
Science Citation Index	Scientific literature	Includes health care and nonhealth care references
Dissertation Abstracts International	Unpublished dissertations	Wide subject background
Computerized Databases		
MEDLINE	Biomedical Nursing	Journals and monographs English and other languages
CINAHL (Cumulative Index to Nursing and Allied Health)	Nursing Allied health Biomedical (selected) Popular (selected)	Focuses on nursing references
ERIC (Educational Resources Information Center)	Education literature	Includes journal articles and papers from presentations
MIC (Mechanized Information Center)	U.S. government publications	Abstracts or summaries of information also available

librarian or the researcher, the first step is to identify words that identify the topic of interest. These key words are entered into the computer, and the computer searches the specified database for the words. The databases arrange information according to descriptions (or key words) that define specific topics. Descriptors are arranged in a thesaurus of terms called Medical Subject Headings (MESH) (Sinclair, 1987). The MESH terms are arranged alphabetically from general to specific concepts and can be combined.

A computerized bibliographical search is most useful when two or more concepts are tied together. The search can draw a relationship between concepts. To further narrow the search, concepts that are to be excluded can be identified. When there has been a great deal of material published on a topic, additional terms may be needed to narrow the search. For example, a search based on "pain" yields many references, whereas a search that adds "postoperative" yields a smaller list of journal articles. The further addition of "spinal fusion" yields an even smaller and more specific list of journal citations for a study about postoperative pain after spinal fusion.

If a librarian is going to complete the computer search for the researcher, it is important for the researcher to have a dialogue with the librarian. Together, the librarian and the researcher identify MESH terms that might yield relevant citations. A MESH term search is comprehensive because all articles related to the subject are listed. A non-MESH term is searched only for inclusion of the specific term in the article. Charges for computerized searches and the length of time required to complete the search vary among institutions.

Depending on the library, the researcher may conduct a search of the available computer databases with little or no assistance from a librarian. A researcher-generated literature search offers two distinct advantages. First, the researcher can have immediate access to search information; second, by transferring the literature search to a computer disk, a computer-based professional library can be started. Although the researcher may actually conduct the search, the reference librarian is a valuable asset in finding the right combination of words and concepts to get the most out of a computer search. Again, cost and length of time to complete the search vary. Many libraries offer training sessions in how to access and search computer databases as a service to library users. With the background provided in the library-sponsored class and the availability of a librarian for questions and guidance, many researchers have learned to conduct computer searches independently, at a much lower cost.

An increasing number of researchers are conducting literature searches using non-library–based computer networks or personal computers. Existing databases and online resources can be accessed through an organization network or through a personal computer that connects to a modem and telephone line. Researchers who use these computer resources to locate the literature have around-the-clock access to multiple libraries and reference sources.

To search the CINAHL or MEDLARS computer database from a personal computer or network, a communications software program or access via the Internet is needed. For example, Grateful Med is a software program that interfaces with the MEDLARS databases. The Grateful Med software automates the process of searching the database online (Nicoll, 1993). After the researcher identifies a search strategy on the input screen, searches can be conducted by subject, journal, and author. The result of the search is a list of references and abstracts that the researcher can print, save to a file, or place an order to receive specific articles by mail or FAX. As with most online computer services, the online time is generally charged by transaction as well as by actual time connected to the computer. There is an additional cost for the articles ordered.

The Internet is probably the best known of the computer networks and is a composite global communication network that connects university, business, military, and science computer systems worldwide (Wright, 1996). To access the Internet, the researcher or computer user pays a fee to a commercial provider. Fees are generally a flat monthly fee plus long distance telephone charges (for the modem).

One of the many communication services accessible on the Internet are LISTSERVs. A LISTSERV is an electronic discussion service for special interest groups that delivers discussion text into the user's electronic mailbox (Wright, 1996). Once a user subscribes to a LISTSERV, information from the other interest group subscribers is transmitted into the user's mailbox whenever information is generated in the LISTSERV. For example, "NurseRes" is a LISTSERV group that allows nurse researchers to discuss research topics. During the literature review phase of a study, the researcher may use NurseRes to identify ongoing research in the same area of the proposed study or to obtain help in locating specific references or resources.

REFERENCE LISTS AND EXPERTS

Final sources of potential literature include the list of references at the end of an article and experts in the topic of interest. Reference lists, especially those at the end of a review article or book, provide a wealth of published information that aids in locating appropriate literature. In some cases, the reference lists provide pertinent, classic studies of which the researcher might not have been aware, thereby preventing errors of omission.

Individuals with expertise in a particular topic or subject area are also potentially rich resources. Experts are likely to be aware of new developments in the area of interest, be well read on the topic, and may be aware of other researchers conducting similar research or research on the same topic. These experts can help the beginning researcher identify pertinent literature and research that will be of use in the proposed study. Experts are often located by identifying authors that have several publications or presentations in a particular area of interest or study.

READING THE LITERATURE

Once the journal articles have been identified, either by hand-searching indexes or by carefully reviewing computer-generated bibliographies, the next step is to locate the articles. If the articles were requested from an online computer search, the researcher simply needs to await the arrival of the designated articles. Otherwise, the researcher needs to go to a university or hospital library and locate the articles of interest.

Each library keeps a list of current holdings—those journals subscribed to at present as well as journals subscribed to in the past. If the library carries the journal, the researcher needs to locate it and begin reading the article of interest. If the library does not carry the journal, the article can often be obtained through interlibrary loan, a sharing system among many libraries.

When reading the literature, the researcher should keep a few guidelines in mind. Whenever possible, primary sources rather than secondary sources should be reviewed. A primary source is a report on research written by the person who conducted the study. A secondary source is a summary of the study written by another person, usually as part of an article citing the original study, or as a summary of studies on a topic. The researcher needs to read the primary source so that independent conclusions can be drawn. Secondary sources are useful for bibliographical information that leads to the primary source.

The date of an article should also be considered. In some areas of study, only slight changes occur over time that would make the results out of date. However, if the research involves rapidly changing information, such as technological changes (for example, computer literacy in nurses, organ transplants), time is an important factor in determining the validity of the research findings. As much as possible, the literature reviewed should be recent (within the past 3 to 5 years).

The emphasis of the literature review should be on research or data-based reports rather than on descriptive articles. In the course of reading the literature, the researcher will find articles that relate directly and indirectly to the study. Emphasis should be placed on information that relates directly so that the background for the study is clear. When new approaches are being researched, however, indirectly related articles are sometimes needed to provide a logical framework for the study. For example, a study may propose to assess sterile versus clean technique in packing deep wounds in the home care setting. In the absence of any research articles on this specific subject, indirectly related research on sterile versus clean technique in urinary catheterization could be used to provide a framework.

In addition, studies that both support and do not support the researcher's ideas should be included. The researcher needs to remember that the purpose of the literature review is to ensure a good understanding of the topic of interest. By including both types of research in the review, the researcher is able to view the proposed study as critically as possible.

ORGANIZING THE LITERATURE REVIEWED

At the beginning of the literature review, it is essential to decide on a method for abstracting and organizing information from each resource. A consistent format benefits the researcher by providing a way to integrate and synthesize the information so that how the proposed study will fit into the body of previous research is clear. In addition, a well-devised system for gathering and organizing information facilitates the retrieval of data and the written summary.

There are numerous systems and formats for gathering the necessary information from research articles. Regardless of the system or format used, the researcher should be sure to include a full bibliographical citation and to record specific information about the study (for example, problem statement, hypotheses, sample characteristics, research tools). The following sections provide additional information on organizing the information that is gathered.

Bibliographical Citations

The researcher needs to identify a complete bibliographical citation format at the outset of the search and use the format consistently (see box). There are several advantages to recording complete and accurate citations. The researcher can retrieve materials quickly and easily if the need arises. Also, compiling the reference list for the proposal and for publication of the study is made easier. Then, once published, the readers of the research can locate referenced articles with little difficulty.

The value of accurate and complete citations cannot be overemphasized. In a study

➤ Elements of a Citation

JOURNAL ARTICLE CITATIONS

1. Author's last name and initials
2. Title of the article
3. Name of the journal
4. Year of publication
5. Volume and issue number
6. Page numbers on which the article appears

BOOK CITATIONS

1. Author's last name and initials
2. Chapter title and book title
3. Year of publication
4. Name of publishing company
5. Editors and edition (if any)

OTHER CITATIONS

Conference proceedings, magazine articles, technical or research reports differ in the information that is included in citations. Refer to a publication manual. The American Psychological Association (1995) publishes such a manual.

---

by Foreman and Kirchhoff (1987), 112 references in nursing journals were analyzed for accuracy. They found that approximately 38% of the references cited were in error, with 4.6% of the errors being severe enough to prevent retrieval of the resource. Although the majority of the errors did not prevent location of the reference, errors did make retrieval more time-consuming.

Recording Information

The researcher needs to identify a method for recording information obtained from each article. Although no single method is superior to another, common approaches include the use of summary tables, index cards, and photocopying articles. Researchers need to identify a method that works well for them and to use the method consistently as the literature is reviewed.

SUMMARY TABLE

A summary table is helpful for organizing a large amount of information (Table 17–2 provides an example). Holm and Llewellyn (1986) suggested that a summary chart include bibliographical citations and the clinical affiliation for the researcher, variables studied, sample selection and characteristics, methods, results, and researcher's conclusions. Bush (1985) suggested that a summary table also include the relevance of the reviewed study to the proposed research. Headings can be modified to fit the focus of any particular proposed study, and statistics can be included if they are significant to the study.

A summary table can serve as the organizing framework for the researcher's thinking and provides an efficient way of getting started because it clarifies the information significant for recall. The summary table cannot, however, substitute for additional note-taking about the reviewed study. Rather, the table forces the researcher to make decisions about the value of the information as it is collected. As a result, the material is carefully analyzed for its relative contribution to the scientific literature and how it fits into the proposed study.

The summary table can also help the researcher prepare the review of the literature for oral or written presentation. The table format makes clear which major themes have emerged, how studies group together naturally, which concepts and variables have been considered, which populations have been studied, which instruments and methods have been used, what questions have been answered, and what hypotheses have been supported. More importantly, the summary table provides clues to populations that have not been examined, methods and instruments that need to be developed, gaps in available information, and questions that have not been asked (Polit & Hungler, 1997).

INDEX CARDS

Many researchers find 5- by 7-inch index cards ideal for taking notes and summarizing information from an article. A single citation is put on each card, leaving space for notes. As with a summary table, the same type of information should be included on each card to ensure that the same infor-

Table 17–2

Recording Summary of Research Studies

Citation and affiliation researcher	Concepts studied and variables	Sample, selection, characteristics	Methods and instrumentation	Results	Researcher's conclusion and critique	Relevance for proposed study

mation is gleaned from each resource. The cards can then be sorted easily into content areas and ranked according to how the citations will appear in the written review of the literature. As with the summary table, the index cards can greatly facilitate preparing the literature review for oral or written presentation.

PHOTOCOPYING

The common practice of photocopying articles can also be an advantage during the literature review process. The researcher may find that having a copy of detailed or especially helpful articles may be useful later in the research process. In addition, photocopying permits working on material when libraries are closed and makes rereading an article for added information or detail much easier. Many researchers underline or highlight specific points within an article to make retrieval of necessary information easier. However, copying an article does not substitute for careful note-taking or critical evaluation of the article; it merely makes the article more accessible.

Some articles the researcher may especially wish to copy are "classics," or references that are commonly cited in the literature on the research topic. Other studies might be particularly relevant to the proposed study because they present a clear statement of a theoretical framework that fits the study, because a similar population was used, or because a particular method or instrument useful for the study is identified. Yet other studies might include multiple tables, figures, and graphs that are important but too tedious to record in notes (Holm & Llewellyn, 1986).

When photocopying an article, the researcher needs to be sure that complete bibliographical information is obtained. Not all journals print complete information on each journal page; therefore, the researcher needs to verify citations and add information as needed at the time the article is copied. It is a painful (and time-consuming) lesson to return to an article that was copied to find that the full citation is not present.

ABSTRACTING THE INFORMATION

It is important to determine how previous research relates to the proposed study and what information it offers to discuss the study critically. An organized and consistent system should always be used when summarizing research articles (see box).

Non–research-related literature should also be summarized to include information clearly and concisely. For example, if the literature deals with a procedure, the steps of interest should be clearly noted. Non–research-related literature can be useful in providing background information on approaches to or opinions on the topic under investigation. Non–research-related literature does not replace research literature; it provides support for the relevance of the research.

There are several computer programs

➤ Abstracting Research Articles

Research articles should be summarized to include the following:

1. Problem statement of the study
2. Description of the subjects, methods used, where the study was implemented, when the study was completed
3. Short critical review of the results. Use exact quotes rather than paraphrasing to avoid later questions regarding meaning and to avoid plagiarism.

available for reference management, including Endnote Plus, Reference Manager, and ProCite. References can be imported into Endnote Plus, and then within a word processing program (Word or WordPerfect), references can be pasted into a manuscript. With a few additional computer keystrokes, a list of references cited in the manuscript can be formatted. If a different format is needed later, the references can be reformatted.

CRITICALLY EVALUATING THE RESEARCH LITERATURE

A research literature review should include information about the study and a critical review of the results. A critical review is an objective evaluation that determines the strengths, weaknesses, and potential usefulness of the research. The research is evaluated in light of the proposed study, particularly addressing whether it supports or does not support the study. Although the focus is on evaluating previous research for its usefulness to new research, the guidelines presented herein are also helpful in determining how the results of completed research can be applied in nursing practice. Guidelines for evaluating research for its utility in practice are addressed in Chapter 3.

If the researcher has given careful consideration to what to include in the search and has diligently and consistently followed the framework, a pattern should emerge as information is recorded. It should become clear how information fits together, where the gaps are in the literature, and how the proposed study fits into the picture in an attempt to fill some of those gaps (Polit & Hungler, 1997).

A critical review of research literature determines the adequacy of each section of the research report. Reading the research literature may be a new skill for the beginning researcher. The following guidelines as well as those in other references (Girden, 1996; Rankin & Esteves, 1996; Burns & Grove, 1997; Polit & Hungler, 1997) can help the researcher begin to build the necessary skills. However, the best way to build the needed skill is to actually read and evaluate the research.

Research reports are written with the same basic information so that the reviewer is able to evaluate each part, regardless of the type of research. Areas to consider when evaluating a study include problem statement, literature review, conceptual framework, research questions or hypotheses, methods, results, and conclusions. Questions and issues that the reviewer should address when evaluating the research literature are included in the following discussion (see box).

Problem Statement

The problem statement should be stated clearly and concisely. It should contain information about the dependent variables (the response or behavior predicted in the research) and independent variables (the treatment implemented by the researcher to create the response or behavior) in the study. Found early in the research report, the problem statement is frequently followed by an explanation of the significance of the problem or why the research was conducted. The problem statement is important because it provides the focus of the study and the rest of the report flows from it and is judged in relation to it.

Review of the Literature

A review of the literature follows the problem statement. Although the literature review is likely to be short in a journal article, the literature providing a background for the study should be reported. The literature presented should be pertinent to the study, should be current, and should include concepts relating to all variables. The review also should include a summary of previous research on the topic. If previous research has not been done, this should be indicated in the article.

Conceptual Framework

Closely related to the literature review and occasionally reported as part of the literature review in a published article is the conceptual framework. The conceptual framework identifies how the research links to previous research and theory. In some cases, the variables are defined in the conceptual framework; if so, the definitions

> ### Questions to Ask When Evaluating the Research Literature

> #### PROBLEM STATEMENT
>
> What was studied? What are the dependent and independent variables? Why is the problem important?
>
> #### REVIEW OF THE LITERATURE
>
> Does the literature relate to the study? How? Is the literature recent? Current? Is previous research included?
>
> #### CONCEPTUAL FRAMEWORK
>
> How does the study relate to previous research? Does the study fit with current knowledge?
>
> #### HYPOTHESIS/RESEARCH QUESTION
>
> What relationship was tested? Can the question be answered by the data collected?
>
> #### METHOD
>
> **Sample.**   How were subjects chosen? How do they relate to the population?
>
> **Treatment.**   How was the treatment assigned to the subjects? How and where was the treatment carried out?
>
> **Instruments.**   What instruments were used? Are the instruments valid? Reliable?
>
> **Data Analysis.**   How were data analyzed? Are the statistical tests appropriate?
>
> #### RESULTS
>
> What did the researcher find? Were all hypotheses addressed?
>
> #### CONCLUSIONS
>
> What meaning did the researcher draw from the results? Do the results make sense? Are there limitations in using the results? What recommendations did the researcher make for practice? For further research?

should be clear. The framework flows directly from the problem statement and literature review. If the relationship is unclear, the research may not be cohesive.

Hypotheses

Hypotheses or research questions are directly derived from the problem statement and flow from the conceptual framework. Each research question or hypothesis states one idea or specific relationship. If more than one relationship is being tested, more than one hypothesis or research question needs to be stated. Also important is whether the question can be answered by gathering data. If the question cannot realistically be answered, the research is of minimal value.

Method

A larger segment than those previously addressed is the method section of the report. Critical evaluation of the method used in the study helps determine the generalizability of results and how closely the previous research will support the proposed study. In the method section, several aspects must be evaluated.

SAMPLE

The sample should be clearly described—who or what was studied and how participants or events were chosen for inclusion must be explained. Demographic characteristics (age, gender) that may be relevant to evaluating results should be provided in some detail. An ideal sampling method is random selection. If random selection is used, study results have a far greater probability of being applicable to all patients in that population. If a convenience sample is used, how the sample is chosen is important to determine bias that could limit generalizability of results. A number of clinical studies use convenience samples because of the constraints of conducting research in a clinical setting.

ASSIGNMENT OF TREATMENTS

Closely related to how subjects are chosen is how treatment methods are assigned to subjects. Like random selection of subjects, random assignment of treatment is preferred over other approaches, which might contain bias (prejudice). Although random sampling may not be possible, random assignment to treatments may, however, still be possible. The reviewer must read the description of the sample selection and the method of allocating treatments carefully. Then, any factors that could limit or bias the results and implications of the study must be identified.

DATA COLLECTION INSTRUMENTS AND METHODS

Instruments and methods should measure the variables that are being examined. Reliability (consistency of the measurement) and validity (whether the instrument actually measures the behavior of interest) of instruments should be addressed; methods should be consistent among all subjects. In most studies, data other than that needed to support the research hypothesis are also collected. Other data are collected to measure variables (extraneous) that might also be important. These extraneous variables often confound the relationship between the dependent and independent variables in the study and must be controlled either in the research design or through statistical procedures (Polit & Hungler, 1997). The reviewer should be alert for extraneous variables that have not been identified or controlled by the researcher. Generalizability and applicability of study results can be affected by extraneous variables.

DATA ANALYSIS

Finally, the method section should describe how the data were analyzed. Methods used for analysis must be appropriate for the data. This can be difficult for the beginning reviewer with minimal background in statistics and data analysis. A statistics book can help in determining whether the tests applied are appropriate. In addition, help can be obtained from an experienced colleague or researcher.

Results

A report on the results of the research logically follows the discussion of the method.

All important results and data that answer the research question are presented. The results section of the report should offer the findings in an organized manner and discuss them in relation to previously identified research and theory. The results section of a research report deserves close attention because this is the outcome of the research.

Conclusion and Recommendations

The discussion section follows the results and gives the researcher's interpretation of the findings. Conclusions are drawn from the study and recommendations for future research are suggested. Conclusions drawn by the researcher should seem logical to the reviewer and be within the scope of the study. The researcher should also recommend how the results can be used in nursing practice. Implications for practice should be realistic and acknowledge any limitations in the study that would affect the generalizability of the results to similar populations.

SUMMARIZING THE LITERATURE REVIEWED

As discussed previously, the tangible result of the review of the literature is a written summary in the research proposal and report. The purpose of the written summary is to provide a background of pertinent studies and related knowledge into which the proposed study fits.

The written summary should be more than a condensed version of previous studies. It should be a discussion of the previous research, with differences in results pointed out and the strengths and weakness of studies noted. Findings that do and do not support the proposed study should be included in the summary, just as they were included as part of the literature reviewed. The summary of the literature should clearly indicate how the proposed study differs from previous studies and how the study fills gaps in the general body of knowledge.

Figure 17–2 illustrates the steps to follow in looking at the literature. Further discussion of the written literature review is included in Chapters 24 and 27.

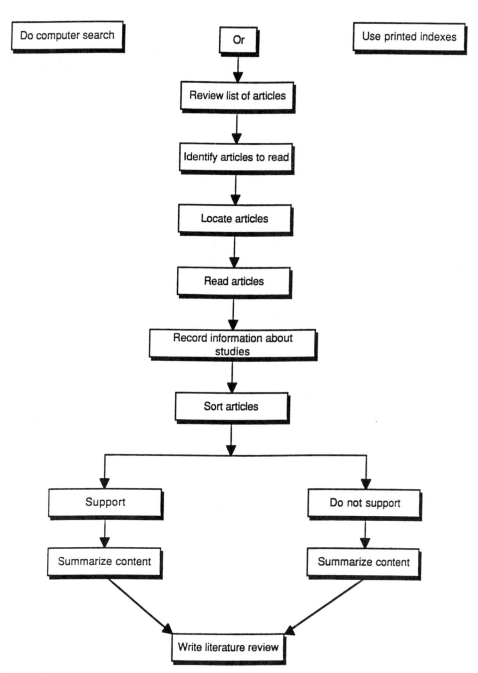

Figure 17–2
Literature review process.

SUMMARY

The purpose of the literature review is to clearly identify the underlying concepts, theories, and previous research findings that provide a basis for the proposed study. Accomplished early in the research process, the literature can yield support for ideas, uncover potential problems or issues, and provide methods that can be used or adapted. Although it is sometimes a time-consuming task, an organized and critical review of the literature provides a strong basis for the proposed research.

REFERENCES

American Psychological Association (1995). *Publication manual of the American Psychological Association* (4th ed.). Washington, DC: Author.

Burns, N., & Grove, S. (1997). *The practice of nursing research. Conduct, critique, & utilization* (3rd ed.). Philadelphia: W. B. Saunders.

Bush, C. (1985). *Nursing research*. Reston, VA: Reston.

Foreman, M., & Kirchhoff, K. (1987). Accuracy of references in nursing journals. *Research in Nursing & Health, 10,* 177–183.

Girden, E. (1996). *Evaluating research articles from start to finish*. Thousand Oaks, CA: Sage.

Holm, K., & Llewellyn, J. (1986). *Nursing research for nursing practice*. Philadelphia: W. B. Saunders.

Nicoll, L. (1993). Keeping abreast of the literature electronically. *Nursing Research, 42,* 315–317.

Polit, D., & Hungler, B. (1997). *Essentials of nursing research: Methods, appraisals, and utilization* (4th ed.). Philadelphia: J. B. Lippincott.

Rankin, M., & Esteves, M. (1996). How to assess a research study. *American Journal of Nursing, 96* (12), 32–37.

Schira, M. (1992). Conducting the literature review. *The Journal of Neuroscience Nursing, 24,* 54–58.

Schira, M., & Pass, A. (1991). Looking in the literature. In K. Kirchhoff & M. Mateo (Eds.), *Conducting and using nursing research in the clinical setting* (pp. 123–134). Baltimore: Williams & Wilkins.

Sinclair, V. (1987). Literature searches by computer. *Image: Journal of Nursing Scholarship, 19,* 35–37.

Wright, K. (1996). The Internet and nursing: A vital link. *Medsurg Nursing, 5* (3), 209–211, 213.

The Conceptual Framework

Madeline H. Schmitt

As discussed in Chapter 2, continuous quality improvement (CQI) and total quality management approaches share some commonalities with research. Both have the goal of improving patient care through increased knowledge. Both acquire this increased knowledge through a systematic process of inquiry that includes (1) literature review, (2) the collection of data through such means as chart review, observations and interviews, self-report measures, and epidemiological data, (3) sampling strategies, (4) analysis of data using either qualitative or quantitative methods, or both, and (5) interpretation of the findings, leading to the next cycle of data gathering. The plan/do/check (study)/act (PDCA or PDSA) cycle (Langley, Nolan, Nolan, Norman, & Provost, 1996) describes the general pattern of inquiry for both quality improvement approaches and research. In Chapter 2, it also is noted that CQI approaches and research can build on one another and that, together, they make a complete framework for improvement of patient care over time.

So what distinguishes CQI approaches from research and how are they linked together?

Conceptual activities generally play a much stronger role in research than they do in CQI approaches to patient care. Concepts, the process of conceptualization, and conceptual and theoretical frameworks all are central to each phase of the research process, from defining the research questions to interpreting the results of the research (Schmitt, 1988). This chapter discusses the role of conceptual and theoretical frameworks in conducting nursing research in the clinical setting. Such a discussion first requires an understanding of concepts and the process of conceptualization, both generally and as they apply to nursing practice. A discussion of the role of conceptual activities in each stage of the nursing research process follows the discussion of concepts and conceptualization, and the description of conceptual and theoretical frameworks of various types. Finally, comparing the role of conceptualization processes in research to those in quality improvement approaches illustrates how they build on one another and, together, make a complete framework for improving patient care and health care.

CONCEPTS AND THE PROCESS OF CONCEPTUALIZATION

Walker and Avant (1988, p. 20) define a concept as "a mental image of a phenomenon; an idea or a construct in the mind about a thing or an action." The mental image consists of the cluster of characteristics or properties that describe the concept. We think in concepts when we observe similarities in the characteristics of objects, events, or processes and give them the same name or label. Assigning labels helps us to link similar phenomena that occur in different times and in different places. Thus, the mental process of thinking in concepts, called conceptualization (Stein, 1984), helps us to organize and order the world around us.

Concepts and their characteristics can range from being very concrete to very abstract. The greater their concreteness, the easier they are to understand, because concrete concepts and concrete characteristics are observable. The concept of "a glass" is relatively easy to understand because it is an observable object with a particular shape and observable characteristics such as that it holds liquid and is used to drink from. Objects from different times and places can be linked and labeled as "glasses" if the objects observed possess these properties.

Concepts may share properties with other concepts. Distinguishing between concepts requires the ability to recognize what properties are shared and what properties are different. Some concepts may be closely related because they have many characteristics in common, and these may be categorized together by a broader concept label. Distinguishing between a glass and a cup means being able to identify differences between the two objects (for example, one has a handle, one does not, and one usually holds hot liquid, the other does not) that have numerous similarities (for example, both hold liquid and are used to drink from). These concepts may be categorized together under a broader concept, such as "drinking utensils," which also may include bottles, flasks, and chalices. Understanding the con-

cept of a glass and other drinking utensils also may be enhanced by knowing about the situational context associated with different types of glasses (for example, a wine glass, a water glass, a paper cup, a chalice).

The concepts of "a drinking glass" and "a window glass," on the other hand, share few characteristics. What they have in common is that they both may be made of "glass." As such, glasses and windows share the observable characteristics that glass typically possesses, such as their transparency, capacity to break, and sharpness when broken. They could be categorized together using a more general concept, "glass objects." However, thinking of a drinking glass in the more general way of "a glass object" does not assist in understanding its usefulness as an object to drink from. The context of situations determines when it is more important to focus on the similarity of objects being "glass" and when it is more important to focus on characteristics that make glass things different from each other.

The concept of glass is an example of a more abstract concept. It may be defined by the aforementioned observable characteristics, but it is fundamentally defined by other, more abstract characteristics, such as its chemical composition and the processes by which it is made. Dictionaries provide a simple definition of the characteristics of glass: "a hard, brittle, noncrystalline, more or less transparent substance produced by fusion, usually consisting of mutually dissolved silica and silicates that also contain soda and lime" (Stein, 1984, p. 559). A glass scientist would be even more precise in the description of its composition, process of formation, and physical properties. Knowing these more technical characteristics may not be important to laypersons in everyday circumstances, but they are important to people in technical occupations who are concerned with determining the uses and limitations of glass under a variety of specific circumstances.

Concepts cannot be studied directly. They can be studied only through use of techniques that measure their characteristics validly and reliably. The study of glass and its capabilities requires the development of physical measurements that will validly and reliably assist in determining whether an object is glass through analysis of its chemical composition, because the presence of soda and lime in glass, for example, is not observable. Other techniques can be used to assess such characteristics as its transparency, hardness, and tendency to break under heat and physical stress.

CONCEPTS IMPORTANT TO THE PRACTICE OF NURSING

The study and improvement of nursing practice begins with the identification, definition, and measurement of concepts that are central to the concerns of nurses. There are three broad, general concepts that are important: nursing care problems, nursing interventions, and nursing outcomes. Nurses are approaching the task of defining nursing care problems, nursing interventions, and nursing outcomes in two different ways.

Nursing Classification Systems

Classification efforts are motivated by the desire to define the domain of nursing knowledge and develop a nursing "language" for identification and description of nursing problems (also called nursing diagnoses), interventions, and outcomes. Numerous nursing classification systems address one or more of the three broad concepts (Carpenito, 1995; Iowa Intervention Project, 1995; Bowles & Naylor, 1996; McCloskey & Bulechek, 1996; Maas, Johnson, & Moorhead, 1996; Snyder, Egan, & Nojima, 1996; Johnson & Maas, 1997). Within these broad classifications, many more specific concepts have been identified, defined by their characteristics and, in some instances, subclassified into types of nursing diagnoses, types of nursing interventions, and types of outcomes. The process of identifying and defining these concepts has incorporated many methods, including literature searches, expert interviews, and focus groups. Although these identification and classification activities have incorporated some content and concept analysis activities, developers acknowledge that the classification efforts often have not incorporated research that would enhance the understanding of the characteristics of these concepts and their interrelationships. The classification systems primarily represent knowledge pertaining to nursing problems, nursing interventions, and nursing outcomes as it exists in the nursing literature.

Even though this classification work is still evolving, recently efforts have been made to link the nursing problems, nursing interventions, and nursing outcomes classification systems (for example, Johnson & Maas, 1997). In addition, the International Council of Nurses (ICN) has begun a project to develop a unitary classification of nursing diagnoses, interventions, and outcomes that would integrate the content of the diverse classification systems presently available (ICN, 1993).

The concepts in these classification schemes are ones that nurses recognize as important and think they understand; however, nurses are realizing that familiar concepts often need further development and refinement of meaning, both as general concepts and as concepts applied more specifically in varied practice situations. Research is needed to develop this greater clarity. Furthermore, there are many problems, interventions, and outcomes in nursing practice that are, as yet, poorly identified and need to be described in terms of their characteristics before they can be studied in relation to each other. Concept development research addresses these needs.

Concept Analysis

In concept analysis research, the investigator has the explicit agenda of developing or refining the meaning of a concept. Morse (1995) has identified concept analysis as one of the priorities for contemporary nursing research. This work is important because the quality of conceptualization affects all aspects of the research process; most importantly, concepts are the building blocks for conceptual and theoretical frameworks. Several different approaches to concept analysis that use data obtained from literature reviews and qualitative research methods are listed in Table 18–1. Research reports of concept analyses are becoming more prevalent in the nursing literature (for example, Morse, Solberg, Neander, Bottorff, & Johnson, 1990; Morse, 1995; Sebern, 1996; Henson, 1997).

Fatigue as an Example of a Concept Important to Nursing Practice

Fatigue is one of the many concepts that have been identified as important to nurs-

Table 18–1
Types of Concept Analysis

TERM	DEFINITION
Concept identification	Used when a new phenomenon of interest is recognized and labeled (Morse, 1995)
Concept development/synthesis	Used when the characteristics of a concept are unclear and the concept needs further development (Walker & Avant, 1988; Morse, 1995)
Concept derivation	Used when a concept is redefined and reapplied from one field to another (Walker & Avant, 1988)
Concept delineation	Used to differentiate characteristics between two concepts that seem to be fused and used as substitutes for each other (Morse, 1995)
Concept comparison	Used when different concepts that do not quite "fit" are used to label a poorly understood phenomenon (Morse, 1995)
Concept clarification	Used when an existing concept thought to be well understood undergoes further refinement (Morse, 1995)
Concept correction	Used when a concept seems wrongly applied to a phenomenon (Morse, 1995)

ing practice. It is part of the broad concept "nursing problems (diagnoses)." More specifically, it is part of a group of problems called symptoms or side effects; their management is one of the important areas of nursing practice. In the latest listing of nursing diagnoses by the North American Nursing Diagnosis Association (NANDA), fatigue is defined as "the self recognized state in which an individual experiences an overwhelming, sustained sense of exhaustion and decreased capacity for physical and mental work that is not relieved by rest" (Carpenito, 1995, p. 379), "a pervasive, subjective drained feeling that cannot be eliminated" (Carpenito, 1995, p. 381).

Fatigue is a more difficult concept to grasp than the concept of a glass because, unlike a glass, it is primarily an internal experience. Although there are some observable behavioral characteristics of fatigue, the occurrence of fatigue can be confirmed only by the self-report of the person experiencing it. There are other concepts that share many of the characteristics of fatigue. Two that are identified in the NANDA diagnosis list are "tiredness" and "activity intolerance." Adequate conceptualization of each concept requires the identification of characteristics that differentiate them.

In the NANDA taxonomy, "fatigue," "tiredness," and "activity intolerance" seem to be differentiated not only by duration and magnitude but also by their causes and response to various forms of intervention. Tiredness is differentiated from fatigue by the idea that tiredness is "transient and temporary" (Carpenito, 1995, p. 381) and can be relieved by rest, whereas fatigue cannot, because it is related to some underlying disease process or treatment for disease. Fatigue can be managed directly only by energy conservation techniques until the underlying disorder is resolved. Activity intolerance is a state of reduced endurance related to physiological deconditioning. It can be resolved through reconditioning activities that build endurance. Current conceptualization of fatigue is incomplete, and it often is difficult to differentiate among these three phenomena in practice.

Since the 1980s, an increasing number of publications have been about conceptualization and measurement of fatigue. One of the most current overall conceptualizations has been developed by Piper and is depicted in Figure 18–1 (Oncology Nursing Society Education Committee, 1996). The inner circle lists six general dimensions that define the fatigue concept; the boxes surrounding the circle depict 14 risk factors contributing to its occurrence. The experience of fatigue with regard to the six dimensions may be different depending on the cause and situational context of fatigue. For example, the experiences of fatigue by cancer patients related to their disease or to treatment may differ from each other, and from fatigue as-

Integrated Fatigue Model

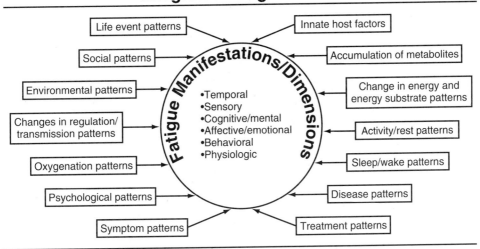

Copyright 1995 Barbara F. Piper, DNSc, RN, OCN, FAAN   Reprinted with permission

Figure 18–1
Piper's integrated fatigue model. (Copyright 1997, Barbara F. Piper.)

sociated with childbearing, or from chronic musculoskeletal disorders such as arthritis.

There are some concepts that are distinct from fatigue but with which fatigue shares some characteristics. Piper (1997) notes that there are similarities between the sensations of fatigue and pain and between some of their proposed physiological central and peripheral nervous system causes. Another example is the concept of dyspnea. Both dyspnea and fatigue are symptoms describing the subjective experience of persons that can be characterized by temporal, sensory, behavioral, and other dimensions. Both are associated with the nursing diagnosis of impaired gas exchange (Carpenito, 1995), so they may share some causal physiological factors, and both may have negative effects on functional status and physical performance (activity intolerance). These similarities have been noticed, and dyspnea and fatigue, along with pain, have been classified together under the more general concept of "unpleasant symptoms" (Gift & Pugh, 1993; Lenz, Suppe, Gift, Pugh, & Milligan, 1995).

Thus, to be clear about the conceptualization of fatigue, it must be understood that it can be conceptualized more generally as one of many unpleasant symptoms for which nurses want to be able to intervene to reduce, to be able to distinguish it from other, similar concepts, and to understand its more specific manifestations in particular illness circumstances. These levels of conceptualization are summarized in Table 18–2.

CONCEPTUAL AND THEORETICAL FRAMEWORKS

The purpose of research is to expand the body of knowledge that identifies, describes, and explains the order of the empirical world (Batey, 1977). Concept analysis, as discussed previously, is a means to identify phenomena of interest to nursing.

Descriptive Research

The purpose of descriptive research is to obtain data on the magnitude of the phenomena. Clear conceptualization is fundamental to accurate estimates of magnitude. For example, in order to describe how common and serious a problem fatigue is in a variety of disease and treatment situations, one first has to identify what is meant by the concept of fatigue (the conceptual framework) and develop measurement consistent with that definition. A nurse researcher may define fatigue by only a single dimension (for example, cognitive/mental) and use

Table 18–2
Levels of Conceptualization of Fatigue

More abstract and general

Fatigue as one of several "unpleasant symptoms"

Temporal
Sensory
Cognitive/mental
Affective/emotional
Behavioral
Physiological

Tiredness ◄——— General dimensions of fatigue ———► Activity intolerance

Temporal
Sensory
Cognitive/mental
Affective/emotional
Behavioral
Physiological

Manifestations of fatigue in specific situations

In childbearing   In radiation treatment   In arthritis

Temporal
Sensory
Cognitive/mental
◄——— Affective/emotional ———►
Behavioral
Physiological

More specific and concrete

a measure of mental fatigue because that is the aspect of fatigue that he or she is most interested in. However, the findings related to the magnitude of the problem of fatigue will be limited by that definition and measurement. Or, one may define fatigue multidimensionally and study a broader set of manifestations of fatigue. In this instance, findings may show that some dimensions of fatigue occur more frequently in a disease situation than others and that the magnitude of the problem depends on the dimensions studied.

This result helps illustrate how a nurse researcher may move from the study of a single concept to the study of relationships between concepts. A question suggested by the findings is whether study of other types of disease situations would reveal a different pattern of occurrence of fatigue dimensions than the first disease situation studied. In other words, does the experience of fatigue vary by the type of disease situation? When one begins to pose questions involving two or more concepts and their

relationship, for example, between the type of disease and the dimensions of fatigue, one has moved to exploratory research.

Exploratory Research

Exploratory research examines the relationships between (or causes of) phenomena. In this instance, clear definitions of both the concept of fatigue and the concept of disease, as defined for the purposes of the particular study, are needed, as is a statement that one is interested in the relationship between these two phenomena. Documenting that the experience of fatigue varies by disease generally lets the nurse know when to look for fatigue as a potential nursing diagnosis. Another relationship that may be of interest to the nurse is one focused on the relationship of treatment to the experience of fatigue. Knowing that fatigue is related to receiving certain types of treatment also helps the nurse identify potential nursing diagnoses. Another type of exploratory research of central importance to nursing is the relationship between the magnitude of the symptom (for example, fatigue) and the nurse's intervention to reduce the level of symptom experience. Research findings that show certain interventions appear to reduce fatigue help direct the nurse toward specific interventions in the future.

The relationships of interest in a study often are depicted in research articles in the form of pictorial models. Figure 18–2 shows the three simple exploratory, conceptual frameworks (or models) discussed in the preceding paragraph. The one depicting a relationship between type of disease and fatigue and that showing a relationship between treatment factors and fatigue each replicates small pieces of Piper's integrated fatigue model shown in Figure 18–1. Piper's model is a more complex conceptual framework in that it depicts the idea of relationships between fatigue and many different risk factors or causes (mechanisms) of fatigue.

Conceptual frameworks, like concepts, can vary from concrete and specific to abstract and general. For example, in model 2, in Figure 18–2, it is more abstract to show that treatment factors are related to fatigue than to show that, for example, radiation therapy is related to temporal, behavioral, and emotional aspects of fatigue. Likewise, with model 3 in Figure 18–2, it is more concrete to say that an energy management nursing intervention (McCloskey & Bulechek, 1996) is related to the temporal and sensory dimensions of fatigue than to say that nursing intervention is related to fatigue. One could be even more specific by specifying what type of energy management intervention is of interest (for example, increased rest or exercise) and what aspects of the temporal and sensory dimensions of fatigue are of interest (for example, onset, duration, and severity of the subjective symptom). The more specifically the concepts are defined, the clearer it is to the

researcher exactly what he or she is studying, and the clearer it is to the reader of research reports exactly what has been studied. Conversely, the more abstract the level of the statement of relationship, the more difficult it is to know exactly what is being studied, because the concepts involved can be defined in multiple ways. The value of a conceptual framework is that it directs attention to the specific phenomena of interest and focuses attention on particular types of relationships. Conceptual frameworks can be developed from observations and research findings; they are a way for the researcher to summarize what concepts are thought to be related to each other. On the other hand, research findings may be perceived as "fitting" an existing conceptual framework that provides a way to organize and order the findings in relation to each other. However, conceptual frameworks often are limited by their generality and by the lack of specificity in what the nature of the relationship is believed to be.

Theoretical frameworks are more refined types of conceptual frameworks. They are distinguished from conceptual frameworks by including more specific statements of the nature of the relationship between concepts. Instead of simply stating that there is a relationship between two concepts, such as nursing intervention and fatigue, theoretical frameworks indicate the type and amount of relationship believed to exist. For example, regular exercise is a nursing intervention that affects fatigue in breast cancer and rheumatoid arthritis (for example, Mac Vicar & Winningham, 1986; Neuberger et al., 1997). Instead of simply stating that the nursing intervention consisting of an exercise program is related to fatigue, a more specific theoretical statement about this relationship could indicate that women with breast cancer (or rheumatoid arthritis) who participate in a regular exercise program (for example, low-impact aerobic exercise) compared with those who do not experience less fatigue (on the temporal, emotional, and behavioral dimensions). This example consists of a single theoretical statement. Such a statement usually takes the form of a hypothesis in the research study. Theoretical frameworks usually consist of a series of specific statements linking several concepts in a logical set of specific relationships.

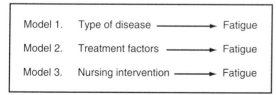

Figure 18–2
Simple conceptual models of fatigue.

Model 1. Increased exercise → Decreased fatigue

Model 2. Increased exercise → X (? Mechanism) → Decreased fatigue

2a. Increased exercise → X (? Mechanism)

2b. X (? Mechanism) → Decreased fatigue

Figure 18–3
Simple theoretical models of fatigue.

Explanatory Research

When a researcher proposes an explanation of why two concepts are linked, he or she has moved to explanatory research. For example, the researcher may want to explain why exercise reduces fatigue. Knowing why exercise reduces fatigue may help the nurse to be more precise in the design and implementation of the intervention and to understand why the intervention might not work in some circumstances. At present, the mechanisms by which exercise may reduce fatigue are unknown. Figure 18–3 schematically displays both the simpler exploratory model (model 1) and the more complex explanatory model (model 2). Model 2 actually is made up of two theoretical statements linked together into one complex statement. Models 2a and 2b show the simpler statements that are parts of model 2. Model 2 is the core model for studying interventions and outcomes in clinical settings.

LEVELS OF THEORETICAL CONCEPTUALIZATION

A well-stated theory provides an excellent guide for the conduct of research in clinical settings. The relevance of a well-stated theory to research and to practice is apparent, because the concepts in the theory are meaningful to practicing nurses. A second requirement of a good theory is that the concepts in the theory can be measured. This makes the ideas in the theory testable. The usefulness of theory to practicing nurses has been questioned because many of the early "theories" in nursing do not have these properties of meaningfulness and testability in the clinical setting, creating a theory-practice "gap" (Pryjmachuk, 1996). That is, nursing theories created outside of the context of practice are forced into the practice situation from a "top-down" perspective, regardless of their relevance (Morse, 1996). A listing of the types of theories discussed and debated in current nursing literature is provided in Table 18–3, arranged from the most abstract to the most concrete. The next sections describe these types of theories and their contribution to the conduct of research in clinical settings.

Metatheory

Metatheoretical conceptualizations and grand theory conceptualizations are among the earliest developed and are the most abstract. Metatheoretical ideas are theoretical ideas about theory. The most prominent metatheoretical conceptualization in nursing is one adopted by the National League for Nursing (Torres & Yura, 1974), which identifies four very general and abstract concepts and their relationships as fundamental to any theory in nursing. The four concepts are nursing, environment, person, and health. Whereas this combination of concepts may delimit the broad domain of nursing theory, the concepts are so general they may be defined in many different ways at many different levels. For example, with some imagination, one could "fit" the broad concepts of environment and health to the specific intervention of low-impact aerobic exercise to reduce fatigue. In this example, "reduced fatigue" would be the manifestation of health. However, if one had started with the broad concept of health, one would

Table 18–3
Levels of Theoretical Conceptualization

Metatheory
Grand theory
Middle range theory
Prescriptive theory
Informal theory

not have been guided through logical deduction to focus attention on reduction of fatigue, because "reduced fatigue" is only one of the numerous kinds of health. In other words, such broad metatheoretical ideas offer no guidance in specific nursing studies.

Grand Theory

Grand theories in nursing, often called "nursing theories" or "nursing frameworks," are conceptual frameworks created by nursing theorists that are less abstract than metatheoretical concepts but that are still too abstract to guide specific nursing research studies. Nevertheless, they provide a useful vocabulary of concepts for thinking about nursing. An example is Orem's self-care theory (Fawcett, 1995). This conceptual framework places emphasis on the ability of persons to engage in self-care for health and sees the nurse's role as one of fostering self-care activities. It is one way to conceptualize what nurses value and do.

If one conceptualizes fatigue during an illness and nursing intervention using the language of Orem's self-care model, fatigue would be a specific example of a "self-care deficit" related to "universal self-care requisites" (for example, the need for a balance between activity and rest) and "health deviation self-care requisites" (for example, treatment and disease factors) (Schmitt, 1988). Nursing interventions are "nursing agency." As with the metatheoretical concepts, terms like "self-care deficit" and "nursing agency" may be defined and relationships between the terms stated as propositions. Nevertheless, if one starts with the concepts of "self-care deficit" or "nursing agency," one would not be led through logical deduction to direct one's attention specifically to the phenomenon of "fatigue" or to the nursing intervention of "exercise." Linking the idea of nursing agency with fatigue would give little direction to testing a specific intervention. However, once the specific concepts of interest and their relationships are identified, they can be categorized under the broader concepts and relationships.

Rather than testing a conceptual framework, most research reports containing nursing conceptual models have "fitted" the specific research concepts into the nursing conceptual framework. Despite the limitations of conceptual frameworks, they have guided nursing research by suggesting broad domains in which research might be undertaken (Schmitt, 1983). Orem's ideas about self-care have helped to stimulate research in this broad aspect of nursing practice.

Because of the difficulty of translating abstract concepts into specific and measurable aspects of nursing practice, metatheoretical and grand theoretical ideas have been labeled by nurses as philosophies rather than theories (for example, Morse, 1996). At times the use of particular models in nursing curricula or in nursing practice situations has been confusing to nurses. Rather than facilitating communication and knowledge building, adoption of such nursing models sometimes increases the difficulty of communication between nurses because they need to translate the language of one nursing model into the language of another. Some concepts from nursing conceptual frameworks, such as Orem's, have been adopted into the NANDA nursing diagnosis list (Carpenito, 1995). For the most part, however, rather than the models providing tools for nurses to use in analyzing practice problems, nurses have had to "fit" their practice ideas into the nursing conceptual models.

Middle Range Theory

Middle range theories contain concepts that are more specific and closer to observed data than the metatheoretical or grand theoretical models (Good & Moore, 1996). In addition, the concepts in middle range theories are measurable; therefore, these theories are testable. The models shown in Figure 18–3 are examples of simple middle range theoretical statements. Note that the concepts in the statements can be measured and the truth of the statements can be tested. For model 1, exercise may be measured by the implementation of a specific exercise program; fatigue may be measured by administering an existing self-report instrument reflecting specific dimensions of fatigue (Piper, 1997). In order to test the statements in model 2, the researcher also must identify a causal factor that intervenes between exercise and fatigue and obtain measures of that factor. To support the theory, the data need to show that the exercise program affects the causal factor and that change in that factor leads to changes in the level of fatigue.

Piper's integrated fatigue model in Figure 18–1 suggests the range of causal factors that affect fatigue. Some of these causes can be measured currently (for example, activity/rest patterns, sleep/wake patterns). An investigator might propose that exercise improves sleep patterns and that improvement in sleep leads to reduced fatigue. Testing the model would require that the researcher know something about the field of sleep research in order to be able to measure sleep/wake patterns as well as exercise and fatigue. If the measures of the concepts are related in the ways proposed, the investigator will have evidence to support the theory and will have evidence for the value of the particular exercise intervention. If the data do not support the theory, the investigator would need to decide why; for example, was the theory wrong, was the intervention too weak, or was the measurement poor? The answers help shape the next cycle of research.

Because nursing is a practice discipline with a holistic focus, many of the theoretical ideas incorporated into the testing of middle range theories in nursing have come from other disciplines. Relevant results obtained from research outside nursing can contribute to the development of theory and clinical research that informs nursing practice. Likewise, what nurses learn from the outcomes of intervention can contribute to refinement of theory. To design effective interventions, nurses need to be familiar with the relevant research conducted by others. For example, many causes of fatigue, such as radiation treatment for cancer, are poorly understood. Because few nurses are knowledgeable about theories of physiological mechanisms leading to fatigue and because few nurses have the laboratory research skills required to test these theoretical ideas, this kind of research is beyond the ability of most nurses to conduct.

Physiological mechanisms associated with disease or treatment also may underlie changes in sleep/wake patterns, which then may produce fatigue. This is a more complicated theory involving linking two causal factors; testing an exercise intervention related to this theory would require showing how an exercise intervention alters the underlying physiology, ameliorating sleep/wake problems, thereby reducing fatigue. This would be a more complete explanation of how fatigue is produced, potentially leading to refinement of the intervention as well as improved theory. However, until more specific concepts of the physiological processes are proposed and measured, this part of the theory would remain hypothetical.

Although middle range theories provide excellent conceptual guidance needed for developing clinical nursing interventions, only a few of these kinds of theories exist in nursing. One is the self-regulation theory of coping with stressful events, developed and refined in practice settings in collaboration with students and nursing staff over many years (Johnson, Fieler, Jones, Wlasowicz, & Mitchell, 1997). This theory incorporates cognitive psychological concepts and theoretical processes. It contains theoretical explanations for how patients' ability to cope with treatments and procedures is affected by provision of concrete, objective preparatory information, involving sensory information such as what patients will see, hear, taste, smell, and feel along with the causes of these sensations, and temporal and environmental descriptions of when and in what context certain events will happen. Informational interventions based on this theory have been shown to improve patients' coping while they experience many different types of health care treatments and procedures. This research program provides an excellent model for how middle range theory can influence the development of effective nursing interventions for a specific aspect of nursing practice and how findings from testing those interventions can result in the refinement of the theory that supports nursing practice. Many nurse researchers believe that as a profession, nurses are just entering a phase of increased development and testing of middle range theories in nursing (Lenz et al., 1995; Good & Moore, 1996).

Prescriptive Theory

Prescriptive theories include general theoretical statements, that is, principles, about how nurses ought to practice to achieve desired outcomes. Prescriptive theories are closely related to, but more general than, clinical practice guidelines (Wooldridge, Leonard, & Skipper, 1983). Both should be based on evidence from research guided by middle range theoretical propositions. The general research question to be answered in research using such theories is "If nurses practice according to these principles, are the outcomes of nursing practice improved?"

A prescriptive theory of the use of exercise during illness to reduce fatigue would be built on a theory about how exercise reduces fatigue, research testing that theory in a variety of illness situations, and a belief that implementing exercise interventions according to principles derived from the theory and research will accomplish nursing practice goals. Johnson et al. (1997) provide several principles for the effective implementation of concrete, objective information to enhance patient coping with health care procedures and treatment consistent with self-regulation theory. An example is "When attention is focused on the concrete, objective features of a stressful healthcare experience, coping is directed at problem solving and actions taken to deal with the situation are directed at achieving positive effects on functions" (Johnson et al., 1997, p. 17). In another example, Good and Moore (1996) propose a prescriptive theory for acute pain management derived from the Agency for Health Care Policy and Research acute pain management guidelines.

Informal Theory

Informal theory and related terms, such as "the reflective practitioner," "action research," and "action science," have received attention in recent literature related to the theory-practice gap (Kim, 1994; Pryjmachuk, 1996; Rolfe, 1996, 1997). Informal theories are mental constructs of practicing nurses. They are created when, rather than perform nursing care in an intuitive or routine manner, nurses engage in active reflection as part of their practice. Informal theories are a combination of informal knowledge gained in a particular patient care or institutional situation, past paradigm cases, and formal, research-based theory. This combination of knowledge is formulated into hypotheses about appropriate clinical interventions. These hypotheses are tested through interventions in the immediate clinical situation, and they are revised quickly as part of the reflection on the outcome of the intervention (Rolfe, 1997). A

new round of intervention is triggered by the revised hypotheses, generating new feedback and so forth in cycles motivated by the desire to improve practice. This process is called action research or action science because, while in the practice situation, the nurse uses a process similar to formal research, in which hypotheses are formulated, tested, and revised based on the data gathered.

Formal theoretical ideas, if known, are used by nurses as part of the informal theory process that helps shape the intervention. How informal theory can influence nursing practice, be changed by reflective practice, and be informed by formal theory is illustrated in a story shared by a nurse and recounted by Morse (1996). A nurse trying to show caring toward a father whose child was being resuscitated in the trauma room after being hit by a car on her bike, approached and touched him, and in her words to him indicated that she would be glad to give him a hug. The effect of her words was for him to collapse to the floor. Morse notes that the nurse was very disturbed by the negative outcome her intervention had on the father. This situation suggests that the nurse was acting based on an informal theory that the situation was one calling for a caring action in the form of acknowledging the father's emotional state and the need for emotional support. When the father did not respond to the intervention as expected, a disjunction was created between the intended outcome of the nurse's action and the actual one. It created an opportunity for reflective practice and a reformulation of the informal theory guiding the nurse in responding to such situations. Morse suggests that conceptually recognizing the situation as one in which the father was "enduring" could have changed the nurse's response. People who are enduring cope by suppressing all emotion and stay focused on the present. The offer of a hug caused the man to focus on his emotions and led to his collapse. One of the principles derived from Johnson's theory and research on self-regulation also suggests that focusing on the emotional response can increase negative emotions (Johnson et al., 1997). Incorporating this research-based knowledge as part of the reflection on the situation could help the nurse in reformulation of the informal theory and change her future response in similar situations.

The emphasis in informal theory is on change in an individual's practice, not on theory creation or testing for the profession. Unlike formal theory, which is tested in research for its general applicability in professional practice, the concepts in the informal theory created by the nurse are highly embedded in the immediate practice situation. Consequently, the informal theory is not generalizable. Usefulness of the theory, based on the evidence from the intervention, is subjectively interpreted and evaluated by the nurse. Conceptually, then, it is the most concrete of the types of theory that have been examined herein.

THE RELATIONSHIP OF CONCEPTUALIZATION TO EACH STAGE OF THE RESEARCH PROCESS

Conceptualization is a key aspect of every stage of the research process. Substantive nursing research cannot be conducted with concepts that are vaguely defined and poorly understood. Initial work may need to emphasize further development of the concept through concept analysis techniques, or further descriptive work may need to be done to establish the scope of the nursing problem.

The research process begins with the formulation of a research problem and statement of a research question or hypothesis. In these statements, the investigator should identify the concepts examined in the study and the relationships between the concepts that are of interest. After reviewing how the concepts have been defined theoretically, measured, and studied by others, the investigator should provide theoretical definitions of the concepts as used in the present study. Next, the researcher should provide a summary and critique of previous theory and research about the concepts. Then the conceptual or theoretical framework guiding the study should be described. This framework should be consistent with the conclusions drawn from the literature reviewed. Often it is helpful, in studies involving multiple concepts, to show the concepts and their hypothesized relationship to each other in a diagram, such as those shown in Figures 18–1 through 18–3. The research problem and research questions should be designed to address a gap in what is known

that is of importance to nursing. The researcher should identify this gap explicitly and discuss the importance of the study to nursing. The fact that there is a gap, by itself, does not make the problem important to study.

Measures of the concepts used should be consistent with the theoretical definitions of the concepts. For example, it would be confusing if, in a study of the impact of exercise on fatigue, the literature review focused on studies involving patients' perceptions of fatigue but the measurement involved biochemical indicators of fatigue.

The conceptual or theoretical framework and research questions and hypotheses should guide the analysis and presentation of results. Findings presented should address the research questions or hypotheses. Often, it is confusing when an author reports findings that are not relevant to the literature review or the research questions.

Finally, discussion and interpretation of the findings should focus on whether they are consistent with what was expected. If the outcomes of the research were unexpected, the investigator needs to examine possible explanations for the discrepancy. The discrepancy may be due to problems in conceptualization, design, measurement, or the specific intervention used. Based on this discussion, the investigator then can propose how the research could be improved in the next cycle.

COMPARING CONTINUOUS QUALITY IMPROVEMENT WITH RESEARCH FROM A CONCEPTUAL PERSPECTIVE

As noted early in the chapter, clinical research and CQI have much in common. How do CQI approaches to improvement of care differ from and complement those of clinical research? The aim of clinical research is to discover more effective interventions to address nursing problems, such as those identified in the NANDA nursing diagnoses list. The improvements of interest in clinical nursing research are those related to patients' physical, mental, emotional, or functional status or those that promote overall health and well-being. CQI approaches focus on improving the *organizational system* of delivery of nursing care, of which clinical interventions are a part. This can be achieved by eliminating nursing care activities that have not been demonstrated through clinical research to contribute to clinical improvement, by substituting nursing interventions that have been shown through clinical research to produce higher levels of desired outcomes than presently achieved, or by altering ineffective and inefficient processes that contribute to undesired variation in the institutional delivery of those nursing interventions. The outcomes of interest in CQI include ensuring that the best nursing interventions available for specific nursing problems are delivered in the least costly manner and in a way that ensures patient, family, and staff satisfaction with the care delivered.

The first step in a CQI process is to identify a problem or area for improvement. After the area of improvement has been studied, an improvement goal is stated. A plan for improvement that contains informal hypotheses about what is causing the problem or acting as a barrier to improvement and what actions or interventions will produce improvement is developed and implemented. Data are gathered and studied to determine whether the change resulted in an improvement, which leads to further informal hypotheses, implementation of additional actions or interventions, and reassessment in a PDSA cycle.

CQI tools can assist in conceptualizing the goals for improvement, the process of care delivery, and the changes needed in those processes of care delivery to produce better outcomes, reduce costs, or increase patient, family, and staff satisfaction. For example, systematic data can help identify an outcome, cost, or satisfaction problem; flowcharts can help to visualize the processes of care delivery; and a cause-and-effect diagram (fishbone diagram) can help identify potential causes of the problem or barriers to improvement, suggesting areas for change (Scholtes, 1992). The conceptualization of the problems, hypotheses about processes, and actions or interventions are concrete and specific to the organizational situation. Theory operates in the situation at an informal level. Because the theoretical ideas about the system, its problems, and findings are embedded in the specific circumstances, they are not generalizable to another situation. However, formal theory and research have an important role in CQI. To the extent that formal theories and the results of clinical research are known, they can be incorporated into the informal theories about what will improve care, be part of the planned change, and contribute to the overall level of quality of care achieved.

When a new intervention is implemented, CQI techniques can identify process problems in the implementation. They can be used to ensure that changes do occur in care system delivery processes, to customize the intervention to the specific institutional situation, and to evaluate whether the intervention results in specific improvements in care at a cost the institution is willing to accept. Johnson et al. (1997) provide an excellent discussion of the use of CQI approaches to guide the implementation of a new, theory-based nursing intervention into a system of nursing care in which the intervention is linked to clinical standards and guidelines.

SUMMARY

Clear conceptualization is fundamental to good research. Concept analysis approaches are becoming an important means for identifying and developing concepts of importance to nursing. In descriptive research, investigators identify the occurrence of a phenomenon; in exploratory research, they explore relationships between the phenomenon and other concepts; in explanatory research, they explain why the relationships between concepts exist. Middle range theory development is the most appropriate level of abstraction to guide the development of useful clinical studies in nursing. A clear conceptual framework is the key to integrating the statement of the problem, literature review, measurement, analysis, presentation, and interpretation of results. Patient care is improved when theory and interventions developed from clinical studies are integrated into the informal theories that guide changes in individual nursing practice and nursing systems.

REFERENCES

Batey, M. V. (1977). Conceptualization: Knowledge and logic guiding empirical research. *Nursing Research, 26,* 324–329.

Bowles, K. H., & Naylor, M. D. (1996). Nursing intervention classification systems. *Image: Journal of Nursing Scholarship, 28,* 303–308.

Carpenito, L. J. (1995). *Nursing diagnosis: Application to clinical practice* (6th ed.). Philadelphia: J. B. Lippincott.

Fawcett, J. (1995). *Analysis and evaluation of conceptual models of nursing.* Philadelphia: F. A. Davis.

Gift, A. G., & Pugh, L. C. (1993). Dyspnea and fatigue. *Nursing Clinics of North America, 28,* 373–384.

Good, M., & Moore, S. M. (1996). Clinical practice guidelines as a new source of middle range theory: Focus on acute pain. *Nursing Outlook, 44,* 74–79.

Henson, R. H. (1997). Analysis of the concept of mutuality. *Image: Journal of Nursing Scholarship, 29,* 77–81.

International Council of Nurses (ICN). (1993). *Nursing's next advance: An international classification for nursing practice (ICNP).* Geneva, Switzerland: Author.

Iowa Intervention Project. (1995). Validation and coding of the NIC taxonomy structure. *Image: Journal of Nursing Scholarship, 27,* 43–49.

Johnson, J. E., Fieler, V. K., Jones, L. S., Wlasowicz, G. S., & Mitchell, M. L. (1997). *Self-regulation theory: Applying theory to your practice.* Pittsburgh, PA: Oncology Nursing Press, Inc.

Johnson, M., & Maas, M. (1997). *Nursing outcomes classification (NOC).* St. Louis: Mosby.

Kim, H. S. (1994). Action science as an approach to development of knowledge for clinical practice. *Nursing Science Quarterly, 7,* 134–138.

Langley, G. J., Nolan, K. M., Nolan, T. W., Norman, C. L., & Provost, L. P. (1996). *The improvement guide: A practical approach to enhancing organizational performance.* San Francisco: Jossey-Bass.

Lenz, E. R., Suppe, F., Gift, A. G., Pugh, L. C., & Milligan, R. A. (1995). Collaborative development of middle range theories: Toward a theory of unpleasant symptoms. *ANS: Advances in Nursing Science, 17*(3), 1–13.

Maas, M. L., Johnson, M., & Moorhead, S. (1996). Classifying nurse-sensitive patient outcomes. *Image: Journal of Nursing Scholarship, 28,* 295–301.

Mac Vicar, M. G., & Winningham, M. L. (1986). Promoting functional capacity of cancer patients. *Cancer Bulletin, 38,* 235–239.

McCloskey, J. C., & Bulechek, G. M. (1996). *Nursing interventions classification (NIC).* St. Louis: Mosby.

Morse, J. (1995). Exploring the theoretical basis of nursing using advanced techniques of concept analysis. *ANS: Advances in Nursing Science, 17*(3), 31–46.

Morse, J. M. (1996). Nursing scholarship: Sense and sensibility. *Nursing Inquiry, 3,* 74–82.

Morse, J. M., Solberg, S., Neander, W., Bottorff, J. L., & Johnson, J. L. (1990). Concepts of caring and caring as a concept. *ANS: Advances in Nursing Science, 3*(1), 1–14.

Neuberger, G. B., Press, A. N., Lindsley, H. B., Hinton, R., Cagle, P. E., Carlson, K., Dahl, J., & Kramer, B. (1997). Effects of exercise on fatigue, aerobic fitness, and disease activity measures in persons with rheumatoid arthritis. *Research in Nursing & Health, 20,* 195–204.

Oncology Nursing Society Education Committee. (1996). [Distance learning video]. *Oncology nursing focus. Lesson guide: Fatigue in patients with cancer.* Pittsburgh, PA: Author.

Piper, B. F. (1997). Measuring fatigue. In M. Frank-Stromberg & S. J. Olsen (Eds.), *Instruments for clinical health-care research* (pp. 482–496). Sudbury, MA: Jones & Bartlett.

Pryjmachuk, S. (1996). A nursing perspective on the interrelationships between theory, research, and practice. *Journal of Advanced Nursing, 23,* 679–684.

Rolfe, G. (1996). Going to extremes: Action research, grounded practice and the theory-practice gap in nursing. *Journal of Advanced Nursing, 24,* 1315–1320.

Rolfe, G. (1997). Beyond expertise: Theory, practice, and the reflexive practitioner. *Journal of Clinical Nursing, 6,* 93–97.

Scholtes, P. R. (1992). *The team handbook.* Madison, WI: Joiner Associates Inc.

Sebern, M. D. (1996). Explication of the concept of shared care and the prevention of pressure ulcers in home health care. *Research in Nursing and Health, 19,* 183–192.

Schmitt, M. H. (1983). Nursing theorists and practice theory. In P. J. Wooldridge, M. H. Schmitt, J. K. Skipper, Jr., & R. C. Leonard (Eds.), *Behavioral science and nursing theory* (pp. 80–115). St. Louis: Mosby.

Schmitt, M. H. (1988). Conceptualization: What is it and why is it important in the research process. *Oncology Nursing Forum, 15,* 221–223.

Snyder, M., Egan, E. C., & Nojima, Y. (1996). Defining nursing interventions. *Image: Journal of Nursing Scholarship, 28,* 137–141.

Stein, J. (Ed.). (1984). *The Random House college dictionary* (Rev. ed.). New York: Random House.

Torres, G., & Yura, H. (1974). *Today's conceptual framework: Its relationship to the curriculum development process* [NLN Publication No. 15-1529]. New York: National League for Nursing.

Walker, L. O., & Avant, K. C. (1988). *Strategies for theory construction in nursing* (2nd ed.). Norwalk, CT: Appleton & Lange.

Wooldridge, P. J., Leonard, R. C., & Skipper, J. K., Jr. (1983). Defining the theory of a practice profession. In P. J. Wooldridge, M. H. Schmitt, J. K. Skipper, Jr., & R. C. Leonard (Eds.), *Behavioral science and nursing theory* (pp. 5–35). St. Louis: Mosby.

Chapter 19

Design of Questionnaires and Structured Interviews

Karin T. Kirchhoff

The most common tool used for data collection is the questionnaire. Because it is so common, most individuals assume that the construction of the questionnaire is easy. Those who have filled out poorly constructed ones know that something is wrong but may not be aware of which rules in questionnaire construction were violated. This chapter details one approach to designing questionnaires that has been used for national and local surveys and has had good response rates. Not all suggestions may work in one questionnaire, but they should be used as guidelines. Even though some of the suggestions may seem obvious, when they are used to critique questionnaires that are received in the mail, it becomes apparent that the offering of these suggestions is warranted.

The purposes of questionnaire construction are many and varied. The content in this chapter can be applied to the simplest data collection purpose or to the most elegant study. The use of the questionnaire can be for research, for quality assurance, for administrative decision making, or for simple collection of data about employees' preferences. Most situations require the development of a form specific to the topic under investigation; in other cases, there may be a standardized form available or a compilation of forms used for specific types of studies. Spilker and Schoenfelder (1991) have compiled a volume of forms that can be used in clinical trials.

This chapter's content applies to questionnaires used for telephone interviews, face-to-face interviews, or mailed surveys. Emphasis is on instances when the researcher is not present—mailed questionnaires—because no one is available to answer the respondent's questions. In telephone interviews and face-to-face interviews, lines should be drawn on the tool to lead the eye for specific tasks. In face-to-face interviews, lists or visual aids can be shown. In deciding whether to use mailed questionnaires versus telephone interviews, the characteristics of the sample should be considered. For example, Harris, Weinberger, and Tierney (1997) found that with inner-city patients, response rates were higher with the telephone-first compared with mail-first method. This is the opposite of what is usually recommended but takes into account the mobility of these patients, and a potential for illiteracy. Otherwise, many of the guidelines are similar.

GENERAL CONSIDERATIONS

There are general considerations for the items included in the questionnaire and the type of data generated that should be addressed (see box).

The type of data needed should be carefully planned, and the analysis intended should be designed before the questionnaire is finalized. Many individuals fail to make decisions about the difference between necessary and "interesting" data. The "interesting" information lengthens the questionnaire and may actually interfere with obtaining the necessary data. The novice may wallow in the data and may find that the "unnecessary" data may not get analyzed. Such data should not then have been collected.

The use of "dummy" tables is helpful in ensuring that all needed data are collected

➤ **Considerations for Questionnaire Development**

1. Types of items should be interesting to the intended audience.
2. Items should not be embarrassing or threatening to the respondent—if so, special care is needed to facilitate response.
3. Task should be easy to complete—circle an item, check a box.
4. Cover letter, introduction, and tone of the questions should have a conversational tone and convey respect for the individuals and their privacy.

DUMMY TABLE EXAMPLE

Table X ....

Numbers of Part-time and Full-time Nurses Desiring Child Care

EMPLOYMENT STATUS	DESIRING CHILD CARE	
	Yes	No
Part-time	# or %	# or %
Full-time	# or %	# or %

(see Dummy Table Example). In the dummy table, the title and the column (for example, Employment Status) and row labels (for example, Yes/No) can be determined. In the cells, the proposed data (for example, the number or percentage of the whole) can be reviewed to determine whether the correct information was collected. For example, if age is collected by category (21 to 30, 31 to 40, and 41 to 50), these data could form the rows of a table. However, if data on the actual age were not collected, the data could then *not* be used for a correlation with an attitude score or for the calculation of the average age of the respondent. In the example, real numbers were not obtained, and only a category was identified. Putting the age into categories after the fact is also possible. Without assessing the planned analysis ahead of time, the analysis may be compromised because the level of data collected was not that required. Further discussion on tables is in Chapter 26.

A properly designed questionnaire reduces respondent burden. The goal of a well-designed questionnaire is that the respondent become engaged in the process, feel that the task is important, and complete the task readily and easily. A well-designed questionnaire balances investigative cost and respondent burden.

Appearance and Format

The initial appearance of the questionnaire is important. How the items are laid out and the overall format contribute to the appearance. The black-to-white ratio is critical. White should clearly predominate. When this ratio is violated, the respondent feels that the task is difficult, even if the questionnaire is only a few pages. The crowding of black on the page, especially by reduction techniques in photocopying, does not fool most respondents into thinking that the task is any less than it is. It is more important to attend to the appearance than to the number of pages. The complexity of a questionnaire is not determined simply by counting the number of pages, although the number of pages is a factor. The ease of the tasks and the spacing between items are more critical concerns. Many investigators think that after reduction, a 5-page questionnaire is less overwhelming as a 3-page small-print reduced questionnaire, but the respondent thinks differently.

The cover letter and the questionnaire need to look "official." People are not motivated to respond if the questionnaire looks like it was printed on a dot matrix printer. Some software packages help developers create official-appearing questionnaires with little effort.

The size of the page is another factor. The default of 8.5- by 11-inch paper is not the only possibility. If the questionnaire is to be printed, many sizes are available. One option is to use a center-fold approach, which gives the appearance of a booklet. How the questionnaire is mailed needs to be considered when selecting paper size. The size of the envelope may be a limiting factor.

Color and Quality of Paper

Although white—or near white—may give the best appearance, a different paper color may be chosen for several reasons. For instance, when the respondents need to be separated by groups, the use of different colors for each group makes the task easier. Color also helps prevent the questionnaire from getting lost on the respondent's desk. Avoid the use of dark colors because black print on them is hard to read. The weight of the paper can give the impression of cheapness if it is too light, or it may require toward more postage if it is too heavy. Questionnaire designers should physically feel paper stock before printing questionnaires and weigh the pages with the envelope to determine whether a slight reduction in paper weight will prevent the need for additional postage.

Spacing

Spacing throughout the questionnaire is important. Spacing between questions should be greater than that between lines within the same question, allowing the respondent to quickly read each question. Also, the spacing between response options should be at least 1.5 lines, especially if the task of the respondent is to circle a number. With single spacing, it is difficult to determine which number was circled. When these suggestions are followed, the overall black-to-white ratio is enhanced as well.

Respondent Code

Another consideration is the place for a respondent code number. Usually an underscore line is placed at the upper right-hand corner on the first page. Although code numbers are essential if follow-up is anticipated, respondents are sometimes troubled by these numbers and have erased or obliterated them. This is particularly true when respondents fear an administrator's reaction to their answers. Some explanation about the use of a code number in the cover letter might alleviate this concern but may not totally if any of the information is at all revealing. When the respondent code number is not placed on the questionnaire, follow-up on the nonrespondents is not possible because the respondents will not be able to be separated from nonrespondents. If follow-up is done without the use of code numbers, everyone will need to get the second and third contact, thus increasing costs.

When respondent codes are not used on questionnaires, different colors can be used to represent separate subgroups. In this instance, response rates can still be determined for the entire sample as well as for each subgroup. Selective follow-up without code numbers could be done on everyone in the subgroup with a low response rate if funds and time permit.

Typeface

The typeface should be chosen carefully for readability and appearance. Script typeface should be avoided. Size of type should be selected with the reader in mind. For example, if the questionnaire is to be read by the elderly, the type should be larger than that required by a middle-aged adult. A good test is to have a few persons similar to the intended respondents answer the planned questionnaire.

SECTIONS OF THE QUESTIONNAIRE

Questionnaires comprise several components. These include the title, directions, questions, transition statements as sections change, and a closing statement (see box).

DESIGN OF THE QUESTIONS
Items

An item consists of a question (or request for information) and possible response op-

➤ **Anatomy of a Questionnaire**

1. *Title.* The title of the questionnaire at the top of the first page should be indicative of the content of the items. Avoid using the unimaginative title "Questionnaire."
2. *Directions.* When directions are complicated, they can be included in the cover letter. However, a summary should still be included on the first page of the questionnaire.
3. *Questions.* Number questions consecutively throughout the questionnaire even if there are several sections. Consecutive numbering lessens the confusion of having several questions numbered "1." Multiple-part questions can be labeled a, b, c, and so on, for the same number.
4. *Transitions.* If there are several different types of information requested, or if the respondent task changes, a transitional paragraph should be inserted at that place. For example: "In the next section, the questions will be addressing your needs for child care. Please circle one answer for every question unless otherwise directed."
5. *Closing.* It is appropriate to thank the respondents for their time at the end of the questionnaire—the use of spacing and bold type can make the statement appear stronger.

tions. First, information about the question is discussed; second, response options are addressed.

Types of Questions

The choice between open-ended and closed-ended questions depends on several factors. The *nature of the question to be answered* by the data from the questionnaire is one factor. Are feelings or facts to be obtained? Feelings, especially if detail is needed, are best obtained in the respondent's own words. Therefore, open-ended questions would be the choice. Facts are more easily categorized. When detail is not desired, closed-ended items are designed. If the desired end is a set of statements from respondents, open-ended questions would be chosen. If a quick count of those in different categories is desired, closed-ended items make the task easier.

Another issue in choosing between open- and closed-ended questions is *how much is known about the possible responses*? If only some information is available, open-ended questions are used. When most of the options are known and the closed-ended responses were chosen, the use of "Other (please specify) _____" gives respondents a chance to answer if their response is outside of the known categories.

Possibly one of the most important reasons used to select between the two options is the *analysis planned*. When dealing with a small number of questionnaires (less than 30), both options are possible. With larger surveys (an entire hospital or institution), the closed-ended questions are preferable from a time perspective.

There are trade-offs with either choice. Richness of responses and freedom of expression are lost with closed-ended questions. Ease of analysis and time are lost when open-ended questions are used unnecessarily. The investigator's burden is different for each. The time spent on designing the closed-ended items can be significant, but the analysis will be relatively quick. Open-ended items are quicker to design but may take significantly longer to analyze. Where the time is spent—earlier in design or later in analysis—may be a factor in decision making.

Response Bias

Response bias means that participants' answers are not reflective of true opinions. Sources of response bias reported by Topf (1986) include (1) carelessness, (2) social desirability (tendency for respondents to give the most socially acceptable answer), (3) acquiescence (tendency to agree), and (4) extremity of response (tendency of respondents to choose primarily $+3$ or -3 answers. "Central tendency" (consistently circling 3 when response choices range from 1 to 5) is another source of response bias. Participants are sometimes careless in responding when they are not convinced of the importance of the study or when the questions, items, or directions are unclear. As a result, they omit items, answer all items the same way, or do not follow directions (for example, they sometimes check three items when only one should be checked). Participant carelessness can be reduced by attaching a cover letter that explains the study's purpose and the importance of correct response. Pretesting the questionnaire to ensure clarity of instructions and items, and using a format that is easy to complete also reduce the likelihood of carelessness. Responses based on social desirability hinder the collection of data that reflect "true" opinions. The tendency of respondents to choose socially desirable answers can be reduced by stating that there are no right or wrong answers, by ensuring confidentiality of responses, or by using a predetermined set of responses. Acquiescence (the tendency to agree with positively worded questions) also affects the quality of collected data. A format using equal numbers of positive and negative words decreases the possibility of answers that do not reflect the respondent's agreement. Examples of positively stated items are (1) I am anxious most of the time and (2) I feel rested after a night's sleep. Negative statements include (1) I am not anxious most of the time and (2) I do not feel rested after a night's sleep. With Likert scales (strongly agree = 1, undecided = 3, strongly disagree = 5), there is a possibility that participants will answer items by always choosing "strongly agree," "strongly disagree," or "undecided." The respondent's tendency to use a set of extreme responses can be minimized if the stated items are half positive and half negative.

Wording of the Questions

Words used should be carefully selected, avoiding slang and words with several meanings. When terms that may not be familiar to the respondent are used, a definition should be provided. Avoid abbreviations if possible, or spell out the abbreviation the first time it is used.

The clarity of the questions and potential responses should be ensured before data are collected. By giving the questionnaire to several people who are similar to the intended respondents, any additional meanings or potential confusion may be drawn from their responses.

GUIDELINES FOR WELL-WRITTEN QUESTIONS

1. Use a conversational tone. The tone of the questions and of the entire questionnaire should be as if the respondent were present. For example,

   Problem:

   Sex

   M .... ——
   F .... ——

   Revision:

   What is your sex? Is it

   Male? 1
   or Female? 2

   Substituting the word "gender" instead of sex in the previous question may be preferable because it avoids some strange responses as well.

2. Avoid leading questions that suggest the expected response. For example,

   Problem:

   Most mothers ensure that their infants receive immunizations as infants. Has your child been immunized?

   Yes 1
   No 2

   Revision:

   Has your child been immunized?

   Yes 1
   No 2

3. Avoid double-barreled questions that ask two questions at the same time. For example,

Problem:

Do you favor legalization of drugs for use in private homes but not in public places?

Yes 1
No 2

Revision:

Do you favor legalization of drugs for use in private homes?

Yes 1
No 2

Do you favor legalization of drugs for use in public places?

Yes 1
No 2

4. Try to word the questions simply and directly without being too wordy. In some questions, the respondent wonders "What was the question?" after reading through wordy sections. A direct approach is more likely to yield the desired information.

5. Avoid double negatives.

Problem:

Should the nurse not be responsible for case management?

Yes 1
No 2

Revision:

Who should be responsible for case management?

The physician 1
The nurse 2
An administrator 3
Other (please specify) _____ 4

6. Do not assume that the respondent has too much knowledge.

Problem:

Are you in favor of team nursing in the operating room?

Yes 1
No 2

Revision:

In the operating room, team nursing is a system of regularly assigning the nursing staff to the same service in contrast to assigning nursing staff to any service as needed.

Are you in favor of team nursing in the operating room?

Yes 1
No 2

WORDING OF RESPONSE OPTIONS

1. Do not make response options too vague or too specific.

Problem (too vague):

How often do you call in sick?

Never 1
Rarely 2
Occasionally 3
Regularly 4

Revision:

How often did you call in sick in the past 6 months?

Not at all 1
1–2 times 2
3–4 times 3
More than 4 times 4

Problem (too vague):

What state are you from? _____

Revision:

In which state do you live? _____
In which state do you work? _____

Problem (too specific):

How many total books did you read last year? _____

Revision:

How many books did you read last year?

None 1
1–3 2
4–6 3
More than 7 4

2. The categories should be mutually exclusive, that is, there is no overlap. This becomes a problem when ranges are given. For example,

Problem:

How old are you?

20–30 years 1
30–40 years 2
40–50 years 3
50 or more years 4

The person who is 30 years of age does not know whether to circle a "1" or a "2."

Revision:

How old are you?

20–29 years 1
30–39 years 2
40–49 years 3
50 or more years 4

3. The categories must be inclusive and exhaustive.

In the previous example, the respondents contacted would need to be at least 20 years old for the categories to be inclusive of all respondents. By using the last response, "50 or more years old," the upper age limit has been exhausted. The only caution in its use would be if needed detail is lost by such a grouping. If only a small frequency is expected in this category, then it may be adequate.

4. The order of options given is from *smaller* to *larger* or from *negative* to *positive*.

As an example: values for "not at all" would be scored with "0" or "1" and the maximum value would be "5." In later analysis and explanation of the findings, it is easier to explain that higher numbers mean more of something. A mean attitude score that is higher than another mean attitude score would then be more positive.

The revised example in the next paragraph illustrates the correct order. If the coding were reversed, a higher score would mean less agreement (or more disagreement).

5. The balance of the options is similar.

Problem:

Do you agree that nurses should receive a higher salary?

Extremely strongly disagree 1
Very strongly disagree 2
Strongly disagree 3
Agree 4
Strongly agree 5

Revision:

Do you agree that nurses should receive a higher salary?

Strongly disagree 1
Disagree 2
Agree 3
Strongly agree 4

To further clarify point 4, if the order of the options were reversed, a high mean on this question would be less agreement. That is very confusing when reporting the finding to others.

6. Limit the number of different types of response options chosen for use in the same questionnaire.

Common response options are

Approve—disapprove
Agree—disagree (*alone* or with *strongly* in front of each for two additional options)
Better—about the same—worse
Very good—good—poor—very poor

Whenever possible, the use of the same response options is preferred. The respondent task becomes more difficult when multiple types of options are used. The respondent feels that there is a constant "changing of gears," and the burden is increased.

7. The number of response options per question should be minimized.

The usual recommendation is four or five. If a neutral middle response is desired, then five responses should be used—the number 3 response would be the neutral middle. With even-numbered responses, the respondent is forced to choose one side or the other (such as in the revision in point 5); feelings of frustration or anger may occur. The respondent may feel that neither agreement nor disagreement is the right answer for him or her. Undecided better reflects the position in that case and the emotional response engendered by the situation may result in the questionnaire not being completed. On the other hand, if decisions need to be made based on the degree of agreement obtained, the surveyor may wish to force the respondent to choose. This type of forced choice should be used judiciously

When more detail or spread-of-ratings is desired, responses could include six or seven options per question. When more than seven are used, the task of discrimination becomes difficult for the respondent.

8. The responses should match the question.

If the question is about how satisfied the patient is with the services, then the options should not be agree/disagree.

ORDERING OF THE QUESTIONS

The appendix at the end of this chapter is a questionnaire that has been used at the University of Utah Hospital for all employees. It is used as an example to illustrate some of the points in this section.

Opening questions are critical questions and should be related to the main topic and the title of the questionnaire. These questions serve to engage the responder to begin the task.

Questions of like format should be together. For example, if there are several clusters of "agree—disagree" questions, these should be grouped, unless there is some reason not to do so, such as when there is a major shift in content or change in task.

When the respondent task changes or when a major change in topic occurs, a transitional sentence or paragraph should precede the change. In the sample questionnaire, the directions for question 6 give an explanation for the new task. Because all possibilities were not able to be considered, the intent of the question was explained.

In the sample questionnaire, the desired respondents were employees with children who were interested in an on-site child care program. Because of the need to separate nonrespondents from those who did not desire the child care program, it was decided to have everyone complete the questionnaire and allow those who did not need to continue responding to quit early. Questions 2 and 3 are examples of filter questions, allowing the desired respondents to be filtered from those who did not need to answer the questionnaire (see box).

The first question in the sample is a funnel question that allows respondents to question 1. a. to continue on to question 3. In this case, only those who do not make child care arrangements (answering 1. b.) need to answer question 2. This "skip sequence" prevents those who make child care arrangements (answering 1. a.) from getting irritated by trying to answer why they do not. Skip patterns can become confusing; the directions should be close to the response option as in 1. a. in the sample. People read from left to right, and this principle is used when the response to be read

---

➤ Example of Skip Patterns in Questionnaires

Question 2. I do not make child care arrangements now because I
a. Have no children requiring child care, and will have none in the future.
Thank you! You are finished unless you wish to comment (page X)
b. Have no children now but may in the future. (*Skip to question #7*)
c. Have satisfactory permanent arrangements.
d. Have arrangements for child care but have some needs.

Question 3. If you currently have other arrangements, would you be interested in using the on-site child care program at the University of Utah Hospital?
a. Yes (*Proceed to question #4*)
b. No
(Thank you! You are finished unless you wish to comment (page X)

Source: Child Care Survey. (1989). University of Utah Hospital, Salt Lake City, UT.

precedes the option to be selected. In this case, the skip directions are given immediately before the option is circled.

Another factor to consider in the ordering of questions is the chronology of events. If this is an issue in the questionnaire under construction, then the order of questions may be partially dictated by chronology. For example, if information about a child is to be obtained, the questions should begin with birth, and then proceed to infancy and childhood.

Sensitive questions should be placed near the middle of the questionnaire, at a point where some rapport with the respondent would have developed. If placed too early, this intrusion could result in a lack of completion of the entire questionnaire. On the other hand if sensitive questions are placed too close to the end, the respondent may feel an abrupt ending in a difficult conversation. Lee (1993) addresses the issue of developing material whose entire topic is sensitive.

Demographic questions should always be at the end. They are the least interesting to the respondent and are completed only if the respondent feels that a commitment has been made to finish the task.

CLINICAL DATA COLLECTION SHEETS

Sometimes the tool is used for recording clinical data rather than for asking questions. Data collection sheets are used in clinical studies to record observations or in quality improvement activities to record compliance with standards.

To reduce the amount of writing, units of measurements should be included where information is to entered (for example, ___ mmHg). The use of checks or circles when the options are known reduces writing and permits fewer errors from misreading handwriting.

When data are to be collected from a chart or in a series of steps, the data entry spaces should be placed in the order they occur. For example, if the order sheet is first in the chart, followed by progress notes, nursing notes, and graphs, the data collection should be ordered in that manner.

The same instructions about pretesting apply to data collection sheets as well. By pretesting, it becomes clear whether the order has been reversed or whether placement of items is optimal.

FOLLOWING THE DEVELOPMENT OF THE QUESTIONNAIRE

Many questionnaires are analyzed by simply counting respondents in categories. If more complex analysis is desired, whoever is assisting with the data analysis should have some input into the process of how the data are collected. If consultation on the proposed analysis is needed, the questionnaire should be reviewed by the consultant before the questionnaire is duplicated and the data collected. Revisions may need to be made solely for analytic reasons.

Pretesting

Once the questionnaire has been developed, it should be pretested on subjects who are similar to the desired respondents. No matter how simple it seems, the pretest usually reveals areas for improvement. It is also helpful to debrief the subjects to find out what they thought about each question and the reason for the answers given. Additional areas for revision may be found.

Plans for an adequate response rate should be made. These include (1) how the questionnaire is to be distributed and returned and (2) how to track and contact nonresponders. Personal delivery and collection of completed questionnaires result in the highest return rates. Mailed questionnaires should include a cover letter and a stamped, self-addressed return envelope. Follow-up on mailed questionnaires includes sorting responses by code numbers, accounting for returned questionnaires, and mailing follow-up material to nonresponders. Linsky (1975) reported on studies done to *increase response rates* to mailed questionnaires. There are two broad categories of factors associated with responses to questionnaires: (1) mechanical and perceptual, and (2) broad and direct motivational. The *mechanical and perceptual* category includes those factors related to ease of responding and advance notification about the questionnaire. Ways in which the researcher can make it easier for respondents to reply include the following: (1) ask the respondents to mark answers by checking or circling the number of the response already printed with each item, (2) use questionnaires that are short (1 to 2 pages) and easy to read (print that is not too small, copy that is not too light), and (3) provide a self-addressed return envelope. To increase the awareness about receipt of the questionnaire, the researcher can precontact the person to whom the questionnaire is being sent (telephone, face-to-face, or letter), print the questionnaire on colored paper, and call or send a follow-up letter or postcard to persons who have not responded. Some *broad and direct motivational* factors that can influence response to questionnaires include the following:

1. A mechanism for ensuring anonymity of respondents
2. A cover letter explaining the importance of the study and of the respondents' role, giving the title and organizational affiliation of the sender, and stating a deadline for return of response
3. Rewards (monetary or study results)

Follow-up plans include developing a timeline for one or more additional mailings or telephone calls. When tracking mailed returns, the investigator can plot the cumulative returns by day. When the return line plateaus, it is a good time to start the next wave of follow-up, whether that is by telephone or by mail. A more cogent cover letter is helpful, explaining the need for all the responses.

Telephone follow-up has the advantage of permitting clarification of the reasons for nonresponse. For example, the first mailing might not have been received, especially in a complex organization. Questions that are answered during the telephone call might permit the respondent to reply.

Calculating the Response Rate

The denominator of the fraction is the number mailed (or contacted) minus the ineligibles. For example, if the intended respondent is an intensive care unit (ICU) nurse and the returned questionnaire (or information received about this person) indicates that she is no longer employed in ICU, then she is ineligible. She should not be counted among those who received mail and were eligible. This advantage in improving response rate by decreasing the denominator gives more incentive to follow-up so that the number of ineligible respondents might be

determined; follow-up also increases the number of responses from eligible participants.

The numerator is the number of returned questionnaires minus those not usable. Sometimes a questionnaire has too much missing data or the respondent has removed the code number. If the questionnaire is not usable, although returned, it should not be included in the numerator.

Coding the Results

This section considers issues in coding quantitative data resulting from surveys. Directions for coding qualitative data are found in Chapter 23.

Plans for analysis should be made with regard to the amount of the data, the intended level of analysis, and the method of analysis planned. With a large data set or with complicated analyses, computation by computer is a necessity. With smaller data sets and when simple counts are planned, a manual system might be faster although more errors are possible.

Entry of the data into the computer can be done in several ways. If the questionnaire is complicated or multiple sources of data are used, it may be easier to enter the code numbers onto paper called *FORTRAN sheets* or coding sheets lined with 80 columns and 24 to 25 rows.

If the questionnaire is precoded and simple (as in the sample questionnaire in the appendix), the numbers circled by the respondent may be directly entered into the column designated on the right edge of the questionnaire. In this case, each subject is a row and each answer is found in one column or set of columns. In the sample questionnaire, a decision was made to enter data only from those questionnaires in which more than the first page was completed.

With precoding, the data entry person can check the column number against the respondent's value to ensure correct placement. Without precoding, a codebook may need to be developed that has columns entitled Variable number, Variable label, Source of the data (for example, question 3), Column number, and Value labels (including the missing data options if a value is not circled). The data entry person would look at the codebook and then the individual questionnaire before entering the value in a column in the computer or on the coding sheet. More errors are probable using this method. Plans for checking for errors should be made, especially if a high degree of accuracy is needed. When spreadsheets are used for analysis, concerns about column width do not occur. Because the variable is entered into a single cell, it does not matter whether it is one digit wide (such as in gender, 1/0) or multiple columns wide (such as with age). Some of the more recent statistical software packages function in this manner (for example, SPSS for Windows).

Also available is *Teleform* (5.0 for Windows 95 or NT), a software package that can facilitate the design of forms, distribute them by FAX, receive the responses by FAX, and then set up the data as an SPSS data file. It can also receive data from scanned forms. Costs, time, and errors are all reduced with this process. The software is available from SPSS; more information is available on their Web page: http://www.spss.com/products/tele/.

The first run of the data should include a count of all the values for each variable. Numbers out of the expected range and illegal values are then detected. For example, a yes/no question coded 1 and 2 would not have numbers from 3 to 8. A "9" might be a legitimate value if the usual convention of 9 for missing data was used. If illegal values are found, the case number with that value needs to be determined. Then, the original questionnaire for that subject needs to be found to determine the correct value, and the value can be corrected. This process is called *data cleaning,* which should be done before any meaningful statistics are calculated.

SUMMARY

In summary, multiple decisions about the questionnaire design, questions asked, and responses anticipated influence the amount and accuracy of the data collected. The response rate partially determines the value of the results to the intended audience.

REFERENCES

Harris, L. E., Weinberger, M., & Tierney, W. M. (1997). Assessing inner-city patients' hospital experiences: A controlled trial of telephone interviews versus mailed surveys. *Medical Care, 35*(1), 70–76.

Lee, R. M. (1993). *Doing research on sensitive topics.* Newbury Park, CA: Sage.

Linsky, A. S. (1975). Stimulating responses to mailed questionnaires: A review. *Public Opinion Quarterly, 39*, 82–101.

Spilker, B., & Schoenfelder, J. (1991). *Data collection forms in clinical trials.* New York: Raven.

Topf, M. (1986). Response sets in questionnaire research. *Nursing Research, 35*, 119–121.

ADDITIONAL READINGS

Dillman, D. A. (1978). *Mail and telephone surveys: The total design method.* New York: Wiley.

Fowler, F. J. (1988). *Survey research methods.* Newbury Park, CA: Sage.

Jagger, J. (1982). Data collection instruments: Side-stepping the pitfalls. *Nurse Educator, 7*(3), 25–28.

Payne, S. L. (1951). *The art of asking questions.* Princeton, NJ: Princeton University Press.

Sudman, S., & Bradburn, N. M. (1982). *Asking questions: A practical guide to questionnaire design.* San Francisco: Jossey-Bass.

Warwick, D. P., & Linninger, C. A. (1975). *The sample survey: Theory and practice.* New York: McGraw-Hill.

APPENDIX: Sample Questionnaire

UNIVERSITY OF UTAH HOSPITAL

CHILD CARE SURVEY
Summer, 1989

	ID # Please disregard this column

We are moving closer to an identified site for a child care program at the University of Utah Hospital. This program would be located in a building about a one-minute walk from the hospital under a covered walkway.

As an aid to our planning process, it is extremely important that we have an idea of how many of our employees wish to enroll their children, and how many children that would total. At the present time, no decisions have been made regarding sick-child care or drop-in care. However, if you have special child care needs please comment on the last page of the survey.

We need *everyone* to respond to this questionnaire, and please be very honest in your evaluation of your potential use of your child care program.

Please complete this questionnaire and return it to the head nurse of your unit or to your supervisor.

Circle *one* answer code number for each question unless otherwise instructed.

Col 1–5

1. Do you have child care arrangements right now? | Col 6
   a. Yes (skip to question #3) 1
   b. No 2

2. I do not make child care arrangements now because I | Col 7
   a. Have no children requiring child care, and will have none in the future 1
   Thank you! You are finished unless you wish to comment (page 3)
   b. Have no children now but might in the future 2
      (skip to question #7)
   c. Have satisfactory permanent arrangements 3
   d. Have arrangements for child care but have some needs 4

3. If you currently have other arrangements, would you be interested in using the on-site child care program at the University of Utah Hospital? | Col 8
   a. Yes (proceed to question 4) 1
   b. No. **Thank you! You are finished unless you wish to comment (page 3)** 2

4. How many children *would* you enroll in the hospital child care program? | Col 9–10

	Circle # of children	Col
—Less than 24 months of age .... 0 1 2 3 4 5+		11
—2 years to 5 years old .... 0 1 2 3 4 5+		12
—More than 5 years and less than 13 years ..... 0 1 2 3 4 5+		13

5. Please place an "x" in the boxes that best represent the days of the week and the times during which you expect to have at least one child in the hospital's child care program. We are attempting to determine the peak times the child care center will be used.

Time of Day	Sun	Mon	Tue	Wed	Thu	Fri	Sat	Col
6 AM–10 AM								14–20
10 AM–2 PM								21–27
2 PM–6 PM								28–34
6 PM–10 PM								35–41
10 PM–6 AM								42–48

6. Do you work rotating shifts (for example, days and evenings?)   Col 49
   a. Yes 1
   b. No 2

7. What is your *primary* shift?   Col 50
   a. Days, 8 hours 1
   b. Evenings, 8 hours 2
   c. Nights, 8 hours 3
   d. Days, 10 or 12 hours 4
   e. Nights, 10 or 12 hours 5

8. What is your *secondary* shift?   Col 51
   a. Days, 8 hours 1
   b. Evenings, 8 hours 2
   c. Nights, 8 hours 3
   d. Days, 10 or 12 hours 4
   e. Nights, 10 or 12 hours 5
   f. No secondary shift 6

9. Would you use the child care program for   Col 52
   a. Both shifts 1
   b. Primary shifts only 2
   c. Secondary shifts only 3

10. During what hours would you like this child care program to be open?   Col 53
    a. 6 AM–12 midnight, seven days a week 1
    b. 6 PM–8 AM only, seven days a week 2
    c. 24 hours a day, Monday through Friday only 3
    d. 24 hours a day, Saturday and Sunday only 4
    e. 24 hours a day, seven days a week 5

11. Are you willing to pay a rate comparable to the current market?   Col 54
    a. Yes 1
    b. No 2

Please write any other comments about child care needs.   Col 55

_____

_____

_____

Thank you very much for filling out this questionnaire. Please return this questionnaire to your head nurse or your supervisor.

CHILD CARE COMMITTEE, UNIVERSITY OF UTAH HOSPITAL

Mary Beth Fairbrother
Director of Nursing
Critical Care Areas

Dan Lundergan
Director of Professional
Services

Lil Henrie
Nurse Educator
Nursing Practice

Chapter 20

Biomedical Instrumentation

Kathleen S. Stone and Susan K. Frazier

Biomedical instruments measure physiological variables or parameters by the application or use of electrical devices. Biomedical instrumentation extends human senses by monitoring minute changes in physiological variables and by amplifying or displaying them so that they can be sensed audibly or visually. For example, the electrocardiogram (ECG) monitors millivolt changes in electrical activity occurring in the heart, amplifies the signal to volts, and displays the signal as an audible sound or displays it on an oscilloscope screen or graphic recorder.

CLASSIFICATION OF BIOMEDICAL INSTRUMENTS

Biomedical instruments are classified into two types, in vivo and in vitro. In vivo instruments are applied directly within or on a living organism and are subdivided into invasive and noninvasive types. Invasive instruments require that a body cavity be entered or the skin be broken for application of the device. The introduction of an arterial catheter and the use of a pressure transducer to monitor arterial blood pressure are examples of invasive biomedical instrumentation. A noninvasive biomedical instrument uses the skin surface to apply the sensing device. An electrocardiogram (ECG) is an example of a noninvasive biomedical instrument. In vitro biomedical instrumentation requires the application of a device outside the organism. For example, a Coulter counter is a biomedical instrument that measures the number of red blood cells in a blood specimen outside the subject's body.

The method of monitoring (that is, invasive versus noninvasive) should be considered when measuring physiological variables. It is preferable to use noninvasive techniques because there are fewer risks to the patient (such as blood loss, compromised arterial blood flow with cannulation, and infection). Consideration must also be given, however, to the degree of accuracy of the data and whether continuous or intermittent data are required. A noninvasive, indirect automated oscillating blood pressure cuff that cycles every minute can be used to monitor arterial blood pressure intermittently. When direct, continuous arterial blood pressure recordings are needed to enhance accuracy, however, invasive biomedical instruments are required. Although in vitro biomedical instrumentation does not pose direct risks to the human subject, consideration must still be given to the sample needed. The question to be asked is "Can the necessary information be obtained in a sample other than blood, such as sputum, urine, or exhaled breath?" Stress levels can be physiologically monitored directly by measuring epinephrine and norepinephrine levels in the blood or indirectly by measuring urinary catecholamines in the urine. Carbon monoxide levels can be measured directly in blood by co-oximetry and indirectly in exhaled air by using an ecolyzer.

CATEGORIES OF PHYSIOLOGICAL VARIABLES DETECTED BY BIOMEDICAL INSTRUMENTS

A variety of physiological variables can be detected by using biomedical instrumentation, and these variables are commonly measured in patients in hospitals, at clinics, and in community or home settings. The monitoring of physiological variables is a component of comprehensive nursing care and provides a wealth of quantitative data that can be used in nursing research. To ensure accuracy of the data when collecting physiological measures with biomedical instruments, the components of the organism-instrument system (including the subject, stimulus, and biomedical instrument) must be considered.

Categories of variables that can be detected with biomedical instruments include the following:

1. Electrical potentials
   - Brain—electroencephalogram (EEG)
   - Heart—ECG
   - Muscle—electromyogram (EMG)

2. Pressures
   - Arteries—systolic and diastolic arterial pressure and mean arterial pressure
   - Veins—central venous pressure
   - Lungs—intra-airway and intrapleural pressure
   - Esophagus—esophageal pressure
   - Bladder—degree of distention determined by pressure in the bladder
   - Uterus—uterine activity determined by monitoring pressure in the uterus
   - Brain—intracranial pressure
3. Mechanical waves
   - Ears—sound waves
   - Heart—heart sounds
4. Temperature
   - Surface
   - Core
   - Ear
5. Gases
   - Lungs—oxygen, carbon dioxide, nitrogen, and carbon monoxide
   - Blood—arterial and venous concentrations of oxygen, carbon dioxide, and carbon monoxide

COMPONENTS OF THE ORGANISM-INSTRUMENT SYSTEM

Subject

Components of the organism-instrument system are detailed in Figure 20–1. Most nursing studies deal with human subjects who have specific demographic and clinical characteristics from which the researcher makes a selection. A demographic profile might portray male subjects aged 20 to 70 years who have undergone coronary revascularization surgery with no history of pulmonary or renal disease.

Some research questions regarding human subjects frequently cannot be pursued because of potential risks and must be examined first in animal models. Consideration must be given to choosing an animal model with a response similar to that of humans so that the applicability of the findings will be appropriate.

Stimulus

Once the parameters for the subjects (human or animal) have been selected, then the

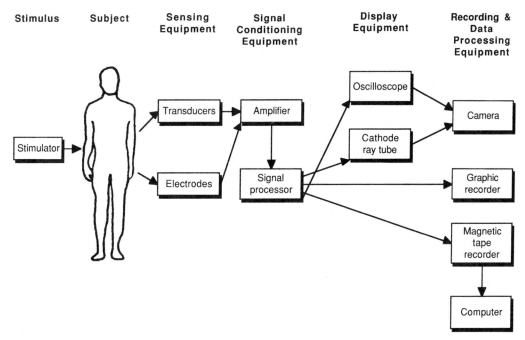

Figure 20–1
Schema of the organism-instrument system. (From Polit, D. F., Hungler, B. P., & Bernadette, P. [1987]. *Nursing research: Principles & methods* [3rd ed., p. 292]. Philadelphia: J. B. Lippincott.)

experimental stimulus is identified so that the physiological response under investigation can be elicited and measured. Various stimuli, such as electrical shock, auditory (environmental noise in decibels), tactile, visual (trauma scene or a flashing light), or mechanical rocking motion), or a nursing care procedure (turning, postural drainage, or endotracheal suctioning) can cause changes in heart rate, blood pressure, and intracranial pressure. In the above examples, the stimulus elicits a response in the dependent physiological variables (in this case, heart rate, blood pressure, and intracranial pressure), which is then measured with biomedical instrumentation. In the experimental study, the stimulus can be altered by changing its duration, intensity, or frequency. For example, the effect of noise lasting for 5, 10, or 15 minutes (duration) can be measured at 20 and 50 decibels (intensity) every 30 minutes (frequency).

Sensing Equipment

TRANSDUCERS

A transducer may be required to sense the change in a dependent physiological variable. This device converts one form of energy into another measures physiological phenomena (for example, pressure, temperature, or gases), while producing an electrical signal in volts proportional to the phenomenon. This conversion is required because a biomedical instrument is an electronic device and responds only to changes in electrical output.

There are many different transducers. For instance, a pressure transducer records displacement. It is placed outside the subject's body and connected to the subject by a needle or catheter inserted into the arterial or venous blood vessel. The attachment to the transducer is completed by pressurized tubing filled with fluid. The tubing is connected to a fluid-filled dome that covers the surface of the sensing diaphragm on the pressure transducer (Fig. 20–2). As the pressure within the blood vessel varies with pulsatile blood flow, the sensing diaphragm is displaced alternately inward and outward. The sensing diaphragm is connected by a wire to a bonded or semiconductor strain gauge.

When the wire on the strain gauge is stretched, the electrical resistance increases; conversely, when the wire is allowed to contract, the resistance decreases.

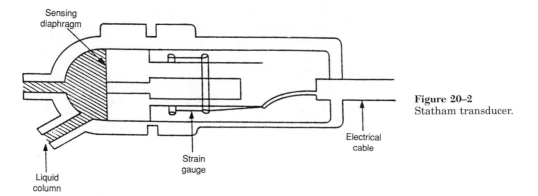

Figure 20–2
Statham transducer.

As the pressure fluctuates in the blood vessel, the pressure change is transmitted to the sensing diaphragm, which bows inward and outward, changing the resistance in the wire. According to Ohm's Law, which states that the Voltage = Current × Resistance, as the resistance in the wire increases and decreases and the current remains constant, the voltage varies proportionally. Through this method, the pressure, or displacement transducer, converts pressure changes into voltage, which then can be measured by a biomedical instrument.

Temperature can be measured with a resistance thermometer or thermistor. A thermistor is a wire whose resistance increases and decreases as temperature increases and decreases. With a thermistor, changes in temperature can be converted to voltage according to Ohm's Law and measured with a biomedical instrument. A thermistor can measure skin surface, rectal temperature, and core body temperature. The small, thin, exposed wire in the tip of a Swan-Ganz catheter is an example of a thermistor.

The principles for measuring pressure and temperature can be applied to measuring the concentration of arterial blood gases. An arterial blood gas machine contains electrodes for oxygen, carbon dioxide, and pH, which are biochemical transducers that convert the concentration of gas pressure and the concentration of hydrogen ions to an electrical signal, both of which are detectable using biomedical instruments.

When using a transducer, a number of issues must be addressed to ensure the accuracy and reliability of the measurement. Blood pressures are measured against a specific reference plane, which is normally the right atrium of the heart. The right atrium is fixed at a point along the midaxillary line at the fourth intercostal space. This point is marked with tape on the subject's body. The subject must be in a supine position when the reference site is determined. Then with a level, the pressure transducer's balancing port is positioned so that it is perfectly horizontal to the subject's right atrium (Fig. 20–3).

Leveling is important because, for each inch (2.5 cm) of difference between the balancing port and the right atrium, the blood pressure varies 2 mmHg. If the subject's position is changed, the position of the transducer must be leveled again. The pressure transducer must then be balanced and zeroed by opening the balancing port and exposing the sensing diaphragm to atmospheric pressure. This procedure sets the strain gauge at zero voltage with respect to atmospheric pressure. Figure 20–4 illustrates this method by examining the strain gauge more closely. To obtain the degree of sensitivity required to measure blood pressure, four strain gauges are mounted to the sensing diaphragm, and these resistances (R_1 through R_4) are connected to form a

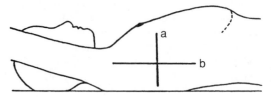

Figure 20–3
Determination of the supine measuring point by use of the phlebostatic axis. Line *a* represents the fourth intercostal space and line *b* is the midaxillary line. (From Kennedy, G. T., Bryant, A., & Crawford, M. H. [1984]. The effects of lateral body positioning on measurements of pulmonary artery and pulmonary artery wedge pressure. *Heart & Lung, 13,* 157.)

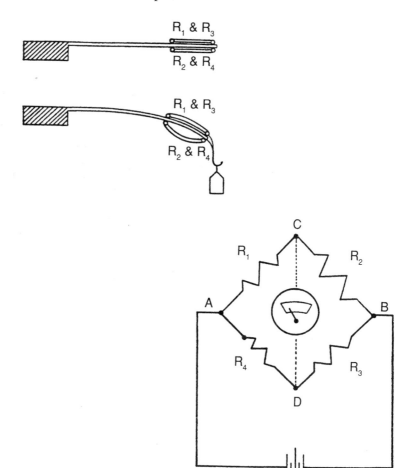

Figure 20–4
Strain gauge transducer.

Whetstone bridge circuit. The gauges are attached so that as the pressure increases, two gauges stretch and two contract; the sensitivity of the transducer is then increased by four. When the balancing port is exposed to atmospheric pressure, the strain gauges are balanced (equal) and the voltage output is set at zero. When the pressurized tubing from the arterial catheter is connected to the pressure transducer, the actual pressure changes occurring in the blood vessel cause the sensing diaphragm to move inward and outward, thereby changing the resistance in the wire and the voltage output. The transducer must then be calibrated against a column of mercury (Hg) or water (H_2O). Known values of pressure in increments of 50 to 100 mmHg, or 50 to 100 cm H_2O, are applied to the transducer to determine whether the output is linear and to verify that the changes in pressure in the blood vessel are proportional to the voltage output. To ensure the accuracy and reliabil-

ity of the research data, the transducer should be calibrated before, during, and after data collection.

The same principles of balancing, zeroing, and calibration apply to temperature and biochemical transducers. For example, to be zeroed, the oxygen electrode of a blood gas analyzer is exposed to a solution with no oxygen and is then calibrated against a solution of known oxygen concentration. The calibration is repeated every 30 minutes to ensure the accuracy and reliability of the data.

RECORDING ELECTRODES

Recording electrodes used to monitor physiological variables are generally surface-type electrodes that obtain bioelectrical potentials from body surfaces. Floating silver-silver chloride electrodes are placed on the skin surface to record electrical potentials. The floating electrode is used to re-

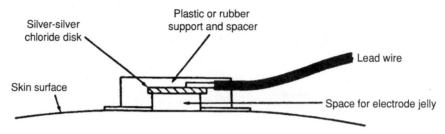

Figure 20–5
Diagram of floating type skin surface electrode. (From Cromwell/Weibell/Pfeiffer, BIOMEDICAL
INSTRUMENTATION AND MEASUREMENTS, 2e, copyright 1980, p. 72. Reprinted by permission of Prentice-
Hall, Inc., Englewood Cliffs, New Jersey.)

move any movement artifact by eliminating
direct contact between the metal in the recording electrode and the skin (Fig. 20–5).

Skin contact is maintained through an
electrolyte bridge of electrolyte jelly or
cream applied directly to the skin surface.
Electrolyte material reduces impedance of
skin contact through surface oils and the
outer horny layer of the skin. Needle electrodes are often used in animals but are
used less frequently in humans.

Signal Conditioning Equipment

Output signals from the transducer or the
electrodes usually occur in millivolts and
must be amplified (see Fig. 20–1). Signals
are amplified from millivolts to volts to
drive the display unit, which could be either
an oscilloscope or a graphic recorder. Most
display units require an input voltage of 5
to 10 volts. Amplification of the signal often
is referred to as "increasing the gain." Once
the signal has been amplified, the frequency
of the signal in cycles per second is modified
to eliminate noise or artifact. An example of
artifact is the muscle movement seen on an
ECG; another example is 60-cycle (Hz) noise
from environmental electrical interference.
Electronic filters control noise or artifact by
rejecting the unwanted signals. Artifact can
be separated, diluted, or omitted by adjusting the sensitivity control on the biomedical instrument.

Display Equipment

After a physiological signal has been amplified or modified by signal-conditioning
equipment, display equipment converts the

electrical signals into visual or auditory output that human senses can detect.

CATHODE RAY OSCILLOSCOPE

A cathode ray oscilloscope displays physiological waveforms on a phosphor screen.
An oscilloscope is actually a voltmeter with
a rapid response time. A beam of electrons
produced by an electron gun has little inertia and is therefore capable of rapid motion.
Horizontal and vertical plates dictate
whether the beam on the screen appears in
the vertical or horizontal plane (Fig. 20–6).

Different output voltages from transducers or electrodes cause the beam of electrons
to be displaced proportionally. An oscilloscope can be used to display a graph of
voltage versus time automatically and repeatedly (Fig. 20–7).

The graphic display of the electron beam
across the phosphor screen is temporary
and is rapidly replaced by incoming voltage
changes. Recordings from an oscilloscope
screen can be converted into a permanent
record by mounting a camera onto the
screen and taking pictures of the display.
The data also may be stored on magnetic
tape and retrieved for future display whenever necessary.

RECORDERS

A permanent recording can be made by
using a graphic recorder, of which there are
several types. The two basic graphic recorders are the curvilinear and the rectilinear.

A curvilinear recorder has a display system in which pens move in an arc and produce a display on curvilinear paper. These
recorders are relatively inexpensive and are
useful for graphic data display. The curvilinear recorder is self-limiting. Because of the

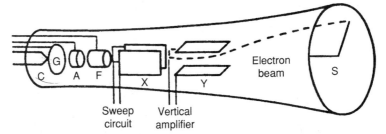

C = cathode (electron emitter)
G = control grid (beam intensity)
A = electron accelerating anode
F = focusing electrode
X = X direction deflecting plates
Y = Y direction deflecting plates
S = phosphor coated screen

Figure 20–6
Cathode ray oscilloscope.

arc of the pen, it is not possible to obtain an exact value. In the clinical setting, graphic recorders are typically of the curvilinear variety. To determine whether a recorder is curvilinear, the recording pen is moved up and down to observe whether the pen sweeps in an arc.

A rectilinear recorder has a display system in which the pens move in a linear mode and produce a display that can be used to determine an exact value. These recorders are considerably more expensive than curvilinear models but are more versatile for the collection of research data.

In addition to the instrument, the method of producing the graph should be considered. Typically, recording pens use ink to produce graphs on the surface of the recording paper or imbedded into the paper. Imbedding ink in paper decreases the potential of smearing copy and possibly losing data. Thermal array recorders use a heat stylus pen and heat sensitive paper. This technique reduces the inking problem; however, a thermal graph fades with time.

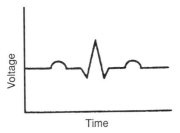

Figure 20–7
Graphic display of voltage versus time using oscilloscope.

Permanent recordings can also be made with a tape recorder by storing data on magnetic tape. This method allows the investigator to replay the experiment at a later time and at different speeds. Output from the signal processor of the recorder can be entered into an analog-to-digital converter and then be read by a computer. Specialized computer software can be used to analyze the data. Data can also be permanently stored on-line during the experiment onto a computer hard disk for later analysis.

CHARACTERISTICS OF BIOMEDICAL INSTRUMENTATION

There are many issues to address in the decision of whether to use clinical biomedical instrumentation or research biomedical instrumentation for data collection. These considerations include the following:

1. Range of an instrument, which is the complete set of values that an instrument can measure (for example, 0 to 100 g for a scale, 1 to 250 beats per minute (bpm) for a cardiac monitor, 0 to 60°C for a thermometer). It is critical that the instruments chosen to record research data have the capability to measure phenomena in the ranges needed. The range of an instrument can be determined by reading the instrument specifications at the back of the equipment manual. Generally, the manual also provides information on the reliability of the instrument within the range specified.

2. The frequency response of an instrument, which indicates the capability of the instrument to respond equally well to rapid and slow components. For example, measuring the action potential of a neuron requires equipment with fast response time, because the total time for an action potential occurs in milliseconds. As a result, to record this type of physiological phenomenon, a cathode ray oscilloscope is required. The response time of the instrument is rapid because there is no inertia in the beam of electrons. A graphic recorder cannot be used to measure a neural action potential because the frequency response is too slow. The inertia of the pen as it moves across the graph paper results in a slow response time.

3. Sensitivity of an instrument, which is the degree of change in the physiological variable that the instrument can detect. For example, one instrument might weigh material within one tenth of a gram (0.1 g), whereas another instrument might weigh the same material within one hundredth of a gram (0.01 g), with the latter instrument being the more sensitive.

4. Stability of an instrument, which is its ability to maintain a calibration over a given interval. Over time, biomedical instruments frequently suffer gradual loss of calibration, called "drift." It is important that a biomedical instrument maintain calibration because the reliability of the data is dependent on an accurate measure. The instruction manual normally specifies the stability of the instrument over time. The manual also indicates how often the manufacturer recommends recalibration. Because loss of calibration, or "drift," is common among biomedical instruments, it is important to check the calibration before, during, and after an experiment to ensure the reliability of the data collected.

5. Linearity of the instrument, which is the extent to which an input change is directly proportional to an output change. For instance, for every one degree of actual change in a subject's temperature, there is a one-degree change recorded on the thermometer.

6. Signal-to-noise ratio of an instrument, which indicates the relationship between the amount of signal strength and the amount of noise or artifact. The higher the signal-to-noise-ratio, the less artifact.

CHARACTERISTICS OF THE MEASUREMENTS OBTAINED BY USING BIOMEDICAL INSTRUMENTS

Different conditions call for different biomedical instrumentation. Not every piece of equipment functions equally well for all circumstances. No matter what the condition, however, there are basic characteristics that should be considered for every biomedical instrument. These features include the following:

1. Validity—the extent to which the biomedical instrument measures the actual parameter of interest (for example, the validity of an arterial blood pressure measurement can be determined by the typical characteristics of the arterial pressure wave that validates the correct placement of the arterial catheter)

2. Accuracy—the degree to which the parameter sensed by the instrument reflects the actual value

3. Precision—the discriminatory power of the instrument (that is, the smaller the change sensed, the greater the precision of the instrument)

4. Reliability—the accuracy of the measurement over time

USING BIOMEDICAL INSTRUMENTATION FOR RESEARCH PURPOSES

There are a number of clinical biomedical instruments used to evaluate patient status. An increasing number of research studies use physiological values from these instruments as research data. There are a number of considerations that require examination before use of these data for research purposes. The use of bedside pulse oximetry as a data collection instrument is evaluated as an illustrative example considering the characteristics of biomedical instrumentation.

Oxygen Saturation

Oxygen is transported to tissues either combined with hemoglobin or dissolved in plasma. Arterial blood gas evaluation of oxygen status (PaO_2) provides a measure of the partial pressure of oxygen dissolved in plasma; however, the PaO_2 represents only about 2% of the total oxygen transported. The primary means for oxygen transport is by oxygen molecules binding with hemoglobin molecules to form saturated hemoglobin or oxyhemoglobin (HbO_2). Clinically, oxygen saturation can be measured by obtaining an invasive arterial blood gas sample and determined in vitro using a co-oximeter. An alternative noninvasive measure of oxygen saturation can be determined by pulse oximetry (SpO_2). A clear understanding of the instrumentation and technique of measurement is vital to ensure that the data obtained with a pulse oximeter are valid, accurate, reliable, and precise.

Measurement of Oxygen Saturation

Measurement of hemoglobin saturation by pulse oximetry integrates elements of optical plethysmography with spectrophotometry. Optical plethysmography generates waveforms from pulsatile blood as the blood moves past sophisticated light absorbance instrumentation. The presence of pulsatile blood differentiates the arterial bed from the venous bed to ensure that the saturation measurement is arterial in origin. Concurrently, spectrophotometry yields quantitative calculations of hemoglobin saturation based on the absorption of multiple wavelengths of light by the hemoglobin molecules. In a pulse oximeter, two light-emitting diodes (LEDs) expose the hemoglobin molecules to two wavelengths of light: a red light (approximately 660 nm) and an infrared light (approximately 920 nm). The status of hemoglobin molecules determines the absorption of the different wavelengths of light by the hemoglobin molecules. Hemoglobin can be saturated with oxygen (HbO_2), reduced or deoxygenated, bound to carbon monoxide, which is called carboxyhemoglobin (HbCO), or oxidized with iron atoms called methemoglobin (Hbmet). A photodetector, placed in opposition to the LEDs, measures the degree of absorption of the red and infrared light by the hemoglobin

molecule. Saturated hemoglobin absorbs a greater degree of infrared light, whereas desaturated hemoglobin absorbs a greater degree of red light. The calculation of hemoglobin saturation by the pulse oximeter is based on the relative amounts of red and infrared light transmitted through the pulsatile blood to the photodetector.

Measurement of hemoglobin saturation may be either fractional or functional. A fractional measurement of hemoglobin saturation is performed by a co-oximeter and is obtained by analysis of an arterial blood sample. The co-oximeter uses four or more wavelengths of light. The fractional oxygen saturation is the ratio of oxygen saturated hemoglobin or oxyhemoglobin (HbO_2) to the total number of hemoglobin molecules. The total hemoglobin includes oxyhemoglobin, hemoglobin available for binding with oxygen or desaturated hemoglobin, and hemoglobin that is not capable of binding with oxygen (carboxyhemoglobin, methemoglobin). The status of total hemoglobin is evaluated with a fractional measurement.

A pulse oximeter provides a functional measurement of hemoglobin saturation. A functional measurement is the ratio of oxygen saturated hemoglobin to the total amount of hemoglobin available for binding to oxygen. This type of measurement does not include evaluation of hemoglobin that is not available for binding with oxygen (carboxyhemoglobin, methemoglobin). For comparison purposes, a fractional saturation value can be converted to a functional value using the following equation:

$$SaO_2 \text{ functional} = \frac{SaO_2 \text{ fractional}}{100 - (\%HbCO + \% Hbmet)} \times 100$$

Validity of Oxygen Saturation Measurement by Pulse Oximetry

The measurement of oxygen saturation by a co-oximeter using four or more wavelengths of light is the gold standard. A number of studies have compared the values obtained by pulse oximetry with simultaneous measurement of oxygen saturation by co-oximeter. In the range of 70% to 100% oxygen saturation, there is a strong correlation between these values (range of correlation coefficients $r = .92$ to .98). Within this range of values, pulse oximetry has been demonstrated to accurately reflect functional hemoglobin saturation. However, when oxygen saturation values are less than 70%, pulse oximetry may provide a falsely high value as a result of the calculation algorithm used in this biomedical instrument. SpO_2 may be a clinically useful indicator of oxygen transport; however, both the clinician and researcher must remember that the use of a functional measurement of oxygen saturation does not reflect tissue oxygen delivery. A high oxygen saturation (SpO_2) value determined by pulse oximetry does not necessarily indicate adequate tissue oxygen delivery. Shifts in the oxyhemoglobin dissociation curve caused by hypothermia, alkalosis, or a decrease in 2,3-diphosphoglycerate can significantly alter tissue oxygen delivery even though the functional oxygen saturation value appears normal.

Accuracy of Pulse Oximetry

Certain clinical and technical phenomena may reduce the accuracy of saturation values obtained by pulse oximetry (Table 20–1). Weak arterial pulsation produced by shock states, hypothermia with shunting of blood flow from the periphery, or increased systemic vascular resistance may result in little to absent light absorption detection by the sensor. The oximeter is not capable of calculating a saturation value if pulsatile flow cannot be detected. Venous pulsation as a result of right ventricular failure or a partial obstruction to venous outflow also reduces the accuracy of SpO_2 values. In the presence of both arterial and venous pulsatile flow, the SpO_2 value may be a composite value derived from light absorbance from both arterial and venous hemoglobin. In this instance, the SpO_2 value provided is lower than actual arterial saturation.

Abnormalities in the blood may produce inaccurate values of oxygen saturation. Anemia may reduce the accuracy of pulse oximetry values, particularly as saturation values decrease. The cause for this inaccuracy is not well understood but may be secondary to the scattering of light in the plasma with a shift in the degree of red light absorbed. In addition, the presence of a significant portion of hemoglobin that is unavailable for oxygen binding (for example, carboxyhemoglobin and methemoglobin) also reduces the accuracy of pulse oximetry measurements. For example, at a carbon monoxide partial pressure of only 0.1 mmHg, hemoglobin is 50% saturated with carbon monoxide. The functional measurement of saturation by the pulse oximeter may indicate very high oxygen saturation, in that the remaining 50% of hemoglobin may be fully saturated with oxygen. This saturation value is further misleading, because the presence of high levels of carboxyhemoglobin increases the affinity of hemoglobin for oxygen and reduces oxygen unloading at the tissues.

Concentrations of certain substances in the arterial blood have been suggested to influence the accuracy of pulse oximetry. The effect of high levels of bilirubin on the accuracy of pulse oximetry is described inconsistently in the research literature. The majority of studies that compared SaO_2 with SpO_2 in the presence of hyperbilirubinemia (bilirubin up to 46.3 mg/dL) suggest that high bilirubin levels do not interfere with the accuracy of SpO_2 when saturation is greater than 90%. Use of systemic dyes has been demonstrated to affect the accuracy of pulse oximetry measurement. Indigo carmine, indocyanine green, and methylene blue absorb light at wavelengths similar to those used by the pulse oximeter (660 nm), and they alter the accuracy of SpO_2 values. Elevated lipid levels either from endogenous

Table 20–1

Factors that Alter Accuracy of Pulse Oximetry Measures

Individual Factors
Inadequate pulsatile arterial blood flow (hypotension, hypothermia, increased systemic vascular resistance)
Venous pulsatile flow
Dysfunctional hemoglobin (carboxyhemoglobin, methemoglobin)
Anemia
Presence of systemic dyes
Hyperlipidemia

Technical Factors
Motion artifact
Ambient light interference
Optical shunt
Optical cross-talk
Electrical interference

lipids or from administration of exogenous lipids solutions, in conjunction with total parenteral nutrition, may produce an artificially lower SpO$_2$ value.

In addition to clinical factors, technical factors may reduce the accuracy of pulse oximetry values. Motion artifact may be interpreted by the photodetector as arterial pulsation. High-intensity, high-quantity ambient light such as that found with heat lamps, surgical lights, or fluorescent lights may reduce the accuracy of SpO$_2$ values. The ambient light may be detected by the pulse oximetry photodetector. In this instance, the photodetector receives information from both the LEDs and the ambient light source. The SpO$_2$ value is then a composite value and is likely inaccurate. An optical shunt may occur when some of the light from the LEDs is transmitted to the photodetector without passing through a pulsatile vascular bed. The degree of red and infrared light received by the photodetector is again a composite of light exposed to hemoglobin and light not exposed to pulsatile blood; thus, the SpO$_2$ value is inaccurate. Optical cross-talk may occur when the pulse oximetry sensor is placed in close proximity to another instrument also using red and/or infrared light. In this instance, the light emitted by the secondary instrument may be received by the pulse oximetry photodetector. The SpO$_2$ value again is a composite that is likely inaccurate. Excessive signal noise (electrical interference) may be received and interfere with signal acquisition. Signal processing may be disrupted with significant electrical interference with resultant delayed values that may be inaccurate.

Bias is a statistical indicator of the accuracy of a measurement and is determined by calculating the mean difference between SaO$_2$ and SpO$_2$. The greater the bias, the less accurate the measurement technique. Bias for pulse oximetry values is reported to vary depending on the degree of hypoxemia; therefore, as oxygen saturation decreases, bias increases. Bias for pulse oximetry measures is reported to range from less than 0.5% to as much as 10%.

Pulse oximetry values in general are reported to have a margin of error $\pm 2\%$ of the actual SaO$_2$ value. This degree of error provides a wide range of potential values if SpO$_2$ values are normally distributed (Table 20–2). The investigator must determine whether measures with this degree of potential error will provide sufficiently accurate data to address the research objectives.

Precision of Oxygen Saturation by Pulse Oximetry

Pulse oximetry can detect a 1% change in oxygen saturation. However, the speed of response by the pulse oximeter is reported to diminish as actual SaO$_2$ values decrease. A statistical measure of the reproducibility of pulse oximetry measures is precision. This value is obtained by calculation of the standard deviation of the bias measurement and evaluates sources of error within the individual. The precision measure is analogous to the scatter of data points. Precision measures for pulse oximetry are reported to be 2% to 4%.

Table 20–2

Range of Pulse Oximetry Values in a Normal Distribution

	RANGE OF VALUES	RANGE IF SaO$_2$ IS 95%	RANGE IF SaO$_2$ IS 90%
Within 1 standard deviation of the mean (68% of population)	$\pm 2\%$	93%–97%	88%–92%
Within 2 standard deviations of the mean (95% of population)	$\pm 4\%$	91%–99%	86%–94%
Within 3 standard deviations of the mean (99.7% of population)	$\pm 6\%$	89%–100%	84%–96%

Reliability of Oxygen Saturation by Pulse Oximetry

Pulse oximetry measures are described as generally consistent over time. Most studies that evaluate reliability of pulse oximetry perform these studies with relationship to consistency of measurement over time using different probe types (reusable versus disposable finger, ear, and nose probes). The development of motion artifact appears to be the primary influence on the reliability of pulse oximetry measures. However, the development of other threats to accuracy also influences the reliability of this type of measurement.

Guidelines to Increase the Utility of Pulse Oximetry for Research Purposes

If SpO_2 values are to be used as research data, the investigator must ensure that these data are valid, accurate, precise, and reliable. The following guidelines help improve the likelihood that these data will be useful. However, the investigators must determine whether SpO_2 will provide them with the information required to answer the research questions or test the research hypotheses.

- Select a pulse oximeter with indicators of signal strength and pulse waveform to ensure that adequate, appropriate signal quality is available.
- Ensure probe type and probe position are optimal to detect arterial pulsation without technical interference from ambient light, optical shunt, or cross-talk.
- Assess the correlation between the apical heart rate and the heart rate detected by the pulse oximeter. These values must be closely correlated.
- Evaluate the individual for the presence of dysfunctional hemoglobin, hyperlipidemia, and anemia before data collection to ensure that these factors are not influencing SpO_2.
- Stabilize the probe so that motion artifact is not a significant confounding factor.
- Analyze the relationship between SpO_2 and SaO_2 regularly. These values should be highly correlated. Calculate the bias and precision to evaluate the accuracy and repeatability of the data.

SUMMARY

The careful selection and use of biomedical instruments to measure physiological outcomes is vital. Examples of instruments used to measure physiological variables and the characteristics of the instruments along with their measurements have been presented in this chapter.

SUGGESTED READINGS

Abbey, J. C. (1978). Symposium on bioinstrumentation for nurses. In J. C. Abbey & M. Mathura (Eds.), *Nursing Clinics of North America: Vol. 13, Bioinstrumentation for nurses* (pp. 559–560). Philadelphia: W. B. Saunders.

Avant, M., Lowe, N., & Torres, A. (1997). Comparison of accuracy and signal consistency of two reusable pulse oximeter probes in critically ill children. *Respiratory Care, 42*(7), 698–704.

Bridges, E. J., & Woods, S. L. (1993). Pulmonary artery pressure measurement: State of the art. *Heart & Lung, 22*(2), 99–111.

Bronzino, J. S. (1977). *Biomedical engineering technology for patient care: Applications for today, implications for tomorrow.* St. Louis: Mosby.

Chulay, M., & Miller, T. (1984). The effect of backrest elevation on pulmonary artery and pulmonary capillary wedge pressures in patients after cardiac surgery. *Heart & Lung, 13*, 138–140.

Chyun, D. A. (1985). A comparison of intra-arterial and auscultatory blood pressure readings. *Heart & Lung, 14*, 223–228.

Cromwell, L., Weibell, F. J., & Pfeiffer, E. A. (1980). *Biomedical instrumentation and measurements* (2nd ed.). Englewood Cliffs, NJ: Prentice-Hall.

Gift, A. G., & Socken, K. L. (1988). Assessment of physiologic instruments. *Heart & Lung, 17*, 128–133.

Glor, B. A. K., Sullivan, E. F., & Estes, Z. E. (1970). Reproducibility of blood pressure measurements: A replication. *Nursing Research, 19*, 170–172.

Gunn, I. P., Sullivan, E. F., & Glor, B. A. K. (1966). Blood pressure measurement as a quantitative research criterion. *Nursing Research, 15*, 4–11.

Hannhart, B., Haberer, J., Saunier, C., & Laxenaire, M. (1991). Accuracy and precision of fourteen pulse oximeters. *European Respiratory Journal, 4*, 115–119.

Hill, D. W., & Dolan, A. M. (1982). *Intensive care instrumentation* (2nd ed.). New York: Grune & Stratton.

Kennedy, G. T., Bryant, A., & Crawford, M. H. (1984). The effects of lateral body positioning on measurements of pulmonary artery and pulmonary artery wedge pressures. *Heart & Lung, 13*, 155–158.

Kirchhoff, K. T., Rebenson-Piano, M., & Patel, M. K. (1984). Mean arterial pressure readings: Variations with positions and transducer level. *Nursing Research, 33*, 343–345.

Levine, S. C. (1985). A review of the use of computerized digital instrumentation to determine pulmonary artery pressure measurements in critically ill patients. *Heart & Lung, 14*, 473–477.

Matthay, R. A., Wiedemann, H. P., & Matthay, M. A.

(1985). Cardiovascular function in the intensive care unit: Invasive and noninvasive monitoring. *Respiratory Care, 30*, 432–455.

Mengelkoch, L., Martin, D., & Lawler, J. (1994). A review of the principles of pulse oximetry and accuracy of pulse oximeter estimates during exercise. *Physical Therapy, 74*(1), 40–49.

Nemens, E. J., & Woods, S. L. (1982). Normal fluctuations in pulmonary artery and pulmonary capillary wedge pressures in acutely ill patients. *Heart & Lung, 11*, 393–398.

Newton, K. M. (1981). Comparison of aortic and brachial cuff pressures in flat supine and lateral recumbent positions. *Heart & Lung, 10*, 821–826.

Polit, D. F., Hungler, B. P., & Bernadette, P. (1987). Nursing research: Principles & methods. Philadelphia: J. B. Lippincott.

Schnapp, L. M., & Cohen, N. H. (1990). Pulse oximetry. Uses and abuses. *Chest, 98*, 1244–1250.

Tittle, M., & Flynn, M. (1997). Correlation of pulse oximetry and co-oximetry. *Dimensions in Critical Care Nursing, 16*(2), 88–95.

Weiss, M. D. (1980). *Biomedical instrumentation*. Philadelphia: Chilton.

West, R. S. (Ed.). (1981). *Using monitors nursing photobook*. Horsham, PA: Intermed Communications.

Woods, S. L., & Mansfield, L. W. (1976). Effect of body position upon pulmonary artery and pulmonary capillary wedge pressures in noncritically ill patients. *Heart & Lung, 5*, 83–90.

Psychosocial Measurement

Magdalena A. Mateo

Psychosocial measurement is the assessment of psychological and sociological variables that influence outcomes. Measurement of patient outcomes is essential for research and practice and can be done through observation (direct or indirect) or self-report (questionnaires, self-rating, and Q-sort). Measurable variables include behavioral changes that occur following participation in educational programs or an intervention, as well as general responses (how a person reacts or feels) to different problem areas. This chapter examines the measurements frequently used in the clinical setting, including observation, interview, and questionnaire. Other assessment tools discussed are scales, diary, Delphi, and projective technique. The chapter also highlights some critical factors that should be considered when making selections from existing tools.

OBSERVATION

Types of Observations

There are different types of observations: direct and indirect, known and unknown, structured and unstructured, scheduled and unscheduled, and complete-observer and participant-observer.

DIRECT VERSUS INDIRECT

Collection of data through direct observation is accomplished as a situation occurs. For example, by observing a patient's return demonstration on self-administration of insulin, the nurse can assess the patient's ability to prepare the injection and the site as well as to administer the medicine. Although it is preferable to observe behavior as situations unfold, there are times when this is not possible. In these instances, the nurse might need to create the event through role-playing. This can be used in situations in which patients must practice certain behaviors, such as assertiveness. The nurse can stage a situation in which the patient practices assertiveness. Afterward, the nurse evaluates the behavior and gives feedback to the patient.

Devices such as closed circuit television and audio and video tapes are used to collect data through indirect observation. Interactions among health care providers, patients, and families can be recorded and replayed later for coding and analysis of content. Group and family therapy sessions are examples of interaction that are often recorded. Other ways of measuring behaviors indirectly include review of records or byproducts of the target behavior (Barlow, Hayes, & Nelson, 1984). For example, by assuming that blood cholesterol levels reflect a person's compliance with changes in eating behavior and exercise, the nurse can assess whether the patient is complying with the diet by testing blood cholesterol level; if the values are lower than those measured before treatment, then the patient has complied.

KNOWN VERSUS UNKNOWN

Although most persons are informed that their behaviors are being observed, there are times when a researcher chooses to examine behaviors without participant awareness. This is done when there is a possibility that awareness might cause alteration in behavior. For example, if the purpose of the study is to observe commonly used suctioning techniques, informing the staff that they are under observation might not give the researcher a true picture of practices in the clinical setting. Staff might alter the usual procedure by using the "ideal" method, particularly when the observer is someone who evaluates their practice.

STRUCTURED VERSUS UNSTRUCTURED

Structured observation means that specific parameters are used for collecting data. In the unstructured method, targeted behaviors are identified and observations are recorded in a descriptive manner rather than by using a checklist. For instance, in observing which role participants assume when they are in a group session, the structured observation evaluates behavior against a checklist that delineates the different roles that a participant can assume, such as (1) leader, (2) silence breaker, (3) scapegoat, or (4) dominant member. In the unstructured method, the general observation guidelines address behaviors manifested by participants and how these behaviors are enacted.

When observing a patient experiencing pain, the nurse uses structured observation if a checklist is used to rate the degree of pain (for example, 0 = no pain, 1 = mild pain, 3 = moderate pain, 4 = severe pain). The nurse uses unstructured observation when collecting data such as the type of behavior that the patient exhibits or what the patient says about the pain experience.

SCHEDULED VERSUS UNSCHEDULED

In unscheduled observation, participants are informed that the event will occur but not when it will occur. This approach is used when role enactment is assessed. Clinical nurse specialist roles as they relate to direct and indirect patient care activities on a given shift are examples of unscheduled observation. The researcher informs the clinical nurse specialist of the plan on the day of observation but not ahead of time. An unscheduled observation increases the possibility of capturing data that represent true daily role enactment.

COMPLETE-OBSERVER VERSUS PARTICIPANT-OBSERVER

Based on the purpose of the study or observation, a nurse can assume a complete-observer or participant-observer role. When a researcher assumes the complete-observer (undetected) role, the person does not participate in the activity and participants are not always aware that observation is occurring. Although this seems ideal for maintaining objectivity of data, there is no opportunity for clarification or confirmation of observations, which can result in incomplete data. When the participant-observer role is assumed by the researcher, however, observation occurs simultaneously with participation. This technique allows the observer to confirm or clarify issues during data collection; however, while doing this, the observer could miss significant participant behaviors. In addition, the observer could have difficulty in deciding when to shift from being participant to observer (Byerly, 1969).

Considerations in the Use of Observation Technique

Observation is valuable and permits the researcher to clarify or confirm data at the time of collection; it is also expensive and time-consuming. Caution must be used when interpreting data, because results are affected by many factors, such as Hawthorne effect, halo effect, observer bias, and differences in rating behaviors. *Hawthorne effect* refers to alteration in participant behavior; participants exhibit outcomes that they believe the researcher expects to see. The *halo effect* occurs when the observer evaluates behavior positively, not because it is good but because the participant exhibits certain likable attributes. When behaviors are not objectively assessed (either because data collectors unknowingly evaluate behaviors based on the desired study outcomes or because they record only selected behaviors), this is called *observer bias* (Polit & Hungler, 1997). Although this can happen with any observer, there is a greater possibility of it's occurring when the researcher collects data.

When several persons are used for data collection, it is important to establish a standard method for observing behaviors and to establish interrater reliability among observers before data collection and at periodic intervals during the course of the study. *Interrater reliability,* also called interobserver or interjudge reliability, is the degree to which two or more independent raters are consistent in observing, recording, or scoring data from a subject (Haller, 1987; Polit & Hungler, 1997).

A commonly used method for determining interrater reliability is to calculate the percentage of agreement between and among raters (Mitchell, 1979; Goodwin & Prescott, 1981). An initial step in establishing interrater reliability is to train observers before data collection (Romanczyk, Kent, Diament, & O'Leary, 1973). Implementing standardized training procedures and a process for evaluating trainers on an ongoing basis are crucial (Castorr et al., 1990). Washington & Moss (1988) identified prag-

➤ Establishing Interrater Reliability: Aspects to Consider

1. Understanding the concept
2. Familiarity with the instrument
3. Use of the tool on at least 10 subjects
4. Observation within a predetermined time period
5. Awareness of interfering variables during observation
6. Scoring and discussion following the observation session
7. Ongoing use of standardized training and process for evaluating rater performance

matic considerations in establishing interrater reliability among observers (see box).

Protection of the rights of individual participants in research is a major ethical concern, particularly when persons are not cognizant of the observation. To obtain consent, subjects should be informed as accurately as possible of the purpose of the study and how the data will be used. Subjects should also be assured that confidentiality of data will be maintained (Levine, 1986). Refer to Chapter 13 for more information on protection of participants in research.

INTERVIEW

Types of Interviews

Interviews can be structured or unstructured, and can occur face-to-face or by telephone (Fox, 1970; Polit & Hungler, 1997). Although individual interviews are common, group interviews in the form of focus groups are used to identify psychosocial issues confronting patients. The telephone interview is often used to readily obtain information for benchmarking efforts. Benchmarking is a process used to compare the performance of an organization with that of similar organizations.

STRUCTURED VERSUS UNSTRUCTURED

A structured format permits the researcher to ask questions in a specific order and assume the same set of responses for all participants. When the unstructured format is used, however, the researcher sets general guidelines to reflect the information that is sought. The questions need not be asked in any specific order and there are no predetermined response sets.

FACE-TO-FACE VERSUS TELEPHONE

Face-to-face interviews imply personal interaction between the interviewer and interviewee. The telephone interview is a commonly used marketing technique for surveying opinions and needs. Telephone interviews can also be used to evaluate care during hospitalization or as a follow-up method for discharged patients.

Considerations in the Use of Interviews

Interviewing is expensive, in both time and money, because of the limited number of respondents that can be reached. To decide whether the interview is the best way to obtain information, the researcher should determine whether the respondents could provide the same information if the questions were mailed to them (Fox, 1970).

If the interview is the option for data collection, the second decision is whether the face-to-face method should be used. Although face-to-face interviews allow the researcher to evaluate a response and alter the line of questioning to obtain the desired level of response, the personal interaction can hinder some responses. Participants can be influenced by the interviewer's personal characteristics or by the way that the interview is conducted. It is, therefore, necessary to establish interview guidelines to minimize bias when gathering data. This can be accomplished through interviewer training programs, which usually consist of the following components: (1) education about the purpose of the study, the questionnaire or data form, recording of responses, and confidentiality; (2) guidelines for interviewing techniques; and (3) practice sessions that include observations of model persons and provision for feedback (Spool, 1978; Collins, Given, Given, & King, 1988). Another factor that influences response is how the interviewer handles the clinician-researcher role conflict (Clinton et al., 1986; Fowler, 1988). Nurses constantly assess patient needs and

intervene; therefore, it is possible that when clinicians interview research participants, they could unknowingly intervene during the interview, thereby prolonging the interview or observation time.

Differences were reported between clinical and research interviews using the five requisites of goals, questions, rapport building, elaboration, and interpretation (Collins, Given, Given, & King, 1988). Goals for clinical interviews are for assessment or intervention purposes, whereas research interviews are for data collection. When clinical interviews are conducted, rapport is established through empathic listening and reflection. When research interviews are conducted, rapport is established by reinforcing acceptable performance through feedback and by role modeling. Questions used in clinical interviews are individualized, elaboration of response is encouraged, and data are interpreted and summarized by the clinician. In contrast, questions used in research interviews are uniform, elaboration is discouraged by selected response choices and specific probes, and responses are recorded with few inferences drawn.

The advantages and disadvantages of telephone interviews for data collection have been reported by Hash, Donlea, & Walljasper (1985). They used telephone survey methods to assess the educational needs of nurses. Interrater reliability among data collectors was established and monitored throughout the project. Training sessions were held to inform volunteers of the telephone interview technique and to standardize the interview process. The advantages cited were (1) lower cost, (2) efficiency of collecting data (3 to 30 calls per hour from a wide geographical sample), (3) ability to immediately respond to questions, (4) low refusal rate, and (5) reduction of interviewer bias. Disadvantages cited were (1) difficulty in detecting misinformation, (2) difficulty in obtaining current telephone numbers, and (3) limited ability to collect additional information.

QUESTIONNAIRE

The questionnaire is a paper-and-pencil approach used to collect data. Participants are asked to respond to a set of printed questions. This data collection technique can be used to collect demographic information (age, sex, educational level, and income) and opinions.

Types of Questionnaires

Based on the types of questions and responses, questionnaires can be open-ended or closed-ended (fixed). Open-ended questions require respondents to complete or explain a statement, whereas closed-ended (fixed-response) questions require participants to choose responses from predetermined choices.

Considerations in the Use of Questionnaires

Questionnaires allow researchers to obtain information from a large number of persons within a relatively short time. This goal is accomplished when issues relative to questionnaire development, participant response bias, and response rates are addressed during the planning phase of a project. Refer to Chapter 19 for a detailed discussion on these important issues.

OTHER TYPES

Scales

There are several types of scales: rating, Likert, rank-order, Q-sort, semantic differential, and paired-comparisons scales. *Rating scales* are used to measure the way a person assigns order to concepts (Fox, 1970). For example, if the researcher wants to find out the degree of importance that employees place on factors associated with job satisfaction, a scale ranging from most important to least important can be used to categorize salary, benefits, or autonomy.

Likert scales are used to determine opinions. The tool comprises a list of declarative statements. Across each statement are numerical values, usually ranging from 1 to 5 (1 = strongly disagree, 2 = disagree, 3 = undecided, 4 = agree, 5 = strongly agree). An example of a Likert scale item is shown in the box.

When using a *rank-order scale*, the researcher asks the person to indicate the degree of importance of certain concepts. For

➤ Example of a Likert Scale Item

	Strongly Disagree				Strongly Agree
Families of patients should be permitted to visit critically ill patients at any time.	1	2	3	4	5

example, the person can be asked to rank five items (time off, work schedule, salary, fringe benefits, and unit assignment) according to the degree of importance (1 = most important, 5 = least important).

The *Q-sort* is an adaptation of the rank-order scale in which the respondent sorts a set of cards into a specified number of piles according to the importance of the statement or word printed on each card (Fox, 1970; Burns & Grove, 1997). Each pile can have only a certain number of cards. For example, the researcher identifies 50 statements that reflect nurse caring behaviors as perceived by patients. Seven piles are designated for sorting cards. The respondent reads the statement on each card and places the card on one of the seven piles. The decision of where to place a card depends on how important the respondent believes the statement to be (see box).

➤ Example of Card Piles and Number of Cards for Q-Sort

Pile Number	Category	Number of Cards
1	Most important	1
2	Next most important	7
3	Less important	10
4	Neither important nor unimportant	14
5	Less unimportant	10
6	Next least important	7
7	Least important	1

➤ Example of Semantic Differential Scale Items

Women				
beautiful _____/ _____/ _____/ _____/ _____/ ugly				
bright _____/ _____/ _____/ _____/ _____/ dull				
anxious _____/ _____/ _____/ _____/ _____/ calm				

Semantic differential scales, which consist of a list of opposite adjectives, are used to measure attitudes or beliefs (Osgood, Suci, & Tannenbaum, 1957). Using a seven-point scale, participants indicate the point on the scale that best describes their views of the concept (see box).

Items of *paired-comparisons scales* are lists of words or phrases. Respondents are asked to circle the letter of the item or statement that is more important to them (Fox, 1970). To eliminate the biasing effect of ordering items, each item is listed twice in the tool, and the order of items is reversed. Although this is ideal, the length of the questionnaire can be cumbersome. An alternative method is to list only selected items twice (see box).

➤ Paired-Comparisons Scale Items Example

Two causes of noncompliance by patients are listed for each item below. Circle the letter of the cause that you believe is more important. Judge each pair separately.

Item 1:
a) Instructions for taking medicine are unclear.
b) Importance of taking medicine is unclear.

Item 2:
a) Wait at doctor's office is too long.
b) No available transportation.

Item 33:
a) Importance of taking medicine is unclear.
b) Instructions for taking medicine are unclear.

Item 50:
a) No available transportation.
b) Wait at doctor's office is too long.

Diary

When information about incidents or behaviors must be recorded over a period of time, persons are sometimes asked to self-record their data on an ongoing basis in a diary format (Barlow, Hayes, & Nelson, 1984; Richardson, 1994). The diary is useful for eliciting experiences related to patient condition. Data can be used as a basis for semistructured interviews for describing a phenomenon (Faithfull, 1992). Diaries can be arranged in different ways. One arrangement is to list behaviors or symptoms the person should be tracking and then have the person respond to the list (see box).

Although the diary can provide more accurate information because persons record the occurrence of events immediately after they happen instead of relying on memory, an increasing awareness can occur and this might trigger some behavioral change in the person. If the purpose of collecting data is to obtain the frequency of a symptom, then more information might be needed to explain changes that are noted. Because the diary can be used to collect data for research, the advantages and disadvantages of its use should be considered (Woods,

➤ Example of a Diary Format

Name: _____
Date: _____
Occurrence of chest pain
Time: _____
Activity before chest pain was felt: _____
The chest pain was:
Mild   _____
Discomforting   _____
Distressing   _____
Excruciating   _____

1981). When using the diary format for research purposes, the data entered permit a retrospective analysis of the sequence of events. On the one hand, this is a distinct advantage when the goal of the study is to determine factors associated with occurrence of symptoms. On the other hand, there are several disadvantages to using the diary for research including the following: (1) it is time-consuming to orient the patient to the diary format, (2) persons who cannot read or write are ineligible to participate, (3) the researcher cannot probe or clarify responses, (4) data analysis is time-consuming, and (5) individual differences in recording data could alter results.

Delphi Technique

The Delphi technique for collecting data seeks expert opinion on specific issues at different times. This is done by distributing successive sets of questionnaires to participants throughout the process. Although two to four rounds of questionnaires are usually distributed, as many as 25 rounds have been reported on (Couper, 1984). Priorities and forecasts are drawn based on responses from the questionnaires.

Administrators in hospitals and schools of nursing were asked through the Delphi technique about the types of research in progress at their institutions and about the sources of funding for those projects (Henry, O'Donnell, Pendergast, Moody, & Hutchinson, 1988). Questionnaires were sent to 432 university hospitals and 129 schools of nursing with graduate programs. As a result of the feedback, the following research priority themes were generated: cost containment, cost of nursing; prospective reimbursement, diagnostic related groups; personnel mix; evaluation of care and programs; nursing care models, interventions; staffing and scheduling; nursing productivity and accountability; environmental and organizational contexts; nursing department structure; and nurse administrator characteristics.

Researchers have modified the Delphi technique for purposes for which it is used. Crisp, Pelletier, Duffield, Adams, & Nagy (1997) reported three modifications of the Delphi technique and ways in which the Delphi method can vary. The three modifications of the Delphi are Classical, Policy, and Decision Delphi methods. In the Classical Delphi—a forum for facts—the investigator asks an unbiased panel of experts to use facts to predict future events (Rauch, 1979). The Policy Delphi—forum for ideas—is used with a panel of lobbyists to define and differentiate views (Rauch, 1979). In the Decision Delphi—a forum for decisions—panel members are not anonymous, and prepared and supported decisions are the outcomes.

Components in which the Delphi method may vary are as follows:

1. Consensus may not be related to general agreement.
2. There are reportedly low levels of reliability and validity.
3. If expertise is needed, the notion of expert and use of one or more panels may vary.
4. The number of rounds (at least two) and the quantity and quality of feedback vary.
5. The role of the researcher and the researcher's objectivity vary.
6. Anonymity of respondents varies.

For further explanation of the Delphi technique, refer to textbooks on measurements.

Projective Technique

Projective techniques are used in assessing a person's underlying motives, needs, desires, attitudes, values, and personality characteristics (Waltz, Strickland, & Lenz, 1991). Persons are asked to respond to ambiguous and unstructured situations, such as sketches, words, pictures, or drawings. Types of projective tests include the Rorschach Inkblot Test, Word Association, Machover's Draw-A-Person Test, sentence completion, play techniques, and role-playing.

Usually, these techniques are used when direct methods of collecting data are unlikely. The use of projective techniques in nursing research is limited because specific skills in psychology and psychiatry are needed to administer the tests and properly interpret the results. For information on the procedures, use, reliability and validity, and special considerations, the reader is referred to *Measurement in Nursing Research* (Waltz, Strickland, & Lenz, 1991).

FACTORS ASSOCIATED WITH SELECTION OF EXISTING INSTRUMENTS

Several factors must be considered when selecting an instrument (Table 21–1).

Does the Instrument Measure the Concept Being Examined?

First, will the instrument measure the *concept being examined*? If the purpose of the study is to determine whether patients are anxious, the researcher should look for an existing tool that has been developed for that purpose. Although the reason for developing a tool does not have to be identical to the reason for the researcher's study, the tool's definition of anxiety should be comparable to that used in the study. For example, if the goal of the researcher is to find out whether patients are anxious before a procedure, a tool measuring a temporary state of anxiety should be used. If the researcher's goal is to determine whether a person is anxious most of the time, however, a tool measuring individual anxiety trait should be used.

What Are the Psychometric Properties of the Instrument?

The second factor that should be considered when selecting an instrument is the psycho-

Table 21–1 ···

Factors to Consider When Selecting an Instrument

Does the instrument measure the concept being examined?
What are the psychometric properties of the instrument?
  Reliability
    Stability
    Equivalence
    Homogeneity
  Validity
    Content validity
    Criterion-related validity
    Construct validity
Is the instrument feasible?
  Instrument availability
  Costs of data collection tools
  Nature of the study sample

metric properties of that instrument. Two basic *psychometric characteristics* that instruments must have are reliability and validity.

RELIABILITY

Reliability is a basic characteristic for an instrument when it is used for collecting accurate, stable, and usable research data. The reliability of a tool is the degree of consistency with which it measures the attribute under investigation (Polit & Hungler, 1995). This is usually reported as a reliability coefficient. The reliability coefficient is determined by the proportion of true variability (attributed to true differences among respondents) to the total obtained variability (attributed to the result of true differences among respondents and differences related to other factors). The researcher takes a chance that data will not reflect true changes in the concept being measured when instruments with reliability estimates of .60 or lower are used.

Three aspects should be considered when determining the reliability of instruments: (1) stability, (2) equivalence, and (3) homogeneity (Burns & Grove, 1997). The *stability* of a tool refers to its ability to consistently measure the phenomenon being studied; this is determined through test-retest reliability. The tool is administered to the same persons on two separate occasions. Scores of the two sets of data are then compared and the correlation is derived. The recommended interval between testing times is 2 to 4 weeks (Burns & Grove, 1997). The time that must lapse between the two points of measurements is important. It should be long enough so that respondents do not remember their answers on the first test, yet not so long that change can take place (Fox, 1970). Interpretation of the test-retest correlation coefficient should be done with caution, because it might not represent the stability of the instrument; rather, it could indicate that change has occurred. For example, change can occur when determining attitudes of nurses toward work schedules, if, for instance, persons who responded to the first test have since gained seniority and are working their preferred shifts. In this case, the second test might be more positive, and the correlation coefficient obtained when the two sets of scores are compared then would represent a change rather than a measure of the stability of the tool.

Equivalence should be determined when two versions of the same tool are used to measure a concept (alternative forms) or when two or more persons are asked to rate the same event or the behavior of another person (interrater reliability). In alternative-form reliability, two versions of the same instrument are developed and administered. The scores obtained from the two tools should be comparable. It is helpful for the researcher to know whether a published instrument has alternative forms; when there is, a decision must be made on which form to use. For example, the Beck Depression test has a long and a short form (Beck, 1978). The researcher might decide to use the short form to test patients with short attention spans or low energy levels. Establishing interrater reliability is important when two or more observers are used for collecting data. Considerations relating to this type of reliability have already been discussed.

The *homogeneity* of an instrument is determined by calculating its split-half reliability, which is obtained by testing a group once. The questionnaire is divided into two halves. Items included in the two sections must be comparable. Responses are tallied in such a way that two sets of scores are acquired from each respondent. The scores are compared and a coefficient correlation is obtained. Another way of determining the homogeneity of an instrument is to use the internal consistency method (to determine whether each item measures the same thing). Internal consistency reliability estimates are calculated by obtaining the Cronbach's alpha coefficient or by using the Kuder-Richardson formula, both of which are described in measurement textbooks.

VALIDITY

It is not sufficient for a tool to be only reliable; it must also have validity. *Validity* is the degree to which a tool measures what it is supposed to measure (Polit & Hungler, 1995). The three types of validity are content, criterion-related, and construct. *Content validity* relates to an instrument's adequacy in covering all concepts pertaining to the phenomena being studied. If the purpose of the tool is to learn whether the patient is complying with a low-sodium diet,

the questions should include a list of all foods that have a high-sodium content. Content experts are vital in the development of valid and reliable tools. Grant and Davis (1997) suggested the use of several criteria in identifying experts. These include publications in refereed journals, research in the phenomenon of interest, clinical expertise, and familiarity with the dimensions being measured. They also suggested the importance of instrument review by a number of subjects from the target population because of their experience.

Criterion-related validity, which could be either predictive or concurrent, measures the extent to which a tool is related to other criteria. Predictive validity is the adequacy of the tool to estimate the individual performance or behavior in the future. For example, if a tool was developed to measure clinical competence of nurses, persons responding to the tool could also be asked the number of medication errors (an objective criterion for clinical competence) they have made. If results indicate that there is a high coefficient correlation (.90), it means that the clinical competence scale can be used to predict the incidence of medication errors. Concurrent validity is the ability of a tool to differentiate the respondent's status at a given time by comparing the result obtained to a criterion. For example, when a patient is asked to complete a questionnaire to determine the presence of anxiety, results of the test can be compared to the nurse's rating of the patient's behavior.

Construct validity is concerned with the ability of the instrument to adequately measure the underlying concept. With this validity, the researcher's concern relates to whether the scores represent the degree to which a person possesses a trait.

Is the Instrument Feasible?

Feasibility is the third factor taken into account in the selection of data collection instruments. Considerations in determining feasibility include (1) availability of the instrument to the researcher, (2) costs, and (3) the nature of the study sample.

Instrument availability indicates whether the researcher obtains permission to use the instrument. Permission can be obtained by writing the author of the instrument or by purchasing a copy of the tool from the pub-

Table 21–2

Standardized Instrument Selection Process

Initial Considerations

What is the purpose?
What is the intended sample?
What is to be measured?
How widely used is the instrument?
Is the manual well written and comprehensive?

Psychometric Considerations

Is reliability acceptable?
Is validity acceptable?

Administration, Scoring, Interpretability

Are administration directions clear?
Are scoring directions and process clear?
Is computerized scoring available?
Is score interpretation clear and compatible with the research question and clinical practice?
Are guidelines offered for clinical feedback? (if appropriate)

Practical Considerations

What are the costs and benefits of use?
Does the instrument make an independent contribution to the assessment or outcome battery?
Are adequate staff, financial, and equipment resources available to use the instrument properly?
What level of staff expertise and training is necessary?

From Meyer, E. C., Edwards, G. H., & Rossi, J. S. (1995). Evaluation and selection of standardized psychological instruments for research and clinical practice. Journal of Child and Adolescent Psychiatric Nursing, 8(3), 24–31.

lishing company. Some organizations require researchers to possess certain qualifications (such as an educational degree, experience in testing, or professional licensure) before granting permission. The Rorschach Inkblot test is an example of a projective test for which credentials are required.

Costs of data collection tools include purchasing the tools and the manual, copying the instruments, and the costs associated with administering, scoring, and interpreting the responses. The manual usually gives information on reliability and validity estimates, a bibliography of studies in which the tool has been used, how the items were developed, and instructions for administering and scoring.

The *nature of the study sample* is an important consideration in choosing a data collection tool. For instance, when assessing pain in patients after surgery, a lengthy interview on the day after surgery could be difficult for patients taking narcotics for pain relief because patients are drowsy or uncomfortable. It is important to consider the challenges that the increasing population of non–English-speaking people presents in using existing instruments. Translation and adaptation of the tool to ensure equivalence of meaning, pilot testing of the translated version, familiarity of respondents to the method (for example, Likert scale) are challenges that confront researchers. It is also important to determine the best way to administer a tool. For example, Bernal, Wooley, and Schensul (1997) reported using visual aids and trained bilingual interviewers to administer a translated Likert-type scale—Insulin Management Diabetes Self-efficacy scale, a self-administered paper-pencil test—to low-literate ethnic Spanish-speaking populations in order to ensure respondents' understanding of test items.

A standardized instrument selection process is listed in Table 21–2.

SUMMARY

Various tools and methods used to assess outcomes of nursing interventions are also used in research. Although the reasons for using assessment tools in practice or research differ, the goal of obtaining valid measurements remains the same. Consequently, care must be taken to ensure that the purpose for which the tool or method was designed is congruent with the concept being measured or examined. Results must be reliable and valid. Appropriate methods for gathering data are the foundation for all accurate and usable information in research and practice.

REFERENCES

Barlow, D. H., Hayes, S. C., & Nelson, R. O. (1984). *The scientist practitioner: Research and accountability in clinical and educational settings.* New York: Pergamon.

Beck, A. T. (1978). *Beck Depression Inventory.* San Antonio: Psychological Corporation.

Bernal, H., Wooley, S., & Schensul, J. J. (1997). The

challenge of using Likert-type scales with low-literate ethnic populations. *Nursing Research, 46,* 179–181.

Burns, N., & Grove, S. K. (1997). *The practice of nursing research: Conduct, critique and utilization* (3rd ed.). Philadelphia: W. B. Saunders.

Byerly, E. L. (1969). The nurse researcher as participant-observer in a nursing setting. *Nursing Research, 18,* 230–236.

Castorr, A. H., Thompson, K. O., Ryan, J. W., Phillips, C. Y., Prescott, P. A., & Soeken, K. L. (1990). The process of rater training for observational instruments: Implications for interrater reliability. *Research in Nursing & Health, 13,* 311–318.

Clinton, J., Beck, R., Radjenovic, D., Taylor, L., Westlake, S., & Wilson, S. E. (1986). Time-series designs in clinical nursing research: Human issues. *Nursing Research, 35,* 188–191.

Collins, C., Given, B., Given, C. W., & King, S. (1988). Interviewer training and supervision. *Nursing Research, 37,* 122–124.

Couper, M. R. (1984). The Delphi technique: Characteristics and sequence model. *Advances in Nursing Science, 7*(1), 72–77.

Crisp, J., Pelletier, P., Duffield, C., Adams, A., & Nagy, S. (1997). The Delphi method. *Nursing Research, 46,* 116–118.

Faithfull, S. (1992). The diary method for nursing research: A study of somnolence syndrome. *European Journal of Cancer Care, 1*(2), 13–8.

Fowler, M. D. M. (1988). Ethical issues in nursing research: Issues in qualitative research. *Western Journal of Nursing Research, 10,* 109–111.

Fox, D. J. (1970). *Fundamentals of research in nursing* (2nd ed.). New York: Appleton-Century-Crofts.

Goodwin, L. D., & Prescott, P. A. (1981). Issues and approaches to estimating interrater reliability in nursing research. *Research in Nursing and Health, 4,* 323–337.

Grant, J. S., & Davis, L. L. (1997). Selection and use of content experts for instrument development. *Research in Nursing and Health, 20,* 269–274.

Haller, K. B. (1987). Interrater reliability: Essential for research and practice. *MCN: The American Journal of Maternal/Child Nursing, 12,* 78.

Hash, V., Donlea, J., & Walljasper D. (1985). The telephone survey: A procedure for assessing educational needs of nurses. *Nursing Research, 34,* 126–128.

Henry, B., O'Donnell, J. F., Pendergast, J. F., Moody, L. E., & Hutchinson, S. A. (1988). Nursing administration research in hospitals and schools of nursing. *Journal of Nursing Administration, 18*(2), 28–31.

Levine, R. J. (1986). *Ethics and regulation of clinical research* (2nd ed). Baltimore: Urban & Schwarzenberg.

Mitchell, S. K. (1979). Interobserver agreement, reliability, and generalizability of data collected in observational studies. *Psychological Bulletin, 86,* 376–390.

Osgood, C. E., Suci, G. J., & Tannenbaum, P. H. (1957). *The measurement of meaning.* Urbana, IL: University of Illinois.

Polit, D. F., & Hungler, B. P. (1995). *Nursing research: Principles and methods* (5th ed). Philadelphia: J. B. Lippincott.

Polit, D. F., & Hungler, B. P. (1997). *Essentials of nursing research: Methods, appraisal, and utilization* (4th ed). Philadelphia: J. B. Lippincott.

Rauch, W. (1979). The decision Delphi. *Technological Forecasting and Social Change, 15,* 159–169.

Richardson, A. (1994). The health diary: An examination of its use as a data collection method. *Journal of Advanced Nursing, 19,* 782–791.

Romanczyk, R. G., Kent, R. N., Diament, C., & O'Leary, K. D. (1973). Measuring the reliability of observational data: A reactive process. *Journal of Applied Behavioral Analysis, 6,* 175.

Spool, M. D. (1978). Training programs for observers of behavior: A review. *Personnel Psychology, 31,* 853–888.

Waltz, C. F., Strickland, O. L., & Lenz, E. R. (1991). *Measurement in nursing research* (2nd ed.). Philadelphia: F. A. Davis.

Washington, C. C., & Moss, M. (1988). Pragmatic aspects of establishing interrater reliability in research. *Nursing Research, 37,* 190–191.

Woods, N. F. (1981). The health diary as an instrument for nursing research: Problems and promise. *Western Journal of Nursing Research, 3,* 76–92.

SUGGESTED READINGS

Baker, C. M. (1985). Maximizing mailed questionnaire responses. *Image: Journal of Nursing Scholarship, 17,* 118–121.

Brinberg, D., & McGrath, J. E. (1985). *Validity and the research process.* Beverly Hills, CA: Sage.

Carmines, E. G., & Zeller, R. A. (1979). *Reliability and validity assessment.* Beverly Hills, CA: Sage.

Couch, A., & Keniston, K. (1960). Yeasayers and naysayers: Agreeing response set as a personality variable. *Journal of Abnormal and Social Psychology, 60,* 151–174.

Cronbach, L. J., & Meehl, P. E. (1955). Construct validity in psychological tests. *Psychological Bulletin, 52,* 281–302.

Fox, R. N., & Ventura, M. R. (1983). Small-scale administration of instruments and procedures. *Nursing Research, 32,* 122–125.

Frank-Stromborg, M. & Olsen, S. (1997). *Instruments for clinical health-care research* (2nd ed.). Sudbury, MA: Jones and Bartlett.

Garvin, B. J., Kennedy, C. W., & Cissna, K. N. (1988). Reliability in category coding systems. *Nursing Research, 37,* 52–55.

Hilbert, G. A. (1985). Accuracy of self-reported measures of compliance. *Nursing Research, 34,* 319–320.

Kirk, J., & Miller, M. L. (1986). *Reliability and validity in qualitative research.* Beverly Hills, CA: Sage.

Knapp, T. R. (1985). Validity, reliability, and neither. *Nursing Research, 34,* 189–192.

Knapp, T. R., & Brown, J. K. (1995). Ten measurement commandments that often should be broken. *Research in Nursing & Health, 18,* 465–469.

Linsky, A. S. (1975). Stimulating responses to mailed questionnaires: A review. *Public Opinion Quarterly, 39,* 82–101.

Lynn, M. R. (1985). Reliability estimates: Use and disuse. *Nursing Research, 34,* 254–256.

Lynn, M. R. (1986). Determination and quantification of content validity. *Nursing Research, 35,* 382–385.

Murphy, C. A. (1993). Increasing the response rates of reluctant professionals to mail surveys. *Applied Nursing Research, 6,* 137–141.

Rew, L., Stuppy, D., & Becker, H. (1988). Construct

validity in instrument development: A vital link between nursing practice, research, and theory. *Advances in Nursing Science, 10*(4), 10–22.

Reynolds, C. L. (1988). The measurement of health in nursing research. *Advances in Nursing Science, 10*(4), 23–31.

Stokes, S. A., & Gordon, S. E. (1988). Development of an instrument to measure stress in the older adult. *Nursing Research, 37,* 16–19.

Tetting, D. W. (1988). Q-Sort update. *Western Journal of Nursing Research, 10,* 757–765.

Topf, M. (1986). Three estimates of interrater reliability for nominal data. *Nursing Research, 35,* 253–255.

Topf, M. (1986). Response sets in questionnaire research. *Nursing Research, 35,* 119–121.

Ventura, M. R., & Waligora-Serafin, B. (1981). Setting priorities for nursing research. *Journal of Nursing Administration, 11*(6), 30–34.

Woolley, A. S. (1984). Questioning the mailed questionnaire as a valid instrument for research in nursing education. *IMAGE: Journal of Nursing Scholarship, 16,* 115–119.

Selecting a Design for the Study

Susan L. Beck

The design of a research study is the glue that bonds the research questions or hypotheses to the research results. Thus, selecting an appropriate design is critical to the investigator's ability to answer the research questions. This chapter defines, dissects, and thoroughly discusses the issues to be considered in research design. Design is distinguished from other commonly used research terms (method and methodology) with which it is often confused. Specific types of design are described and exemplified. Finally, considerations to strengthen the validity and feasibility of the design are addressed.

WHAT IS DESIGN?

Research design is the plan, structure, and strategy of an investigation. It is important to distinguish design from method and methodology—concepts that are often mistakenly substituted for design.

The *method* of a study is the totality of how the study will be carried out. Design is a part of the method, but also included in method are sample, setting, instruments, intervention, procedure, and data analysis. By way of analogy, design might be considered a blueprint, whereas the method is a detailed photograph of the study.

Methodology refers to the study of method and can include research on any of the components of method including design, sample, and instruments. Methodological describes a specific type of design—one used to investigate all or part of a research method.

The research design is a blueprint specifically created to answer the research question and to control variance (Kerlinger, 1986). Control of variance involves taking into account all of the factors that might systematically contribute to individual differences in outcomes and affect the researcher's ability to answer the question at hand. An investigator must therefore consider many factors in designing a study—particularly in the clinical setting. Careful design requires that the researcher step back and ask, "What is the context of this study? What else is occurring that might influence the results?" By answering these questions, the researcher can attempt to design the study to control the effects of the multitude of factors that might confound the results.

Control of variance is a particular challenge in the clinical setting. Patients, families, and hospital staff do not always act or respond as the researcher might expect. What seems like a good idea might be impossible in the real world of a busy patient care unit or clinic. Soliciting the ideas of those involved in the actual clinical setting is essential in the design stage of proposal development. Modifications in design can be made that will increase the feasibility that the study can be implemented. Moreover, key members from the clinical setting become invested in the research at an early stage, when their ideas can be incorporated into the study design. Such collaboration pays off 100-fold as the study is implemented.

ELEMENTS OF DESIGN

Designing a study requires decision making—a task that is sometimes formidable when there appears to be no right solution but only alternatives with their respective advantages and disadvantages. The researcher must identify and operationalize the types and levels of variables and make some important design decisions. These decision points include the following:

1. Deciding how many and which type of subjects to include
2. Selecting and assigning subjects to one or more groups
3. Deciding how many and what type of observations are needed
4. Specifying how many data collection points there will be

The relationship among these elements is represented in the study design, which summarizes the strategy for enacting the study.

Types and Levels of Variables

A variable, as the name implies, is a concept that varies (Polit & Hungler, 1996). Variables can be continuous in nature, for example temperature or weight, or can belong to discrete categories, such as sex or race. Several types of variables may be included in a study: independent, dependent, intervening, preexisting, and extraneous. Each type of variable is discussed in relation to the research design.

The *independent variable* is the experimental condition or event—the presumed cause; the *dependent variable* is the outcome—the presumed effect. In a classical experiment, the independent variable is one that is controlled or manipulated by the investigator in order to evaluate a response, the dependent variable. For example, a study of the effect of method of patient education (the independent variable) on knowledge about self-care behaviors (the dependent variable) might be designed to manipulate the method of patient teaching—a videotape and a self-learning module. The same distinction is used to differentiate variables in nonexperimental studies in which the independent variable is not manipulated. For example, in a study of the effects of age (independent variable) on beliefs about sexually transmitted diseases (the dependent variable), age would not be manipulated per se, but measured so as to assess its influence on the outcome.

Intervening variables occur between the independent and dependent variable. For example, in a study of the effect of the La-Maze method on pain during labor, level of anxiety may be an intervening variable that exerts an influence on the outcome.

Confounding variables are the numerous factors other than the independent variable that might be exerting an influence on the dependent variable (Kirk-Smith, 1996). Such confounding variables could include antecedent, attribute, demographic, or *preexisting variables* such as gender, education, and income, as well as *extraneous variables*, alternative factors that might be contributing to the response. For example, in a study of the effects of progressive muscle relaxation on nausea, it would be important to consider gender as well as the use of antiemetics, which could confound the results. The aim is to minimize the effects of possible confounding variables and maximize the effect of the independent variable.

Design Decisions

In designing the study, decisions must be made as to the number of groups to be studied and the number of observations to be made. Is it appropriate to study one group or does the research question indicate comparing two or more groups? Are observations at one point in time sufficient or is it necessary to compare a prescore to a postscore or to assess trends over time? As these questions are answered, the building blocks of the research design are identified.

The perspective of the study in regard to time must also be considered. In a *retrospective* study, the time perspective is toward the past and the focus is on data that already exist. An example of such a study might be a review of charts from the past 6 months to evaluate patient teaching as evidenced in documentation. A *prospective* study looks to the future and allows for planning and controlling when and what data are collected. It also allows better control over the manipulated or independent variable.

The next set of decisions influences the ability of the study to minimize the effect of possible confounding variables. One simple way is to eliminate the variable from the sample. For example, if the sex of the subjects might influence the results, the study can be designed to include members of only one gender. A second approach is to randomly assign subjects to treatment groups; with a large enough sample, the researcher can assume that the effects of the confounding variables are approximately equally distributed among the groups. Alternatively, the groups can be matched or blocked (divided) on a particular variable such as sex, age, or level of anxiety. The ultimate form of matching is in a study in which each subject is his or her own control and receives all treatments. This design allows control of all preexisting variables and numerous extraneous variables if they remain constant over time (Beck, 1989). Finally, confounding variables can simply be measured and their influence can be evaluated in the analysis of the study.

Illustrating the Design

Just as a blueprint is useful in guiding the construction of a building, a graphic illustration of a research design can clarify the relationships between the elements. Several approaches to illustration are commonly used. In the X and O model (Fig. 22–1), X represents the independent variable and O represents the dependent variable or observation point. In a more complex model with multiple factors, a matrix (Fig. 22–2) is often useful to visualize the dimensions of the study. Finally, a causal model (Fig. 22–3)

Parallel Group Design (True Experimental Design)

O X O

Randomize

O   O

Self-Controlled Design (One-Group Pretest-Posttest Design)

O X O

Crossover Design (Counterbalanced Design)

OX₁OX₂O

Randomize

OX₂OX₁O

O = Observation   X = Treatment

Figure 22–1
Examples of X and O model of research design.

can represent multiple, interrelated variables.

TYPES OF DESIGNS

Research designs are best conceptualized on a continuum (Fig. 22–4) that represents a number of design options that parallel the extent of knowledge about a particular topic. When little is known, it is necessary to begin by asking the question "What is this?" The main purpose of this type of study is to describe phenomena of interest. On the other end of the continuum are experimental studies, designed to test hypotheses about the cause and effect relationships between phenomena. Experiments are designed to ask "To what extent does variable A cause factor B?" Research aimed at assessing causal relationships requires more control of variance to minimize the effects of confounding factors, which might challenge the validity of the cause-and-effect relationship. In between these extremes are designs that search for relationships and that evaluate the strengths of associations between variables (Diers, 1979).

Qualitative Versus Quantitative

It is a common but mistaken notion to classify designs as qualitative or quantitative. These terms more accurately describe research paradigms, approaches, or ways of thinking about research (Cook & Reichardt, 1979). In the qualitative paradigm, the ap-

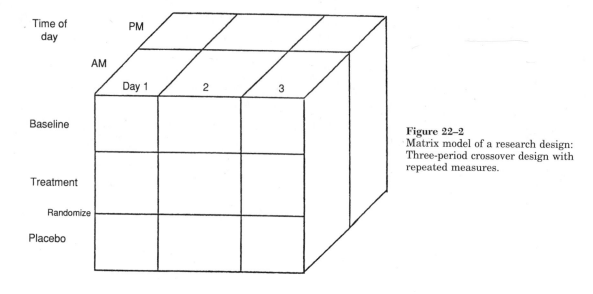

Figure 22–2
Matrix model of a research design: Three-period crossover design with repeated measures.

proach is descriptive, subjective, and naturalistic, whereas the quantitative paradigm seeks facts or causes in a more objective and controlled way.

In a concrete sense, these terms distinguish types of data. Qualitative data consist of words; quantitative data consist of numbers. Although research on the descriptive end of the continuum is more likely to gather qualitative data and vice versa; these distinctions are not absolute. Descriptive research may gather qualitative data, quantitative data, or both; experimental studies sometimes add a qualitative component to the quantitative data of the experiment. For example, a study of patterns of weight in patients receiving interleukins would rely on numerical variables, whereas an investigation of the effectiveness of music therapy on pain might elicit verbal descriptions of the effect. The most important point is that the type of design and the type of data collected must be in concert with the knowledge that is desired.

Specific Types of Designs

Within the continuum of research design lie numerous possibilities; some designs have been described and labeled and others may be unique to a particular study. There is no universal standard for categorizing designs (Burns & Grove, 1997). For simplicity, specific designs can be classified by purpose into four classes: descriptive, correlational, experimental, and methodological.

DESCRIPTIVE DESIGNS

Descriptive designs are used when the primary purpose of a study is to name, char-

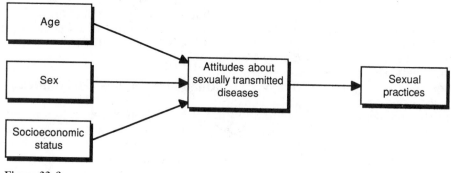

Figure 22–3
Example of a causal model.

Less Knowledge------------------More Knowledge
(about topic)   (about topic)

DESCRIPTIVE _____ **EXPERIMENTAL**

Low Control----------------------High Control
(of variables)   (of variables)

Figure 22–4
The design continuum.

acterize, or thoroughly describe a phenomenon. When little is known and the question of concern is "What is this?", a descriptive study may be termed *exploratory*. In a descriptive design, there is not a designated independent variable but there may be multiple outcomes or dependent variables. Numerous methods can be used to collect data ranging from observation and physiological monitoring to interviews and questionnaires. For example, Hinds and Martin (1988) used a descriptive design to explore adolescents' perceptions of how they helped themselves achieve hopefulness during their cancer experience. Guided by the grounded theory method (Glaser & Strauss, 1967), they used interviews, observations, and reviews of medical records to gather data for the study.

CORRELATIONAL DESIGNS

Correlational designs are used when the purpose of a study is to evaluate the significance of the relationship between or among variables. This type of study most often includes multiple dependent variables; however, an independent variable may be designated if it is thought to predict or influence another variable. In the latter case, the study may be described as *predictive* or *explanatory*. For example, Gass and Chang (1989) used an explanatory type of correlational design to evaluate the influence of individual and situational factors on stress appraisal, coping, and psychosocial health dysfunction in widows and widowers. They used a variety of instruments to operationalize and measure the variables of concern.

EXPERIMENTAL DESIGNS

Experimental designs refer to a class of investigations that test hypotheses about cause-and-effect relationships. There are three essential conditions of a true experi-

ment: (1) there is an independent variable that is manipulated by the investigator who then observes dependent variables for effect, (2) a control group is used for comparison, and (3) the researcher has the ability to randomly assign patients to either the experimental or the control condition. For example, Munro et al. (1988) randomly assigned postmyocardial infarction patients to an experimental (relaxation technique) or control (time/attention) intervention. They measured the effects of the interventions on both physical and psychosocial variables.

When it is not possible to meet all of these conditions, a design is considered to be *quasi-experimental*. Most often, quasi-experiments do not use random assignment to allocate subjects to comparative treatment groups (Johnson, Ottenbacher, & Reichardt, 1995). For example, in a study of the impact of a new oral care protocol on stomatitis, Beck (1979) used a pretest, posttest design. The oral status (dependent variable) of all patients receiving chemotherapy was assessed, a systematic protocol (independent variable) was implemented, and all patients were assessed again. Although there was a manipulated variable, it was not feasible to randomly assign to the control and experimental conditions. Once the nursing staff received education on the systematic protocol, it would have been difficult to prevent a dissipation of the treatment effect to patients in the control group.

METHODOLOGICAL DESIGNS

A methodological design is used when the purpose of a study is to develop and evaluate a specific component of a research method. Such studies might include investigations of a particular design or sampling technique but most commonly have included studies to develop and test an instrument for reliability and validity. For example, Rhodes, Watson, and Johnson (1984) conducted a study to test the reliability and validity of an index to measure nausea and vomiting.

In Table 22–1, an example of how the research design might change in relation to the current state of knowledge of the problem of mucositis in cancer patients is presented. Each of four types of designs are matched to the purpose of the investigation.

Table 22–1 ··

Type of Design and Research Purpose Applied to the Problem of Mucositis in Oncology Patients

TYPE OF DESIGN	PURPOSE OF STUDY
Descriptive	To describe the patterns of mucositis in oncology patients receiving chemotherapy
Correlational	To determine the relation between the absolute granulocyte count and the extent of mucositis in patients with acute leukemia receiving induction therapy
Experimental	To compare the effectiveness of two oral care protocols on the incidence of mucositis in patients receiving radiation therapy to the head and neck
Methodological	To develop and test the reliability and validity of an instrument to measure the status of the oral cavity

Designs for Outcomes Research

Although the use of outcomes as an indicator of patient status is not new, the value placed on outcomes research has increased dramatically. This phenomenon is primarily due to intensified interest in the effectiveness of health care delivery on both cost and quality of care.

An outcome is most commonly defined as an end result of treatment or intervention (Lang & Marek, 1992). A critical element of this definition is the notion of "end result." Thus, in designing outcomes studies, decisions regarding the frequency and timing of measurement are critical (Gottlieb & Feeley, 1995). When is the expected endpoint? What if the phenomena change over time? Which points are appropriate to measure? Which points will be most sensitive to change?

Design decisions parallel those previously discussed and must be based on the research objectives. Outcome studies range from those that define, describe, and mea-

sure to specific tests of causal influences of treatments on patient response (Hegyvary, 1993). Thus, a study to describe an outcome such as functional status in patients receiving radiation therapy would be descriptive in nature; whereas a test of a nursing intervention such as exercise on an outcome such as fatigue would necessitate an experimental approach.

Such decisions become more complicated in studies evaluating the impact of organizational change on patient outcomes. Unlike an experiment with careful control of the manipulated condition, organizational change takes place in a dynamic and often uncontrollable environment. In addition to formative evaluation of the change process, such evaluation studies may require repeated measurement. Measuring designated outcomes at specific windows can allow evaluation over time as specific aspects of the change are actually implemented.

Another important decision in studies of organizational change relates to the selection of outcomes to measure. Common approaches include global measures such as patient satisfaction; such data are often available in health care institutions. Such outcomes, however, are usually skewed in the positive direction and change is not easily detected. Moreover, outcomes such as patient satisfaction are influenced by multiple confounding factors in the health care delivery system. It thus becomes nearly impossible to support the connectedness of the intervention to the change in outcome. As in any strong research design, outcomes should vary and be sensitive to the specific influence of the change. More information on outcomes can be found in Chapter 7, Outcomes Evaluation.

DESIGN VALIDITY

The validity of a research study refers to its "truth value" or "worth." Design is critical to validity in that the design should provide the best pathway to obtain a valid or truthful result. Validity is reflected in the level of confidence that can be placed in the findings of a study.

Although validity has most thoroughly been described in relation to experimental designs (Cook & Campbell, 1979), the concept holds true in all types of research. It can perhaps most simply be explained by how well the researcher can respond to the question "Did you study what you intended or *was it something else?*" To follow through on the previous examples, one might ask Hinds and Martin, "Did you describe the experience of hopefulness or *was it something else?*" To Gass and Chang, one might ask "Did you evaluate the relation between coping and health or *was it something else?*" Finally, one might ask Munro et al., "*Was that the effect of* relaxation response or *was it something else?*"

Many issues must be considered in designing a valid study; in the language of experimental research, these issues are termed *threats to validity* (Campbell & Stanley, 1963; Cook and Campbell; 1979). Table 22–2 presents a list of problems and solutions that can help minimize threats to the validity of an experimental design.

Many of these issues are also relevant to other designs as well.

SENSITIVITY

In studies of the effectiveness of various treatments on outcomes, the sensitivity of the research design is critical. Design sensitivity refers to the ability of the experiment to detect a real contrast or difference between two conditions when one really exists (Lipsey, 1990). The sensitivity of the design depends on six factors:

1. Effect size—how powerful of an effect is the treatment expected to have?
2. Heterogeneity of the subjects—how diverse are the subjects on the variables of interest?
3. Sample size—how many subjects are selected from the population?

Table 22–2

Ten Common Problems and Solutions to Minimize Threats to Validity in an Experimental Design

PROBLEM	SOLUTION
1. Sample size is too small to detect a statistically significant difference.	1. Do a power analysis to plan an adequate sample size before the study is begun.
2. Instruments or measures cannot be depended on to register true changes.	2. Use instruments with known reliability. Do a pilot study. Measure reliability during the study.
3. The way a treatment is implemented may vary from one subject to another.	3. Specify the treatment in a detailed manner. Ensure adequate training. Monitor for protocol violations.
4. Groups may differ on factors that are related to the dependent variable.	4. Select a homogeneous sample or randomly assign between groups and measure variables of concern.
5. The outcome may be influenced by some alternate event that has occurred during the course of the study.	5. Randomly assign subjects to treatments. Try to minimize outside influences. Test for differences in responses before and after event.
6. Subjects become more knowledgeable or experienced during the study.	6. Randomly assign subjects to treatments.
7. Subjects become familiar with a test or instrument by taking it repeatedly.	7. Use alternative forms of a test. Randomly assign subjects to treatments.
8. Different kinds of subjects drop out of a study than those who stay in.	8. Monitor reasons for dropouts. Randomly assign subjects to treatments.
9. Subjects in one group share information with subjects in the other—diffusing the treatment effect.	9. Try to use groups that will not be in contact with each other.
10. Control subjects feel like the underdog and thus artificially affect the results—wiping out the expected difference.	10. Consider a crossover design in which all subjects receive all treatments in random order.

Data from Cook, T. D., & Campbell, D. T. (1979). Quasi-experimentation. *Boston: Houghton-Mifflin Company.*

4. Experimental error—how consistent is the administration of the experimental condition?
5. Measurement—does the measurement approach consistently and reliably measure the outcome of interest?
6. Data analysis—do the statistical tests have adequate power (that is, is there an ability to detect a difference if one exists)? Power is dependent upon the previous factors.

Thus, a design with the greatest sensitivity has a large homogeneous sample, includes reliable and valid measurement tools, carefully controls the experimental condition, and includes appropriate analysis of the data. Moreover, such experiments should be designed to test interventions that have the greatest likelihood of making a difference. These criteria can be summarized in the old rule of thumb: maximize the experimental effect and minimize the error.

FEASIBILITY

The final and perhaps greatest challenge in design construction is balancing validity with feasibility. In clinical nursing research, this challenge is often concretely posed in sampling. It is well recognized that a random sample can strengthen a study, allowing greater generalizability to other populations. However, the nurse researcher is often faced with finding enough subjects who are eligible and able to participate. Random sampling is often impossible. Additionally, constraints of time, money, and human resources place limitations on research. The researcher must be able to identify who will carry out the study and how it will be conducted. Finally, the reality of the clinical setting means that many variables are difficult, if not impossible, to control.

Several steps can be helpful in achieving this balance between validity and feasibility. First, the researcher should maintain a close link with the clinical setting where the study will be conducted. Contacting the appropriate administrators and clinicians early in the proposal development is essential. Their experience and wisdom can yield important suggestions. They should be kept appraised of the development of the proposal.

Second, the proposal should be submitted for peer review by individuals who are experts on the topic. Professional colleagues, nurse researchers in the clinical setting, and faculty from a college of nursing can be helpful in identifying weaknesses in a proposal and suggesting alternatives. Third, the design should be tested by conducting a pilot study. The process of actually conducting the data collection increases awareness of superfluous data and glitches in the data collection process.

Even with these safeguards in place, the researcher must be prepared for numerous challenges in striving to maintain rigor in the final implementation of a clinical study. In the long run, however, a study that is well designed—balancing both validity and feasibility in order to answer the research questions—is a study that is more easily implemented, analyzed, and reported. Thus, taking the time and thoughtfulness to thoroughly and carefully design research is of immense value.

REFERENCES

Beck, S. L. (1979). Impact of a systematic oral care protocol on stomatitis after chemotherapy. *Cancer Nursing, 2*(3), 185–197.

Beck, S. L. (1989). The crossover design in clinical nursing research. *Nursing Research, 38*(5), 291–293.

Burns, N., & Grove, S. K. (1997). *The practice of nursing research: Conduct, critique, and utilization* (3rd ed.). Philadelphia: W. B. Saunders.

Campbell, D. T., & Stanley, J. C. (1963). *Experimental and quasi-experimental designs for research*. Boston: Houghton Mifflin.

Cook, T. D., & Campbell, D. T. (1979). *Quasi-experimentation*. Chicago: Rand-McNally.

Cook, T. D., & Reichardt, C. S. (1979). *Qualitative and quantitative methods in evaluation research*. Beverly Hills: Sage.

Diers, D. (1979). *Research in nursing practice*. Philadelphia: J. B. Lippincott.

Gass, K. A., & Chang, A. S. (1989). Appraisals of bereavement, coping, resources, and psychosocial health dysfunctions in widows and widowers. *Nursing Research, 38*(1), 31–36.

Glaser, B. G., & Strauss, A. L. (1967). *The discovery of grounded theory: Strategies for qualitative research*. New York: Aldine De Gruyter.

Gottlieb, L. N., & Feeley, N. (1995). Nursing intervention studies: Issues related to change and testing. *Canadian Journal of Nursing Research, 27*(1), 13–29.

Hegyvary, S. T. (1993). Patient care outcomes related to management of symptoms. *Annual Review of Nursing Research: Research on Nursing Practice 11,* 145–168.

Hinds, P. S., & Martin, J. (1988). Hopefulness and the self-sustaining process in adolescents with cancer. *Nursing Research, 37*(6), 336–339.

Johnson, M. V., Ottenbacher, K. J., & Reichardt, C. S. (1995). Strong quasi-experimental designs for research on the effectiveness of rehabilitation. *American Journal of Physical and Rehabilitation Medicine, 74*(5), 383–392.

Kerlinger, F. A. (1986). *Foundations of behavioral research*. New York: Holt, Rinehart, & Winston.

Kirk-Smith, M. (1996). How to design an effective research study. *Nursing Times, 92*(28), 40–41.

Lang, N. M., & Marek, K. D. (1992). Outcomes that reflect clinical practice. *Patient outcomes research: Examining the effectiveness of nursing practice* (NIH Publication No. 93-3411). Washington, DC: U.S. Department of Health and Human Services.

Lipsey, Mark W. (1990). *Design sensitivity: Statistical power for experimental research*. Newbury Park, CA: Sage.

Munro, B. H., Creamer, A. M., Haggerty, M. R., & Cooper, F. S. (1988). Effect of relaxation therapy on post-myocardial infarction patients' rehabilitation. *Nursing Research, 37*(4), 231–235.

Polit, D. F., & Hungler, B. P. (1996). *Essentials of nursing research: Methods, appraisal and utilization* (4th ed.). Philadelphia: J. B. Lippincott.

Rhodes, V., Watson, P., & Johnson, M. (1984). Development of reliable and valid measures of nausea and vomiting. *Cancer Nursing, 7*(1), 33–41.

Qualitative Methods

B. Lee Walker

The goal of nursing research is the creation or discovery of knowledge that will enhance nursing practice. In the course of practice, nurses frequently ask questions about events or experiences of which little is known or of which the answers may vary depending on individual perception. In such cases, in which pertinent variables and the relationships among them is unknown, it is not possible to design a research study that will provide causal explanation or prediction. Qualitative research examines events or experiences in context, from the perspective of the individuals experiencing the phenomena. This approach allows the researcher to explore the depth and complexity of a phenomenon, identify and describe its various components and their relationships, and present a picture of the whole, which can enhance and guide practice and aid in the process of theory development.

COMPARING QUALITATIVE AND QUANTITATIVE APPROACHES

Although the terms *quantitative* and *qualitative* are merely descriptions of two types of data (numbers and words, respectively), the methods associated with these terms approach the research process from two different paradigms or ways of viewing the world (Table 23–1). The researcher using a quantitative approach seeks to explain causes and make predictions (Morse & Field, 1995). Stemming from an assumption that there is a reality that may be discovered and manipulated, the researcher investigates the problem deductively, examining variables thought to be pertinent based on either existing theory or the researcher's own interpretation of the phenomenon. Attempts are made to control intervening variables arising from the particular research context to ensure generalizability to other situations or contexts. Data are numbers derived from subjects' responses to paper and pencil instruments developed to measure the variables of interest or from some objective measurement (for example, laboratory analysis of blood, temperature measurements). Bias is controlled by random selection of a large and representative sample of the population of interest. Throughout the process, the researcher attempts to maintain the stance of an objective outsider.

Table 23–1

Contrasts Between Quantitative and Qualitative Approaches

	QUANTITATIVE	QUALITATIVE
Purpose	Seeks to explore causes, make predictions.	Seeks to describe a phenomenon or generate theory.
Sample	Samples are large, representative. Subjects are selected randomly and/or are randomly assigned to group.	Samples are small. Participants are selected purposely, based on their knowledge and/or experience.
Data	Data are numbers, gathered from (1) responses to questionnaires measuring researcher-defined variables or (2) some objective measurement (for example, temperature).	Data consist of (1) words (from interviews, diaries, other written documents), or (2) pictures or other artifacts whose meaning and significance are rendered in words.

In contrast, the qualitative researcher assumes the existence of *multiple* realities, based on the supposition that people construct meaning in relation to the world in which they live and that each individual's reality is in some respects unique. The researcher makes no effort to control variables; rather, all aspects of the problem are explored in depth and any intervening variables identified in the context are considered a part of the phenomenon (Morse & Field, 1995). The description or explanation of the phenomenon develops inductively, derived from participants' interpretation of events in the particular context in which these events are experienced. In clinical nursing research, participants may be patients, caregivers, or family members. Data are collected primarily via interview, but they also may be derived from observation and supplemented by a variety of written or pictorial records. Sample size is usually small, and participants are selected from among persons who are in key positions or have special knowledge of the phenomenon of interest and are willing (and able) to share their perceptions. In the process of selection, reflection on, and refining of the data, the researcher becomes an integral part of final product (Boyd, 1993a). The result is a rich description of the whole phenomenon that identifies the essence of an experience or describes a process.

UNIQUE FEATURES OF QUALITATIVE APPROACHES

Several features related to the roles (of both the researchers and study participants) and

to the research design also serve to differentiate qualitative from quantitative research. In qualitative studies, individuals who agree to take part in a study are regarded as partners in the discovery and verification of knowledge and are viewed as participants in the research process, rather than as "subjects." The interchange between participant and researcher increases the sensitivity of both to the topic under study, creating the potential for a fuller understanding and interpretation of phenomena than might otherwise have been possible. This interaction between researcher and participant, as well as reactions and ideas of the researcher recorded as field notes and memos, becomes part of the study data; in this way, the researcher is made a part of the final product.

In qualitative studies, *decisions* regarding the selection and size of the sample also differ from those in quantitative studies Participants in qualitative studies are selected because they are knowledgeable about or have experienced the phenomenon of interest and are able to share that knowledge with the researcher. In some approaches (for example, grounded theory), ongoing selection of participants is guided by information emerging from concurrent analysis of data. The researcher increases the sample based on theoretical (purposive) sampling, a process in which the researcher seeks to verify hunches or to determine whether emerging theory fits in different situations or with participants with selected characteristics. In other approaches (ethnography), initial participants are chosen because they can provide entry to a group or culture and they assist the researcher by either explaining activities and behavior that the researcher has observed or suggesting other informants who can provide the information and explanations that the researcher seeks. Because any qualitative approach generates enormous amounts of (mostly) verbal data, it is not feasible to have large sample sizes. The number of participants that will be needed can only be estimated before data collection; as collection progresses, sample size is determined by the criterion of "saturation" that is, when the researcher is obtaining the same data from additional participants or other sources, the data are considered saturated and no new information is obtained. (The fact that saturation occurs supports the social/psychological position that although each individual is unique, patterns *do* exist, and that people tend to make sense of their experiences in similar ways.)

CRITERIA FOR CHOOSING A QUALITATIVE APPROACH

The purpose of the research and the state of knowledge in the general field of interest should direct the choice of research approach. A qualitative approach is appropriate when the research question pertains to understanding or describing a particular phenomenon or event about which little is known or when the investigator seeks to generate new theory or to reformulate a conceptualization or gestalt about a known phenomenon or process (this is particularly appropriate when there is some indication that present knowledge or theories may be incomplete or biased) (Morse & Field, 1995; Burns & Grove, 1997). A qualitative method may also be used to identify questions and develop instruments for quantitative research, although such an approach is usually not directed by the philosophic beliefs and values that guide qualitative paradigms (Boyd, 1993a).

Qualitative research is appropriate to address questions such as "What is going on here?" and "How can I explain it?" or to describe how people live or cope with particular experiences, questions that frequently arise in clinical settings. For example, if the researcher wants to understand how patients experience pain or how they cope with the information that they are genetically at risk for the development of cancer, a quali-

tative approach may be the method of choice.

QUALITATIVE METHODS

A number of qualitative approaches are subsumed under the umbrella of qualitative methods. Some of these methods are rooted in theoretical and philosophical beliefs that direct inquiry and guide analysis (phenomenology, grounded theory), others have developed as methods of inquiry in particular disciplines (ethnography, historical research) and provide detailed guidance related to data generation and interpretation. Some approaches often discussed in the context of qualitative methods are probably more accurately designated as data collection methods (focus groups) or guides to data management and analysis (content analysis, case study methods). Descriptive research can generate both qualitative (interview, written comments) and quantitative (survey) data but lacks the foundation and structure that would qualify it as a distinct approach or method. Finally, some texts mention philosophical inquiry and critical social theory in their discussion of qualitative research approaches (Burns & Grove, 1997). Both approaches critically examine data either for the purpose of theory development or ethical inquiry (philosophical inquiry) or to sensitize the researcher to processes within a particular system that serve to maintain and perpetuate the status quo (critical social inquiry). These approaches may use both qualitative and quantitative data in the process of knowledge discovery.

This chapter briefly describes four of the most frequently encountered qualitative research approaches: grounded theory, phenomenology, ethnography, and historical research (Table 23–2). References associated with each discussion provide examples of research studies using that approach and a more in-depth description for those interested in further exploration of the particular approach.

Phenomenology

Phenomenology seeks to understand and describe the experience of interest as it is lived, from the perspective of the individual

Table 23–2

Four Qualitative Research Approaches

	PURPOSE	GENERAL QUESTION ASKS
Phenomenology	Seeks to understand an experience from the participant's perspective	What is it like . . . ? What is the experience of . . . ?
Grounded theory	Seeks to generate theory regarding a process (social or psychological)	What is the process . . . of learning to manage an illness? . . . of integrating some experience into one's life?
Ethnography	Seeks to present a total picture of the culture of interest	What is the daily life of this group like? What are values, beliefs that influence behavior?
Historical	Seeks to understand historical events, ideas, institutions, or people	What happened here and what effect did it have *(on nursing or some nursing function or institution)?*

participant's subjective reality. Phenomenology emerges from the works of philosophers such as Husserl, Kierkegaard, Heidegger, and Merleau-Ponty (Boyd, 1993b), and various phenomenological styles are exemplified in nursing in the works of Benner, (1984, 1985), Parse (1990), Paterson and Zderad (1976), and Ray (1985). The common theme among the various phenomenologies is the concern for human meaning and how those meanings can be translated into information that will lead to more informed and sensitive nursing practice and science (Boyd, 1993b).

The phenomenological approach asks questions such as "What is it like to have a certain experience?" or "What is the meaning of a particular experience to the individual living through that experience?" Fareed's (1996) study of patients' experiences of reassurance provides an example of phenomenological research whose results are applicable in the clinical setting. She asked patients from medical and surgical settings in a general hospital what it meant to them to be reassured. The results highlighted attributes that patients look for in a nurse's behavior, such as knowledge, skills in interpersonal relationships, providing patients with a sense of being cared for, and providing a perceived therapeutic environment. Another example is Nelson's (1996) study of women's struggle to gain meaning as they live with uncertainty following treatment for breast cancer. Her question focused on women's experiences with uncertainty from the time of diagnosis and treatment to the present.

DATA COLLECTION AND ANALYSIS

Data for the two aforementioned examples came primarily from interviews, although Nelson also included photographs taken by the women that provided symbolic representation of their experiences and feelings of uncertainty since diagnosis. In most qualitative studies, interviews are taped and transcribed verbatim. Such studies generate mounds of data, verbal and otherwise, which then must be reduced and synthesized into themes that communicate the essence of the experience. The concern with "wholeness," however, makes phenomenologists reluctant to condense data through segmenting and reassembly of text. Although some segmentation usually occurs in the process of analysis, most approaches to data analysis developed by phenomenological researchers begin with careful reading and re-reading of source material to capture the "essence" of an account, with the aim of gaining an understanding of meaning and actions. A number of researchers have developed guidelines for accomplishing this process while remaining true to the precepts of phenomenological inquiry. Fareed (1996) followed steps outlined by Colaizzi (1975) and provides a detailed description of the process of analysis. Nelson was guided by the writings of van Manen (1990) and Ray (1991). Boyd (1993b) provides a more comprehensive discussion of various guidelines for phenomenological analysis.

Grounded Theory

The purpose of a grounded theory approach is to generate explanatory theory that will further understanding of social and psychological phenomena. The approach emerged from the social psychological theory of symbolic interaction, which is both a theory about human behavior and an approach to inquiring about group behavior (Chenitz & Swanson, 1986). According to symbolic interaction theory, people create their reality by attaching meaning to situations. These meanings (or beliefs) are expressed through symbols such as words, dress, hairstyles, and objects of worship. Although each person's reality is unique, symbolic meanings are shared by groups and form the basis for actions and interactions. In the process of interaction, meanings may change. Grounded theory research focuses on these symbols and interactions, and how they change in particular situations, to develop theories about social processes "grounded" in the lives of those experiencing the process.

The specific techniques referred to as *grounded theory method* were developed by Glaser and Strauss (1967), two sociologists at the University of California at San Francisco. In this approach, initial questions focus broadly on what is happening or how something occurred, then questions are narrowed to pursue specific paths or processes identified from interviews, as concurrent data analysis sharpens the focus of the research. For example, Mishel and Murdaugh (1987) studied the processes used by family members of heart transplant patients to cope with the unpredictability associated with waiting for and receiving a heart transplant. The researchers began by asking groups of family members "What has been happening with you?" and continued the discussion with family members as the patient progressed through the experience. The social psychological process that emerged from the data was that of "redesigning the dream," a process that refers to cognitive and behavioral changes occurring in the family member from entry into the heart transplantation program to some indeterminate period after transplantation. Another example of a grounded theory study is provided by Baker and Stern (1992) who investigated the evolution of readiness to manage one's own illness in a group of adults with a nonfatal chronic illness. The initial interview inquired about the history of the illness, the care received, and what the person did when he or she noticed changes in general health or changes specific to the illness. Consistent with the constant comparative method that is the hallmark of grounded theory, data collection and analysis proceeded concurrently, and questions were changed and new ones added as analysis sharpened the focus of the study. Findings from the study indicated that the key process in self-care readiness was to find meaning in the illness.

DATA COLLECTION AND ANALYSIS

A number of sources provide detailed guidance for the researcher whose study question suggests a grounded theory approach (Glaser & Strauss, 1967; Stern, 1985; Chenitz & Swanson, 1986). As in the case of phenomenology, in grounded theory, much of the data are collected through interviews with people directly involved with the process or phenomenon of interest. However, grounded theory studies may also use other data sources, such as written records or reports from individuals knowledgeable about but not necessarily directly experiencing the process. (In the Baker and Stern [1992] study, for example, the primary nurse caring for each participant was also interviewed to provide another source for verifying the conclusions of the researcher.) Each interview is transcribed and analyzed as soon as possible after its conclusion, and the process of developing categories begins with the first interview. Questions are added and the interview is refocused based on emerging theory. The researcher often returns to previous participants to ask questions that arose from later interviews and to verify emerging interpretations. Subsequent participants are selected and other data consulted as suggested by the emerging social psychological process or theory.

Ethnography

Ethnography is a research approach developed by anthropologists to study cultures. The goal is to present a total picture of a defined group's daily life, complete with beliefs, patterns of activities, and meanings attached to various activities and behaviors. The researcher becomes immersed in the everyday life of the culture being studied, participating in that life to the extent possible, and using multiple methods (interview, observations, written records, pictures, artifacts) to understand how daily life conditions and cultural patterns influence the phenomena that is the focus of the research. The interest or focus of the researcher influences both data collection and interpretation. For example, Leininger's "ethnonursing," a merger of ethnography and nursing research, focuses on how the culture of a particular group influences self-care, health, and nursing care practices (Lackey, 1991).

DATA COLLECTION AND ANALYSIS

In ethnographic research, data comes primarily from interviews and observation but may also include diaries, pictures, and various cultural artifacts. Analytical methods tend more toward description leading to understanding of the culture than toward theory building. Magilvy, Congdon, and Martinez (1994) used an ethnographic design to understand the culture of rural life and aging as the context for providing home care services to frail elderly persons. Data were generated through interviews, participant observation, the examination of cultural artifacts (agency policies, community newspapers, historical documents), and photography. Twenty-six nurses providing home care were considered the key informants, but physicians, home care providers, community leaders, patients, and families were also interviewed, illustrating the diversity of data sources used in an ethnographic study. Interview transcripts, field notes, documents, and photographs were analyzed to identify common categories, patterns, and themes. The researchers identified two patterns, or "circles of care," one embedded in the continuity of care provided to older adults and their families through professional health and social services and the other comprised of informal support from family, friends, and neighbors, such as helping with shopping, assisting with household and personal tasks, and providing companionship. Consistent with rural culture, health care providers caring for elderly persons also became a part of the informal system. The researchers note that support of the informal care system is crucial for maintaining frail elderly persons in their homes and preventing unnecessary hospitalization or institutionalization.

Historical Research

Historical research provides understanding of historical events, ideas, institutions, or people that have influenced the development and practice of nursing. Fitzpatrick (1993) maintains that a solid historical interpretation of the past can strengthen current organizational and political planning, provide prototypes for the development of nursing leaders, contribute to the development of clinical practice, make apparent the contribution of nursing to the history of women, and serve as a socializing agent for new members of the profession. Ideally, a historical study is not just a narrative, but describes patterns or relationships over time to provide a coherent and meaningful historical explanation. The historical researcher is often guided in choice of topic and interpretation by a particular framework. For instance, a sociological approach emphasizes social forces and their influence on people and groups; a political or economic approach uses ideology, such as Marxism or feminism, for analysis and interpretation; a "great person" approach focuses on individuals and their accomplishments and power within a particular social context (Fitzpatrick, 1993).

DATA COLLECTION AND ANALYSIS

The data gathered in historical research are predominantly words, derived from interviews with people who were present or have some special knowledge of the time of interest, and from diaries, narratives, newspapers, and other written records pertinent to the event or period. Photographs and other artifacts also provide the researcher with information. The historical researcher becomes something of a detective while searching for potential sources of data. As data are collected, the researcher is faced with the problem of determining the reliability and validity of the information being gathered. Validity relates to the authenticity of documents and other artifacts. The researcher must verify, for instance, that a document is indeed in a particular person's handwriting or that the paper and style of writing is consistent with the time period under study. Reliability is an attempt to establish truth and depends on correct understanding of the language and customs of the period to produce an accurate interpretation of the data collected. The final product is a narrative that "provides understanding of the interconnectedness among events and moves the process from analysis to synthesis and, finally, to interpretation" (Fitzpatrick, 1993).

Stevens (1990) conducted a historical study to investigate strategies that were successful in promoting the image of nursing during World War II in the hopes of identifying strategies or principles that might be currently relevant. Her sources were primarily news briefs presented to the public in the form of short motion picture news reports (Movietone News) of the war effort at home and events in European and Pacific war zones where nurses were caring for U.S. servicemen. She supplemented this material with historical records, newspapers, plays, and movies that provided a picture of the social and political climate of the time. Her conclusions emphasize the need to present a professional, positive image of nursing in the media to attract capable people who will make a difference in the profession.

Perhaps more pertinent to clinical nursing research is a study conducted by Fairman (1992) analyzing the role of nurses in the development of intensive care units. Among her many sources were narrative accounts of precursors to the modern intensive care units and nurses' roles in their development dating from the Civil War forward, historical developments in the arrangement and delivery of care in hospitals, hospital policies, and advances in medicine. Fairman's historical narrative presents a clear picture of the contributions made by nurses over time to care of the critically ill and to the development and success of intensive care units.

TRIANGULATION

Methods are sometimes combined in a single study to confirm or clarify findings, a design approach known as *method triangulation*. There are two main purposes of method triangulation: (1) to increase the reliability and validity of a study, which occurs when data generated by one method confirm the findings of another method, and (2) to increase the comprehensiveness of a study. Methods can be combined *within* a particular tradition, as demonstrated by

Wilson and Hutchinson (1991), who used two qualitative approaches (a Heideggerian phenomenological approach and grounded theory) in a study of caregivers to discover meanings and ways of being (exploration of phenomena) while generating a conceptual framework (through grounded theory) useful for planning interventions and guiding further research. Methods are also combined *across* traditions (quantitative with qualitative), although there is some disagreement about the appropriateness of combining methods whose assumptions stem from vastly different world views of the nature of reality (Boyd, 1993c). However, Sandelowski (1997) argues that the inclusion of a qualitative component often enhances the clinical significance of study findings. Whereas quantitative measures may indicate that variables are linked, qualitative research, because of its "case" approach, can explain *why* they are linked by identifying the "actual configuration of events that led to specific outcomes in specific cases." Breitmayer, Ayres, and Knafl (1993) provide a convincing argument for using both qualitative and quantitative data generation methods in their report of how families define and manage a child's chronic illness. This study used information from qualitative interviews either to confirm or to refute information obtained from selected self-report instruments (thus increasing credibility) and attempted to identify in the interview data possible explanations for variations in self-report of mood (increasing completeness of the results). The study provides expert guidance on how to design and implement a study using *across method* triangulation.

MANAGEMENT AND ANALYSIS OF DATA

Although the data to be analyzed in qualitative studies consist primarily of words, that analysis calls for the same careful and critical scrutiny that is required in quantitative studies. The researcher must synthesize an enormous amount of data, moving from the concrete to increasing abstraction. Some guidance for synthesis of the data is provided by researchers such as Colaizzi and Giorgi for phenomenological studies and by Glaser and Strauss for grounded theory. However, the researcher, while adhering to the spirit of the qualitative approach guiding the research, must find a useable system for data reduction and synthesis. Miles and Huberman (1994) identify three streams of activity that are common throughout most qualitative analyses: (1) data reduction, (2) data display, and (3) conclusion drawing and verification. These activities are overlapping and iterative or cyclical, rather than separate and discrete steps in the analysis process.

Data reduction consists of selecting, grouping, and summarizing data from transcripts, field notes, and other sources. This activity serves to sharpen, focus, and organize the data to assist in drawing final conclusions. As such, it is an integral part of those final conclusions, because the decisions being made regarding what segments to code, how to group them, or which pieces of data or patterns best summarize the various portions of data are all analytical choices. Figure 23–1 is an example of data reduction. The example presents three segments of text taken from an interview with a woman 6 months after treatment for breast cancer. The researcher labeled both segments as "management strategies" and underlined words and short phrases representing these strategies. The researcher further noted that the "strategies" identified include both active (behavioral) and internal management processes.

The task of the second activity, *data display*, is to develop a system that allows the researcher to view the reduced data in some organized fashion that assists in comparison of groupings and suggests relationships. Reduced data may be displayed as networks, or in columns, charts, or matrices. From this display, the researcher is able to see connections within the data and either to draw conclusions or to proceed with further analyses suggested by the display (Fig. 23–2). Again, the decisions regarding what to display (for example, what goes in the rows and columns of a matrix) or how to arrange elements hierarchically within a network are analytical activities. The process of developing the data display may also lead the researcher back to the original sources to verify the context of a piece of datum before locating it in a particular category, an example of the iterative process of qualitative analysis.

According to Miles and Huberman (1994), *conclusion drawing* is present from the start

Participant 000*	
MANAGEMENT (internal; active)	
it would like explode out and I	*43*
couldn't contain it and what works	*44*
much better for me is to <u>keep it as</u>	*45*
<u>a low level presence in my life</u> and	*46*
to <u>be involved</u> in the breast cancer	*47*
community and go <u>see my friends</u>	*48*
and just have cancer as a fact of	*49*
life rather than to say,	
MANAGEMENT (active)	
then, so I <u>went back to being a veg-</u>	*166*
<u>etarian</u> and I've been drinking all	*167*
my carrot juice, I <u>take Vitamin E,</u>	*168*
my stress approach is every time I	*169*
think oh my God, I'm going to die,	*170*
which happens pretty regularly, I	*171*
<u>go to the gym</u>	
MANAGEMENT (active; internal)	
usually <u>meditate</u> before I go to bed	*257*
and so I have . . . then I have sleep-	*258*
ing and all. I think that there is just	*259*
enough <u>time there for my subcon-</u>	*260*
<u>scious to process things.</u> Things	*261*
are generally better in the morn-	*262*
ing.	*263*
***Used with permission of participant.**	

Figure 23–1
Data reduction.

of data collection, as the researcher begins to note patterns and regularities. Ideally, the researcher remains both open and skeptical, and final conclusions may not appear until data collection is complete, but these "hunches" often influence subsequent participant recruitment and data gathering. In the example, the researcher indicates in the diagram that there may be interaction between some active and internal management strategies (indicated by the broken line in Fig. 23–2) and notes in the *MEMO* that management strategies may serve both to reduce anxiety and to facilitate integration. This beginning data display provides a framework for further analysis that may or may not support the connections depicted in Figure 23–2. Conclusions must also be *verified* as the analysis proceeds. This verification may take the form of return to the interview data or field notes to determine whether a conclusion is actually rooted in

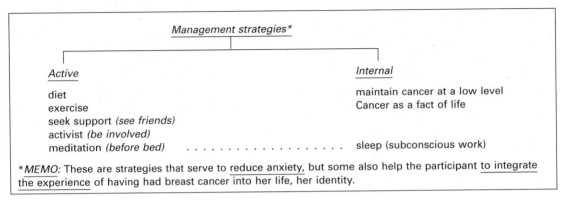

Figure 23–2
Data display.

the data, or it may involve review and discussion with colleagues to develop consensus regarding the conclusions. Ideally, the researcher also returns to talk with at least some of the participants, to verify that they recognize the processes described or that the narrative does capture the essence of their experience. This process of verification is an integral part of the evaluation of any qualitative study.

Although some researchers prefer to accomplish the mechanical tasks associated with data reduction by pasting segments of data on cards or by color coding portions of the text, a number of computer programs offer assistance with these data management tasks, efficiently sorting, storing, and retrieving segments of data while allowing the researcher to move between grouped segments and the original context of each segment. Features of some of these programs also assist in the development of a data display. Weitzman and Miles (1994) provide an excellent review of the varieties of computer programs available to assist in the management of qualitative data. However, although computer programs provide *assistance* in data management, the researcher must make the data reduction and display decisions, and only the researcher can draw the final conclusions.

EVALUATING QUALITATIVE STUDIES

Quantitative studies are judged on criteria related to reliability and validity. However, because qualitative approaches have different rules regarding aims, evidence, inference, and verification, quantitative criteria are not appropriate for evaluating qualitative studies (Sandelowski, 1986). Lincoln and Guba (1985) proposed that four factors be used for assessing the rigor of qualitative studies: credibility, transferability, dependability, and confirmability.

Credibility addresses the truth value of a study and is present when the descriptions or interpretations presented are immediately recognized by people who have had that experience. These "member checks" were used in both the Mishel and Murdaugh (1987) and Nelson (1996) studies as one evidence of the credibility of their findings. Results of a study are also credible when others (researchers or readers), after having read the study, can recognize the experience when it occurs.

Transferability is achieved when findings can "fit" for samples and settings beyond that of the particular study. Mishel and Murdaugh (1987) addressed this concern by recruiting a sample that varied in age, educational level, and role activities in an effort to make their findings applicable to as diverse a group as possible.

Dependability (or consistency) refers to the stability of the findings and the ability to track variance in the data over time. Lincoln and Guba (1985) proposed that auditability be the criterion for evaluating the consistency of qualitative findings. To meet this criterion, the qualitative researcher needs to keep a written record detailing and justifying what was actually done at each step in the research process. This record needs to be complete enough so that another researcher could arrive at similar conclusions by following this "decision trail." The researchers in both the Mishel and Murdaugh (1987) study and the study conducted by Magilvy, Congdon, and Martinez (1994) sought to ensure the dependability of their findings by independent coding and by having researchers not involved in the study follow the decision trail developed throughout the study.

Finally, *confirmability* is the criterion proposed to evaluate neutrality. Because the qualitative researcher is, in a sense, a part of the final product, objectivity is not possible. Only when the results can be confirmed by others not involved in the research is it possible to verify that the findings are not simply the perception of the researcher alone. That confirmability is achieved when auditability, creditability, and fit are established (Sandelowski, 1986). However, Sandelowski (1997) cautions qualitative researchers to avoid concentrating too much on cookbook methods to demonstrate the validity of the research and to focus instead on the "art of their work." The purpose of the research report is not to defend how a qualitative study measures up to the standards and criteria of the quantitative paradigm, but rather to present the unique knowledge stemming from the study in a manner that enhances understanding and practice.

SUMMARY

Although qualitative and quantitative approaches in nursing research differ in basic assumptions and methods, both have the goal of furthering the scientific basis for practice. There are a variety of qualitative approaches, and the choice of an approach depends on the purpose of the research. In general, qualitative investigations address broad questions related to description, discovery, or theory building and, as a consequence, the researcher is concerned with the entire context surrounding the phenomenon of interest, rather than a concentration on specific variables thought to influence that phenomenon. Although the type of data collected and the methods of analysis differ, qualitative research demands the same careful attention to the selection of a design appropriate to answer the research questions and the same assurance of rigor in the conduct of the research and interpretation of results as is required in quantitative studies. When these issues are thoroughly addressed, the clinician has a basis for judging both the accuracy and the applicability to practice of the qualitative research findings.

REFERENCES

Baker, C., & Stern, P. N. (1992). Finding meaning in chronic illness as the key to self care. *Canadian Journal of Nursing Research, 25*(2), 23–36.

Benner, P. (1984). *From novice to expert: Excellence and power in clinical practice.* Menlo Park, CA: Addison-Wesley.

Benner, P. (1985). Quality of life: A phenomenological perspective on explanation, prediction, and understanding in nursing science. *Advances in Nursing Science, 8*(1), 1–14.

Boyd, C. O. (1993a). Philosophical foundations of qualitative research. In P. L. Munhall & C. O. Boyd (Eds.), *Nursing research: A qualitative approach* (2nd ed., pp. 66–93). New York: National League for Nursing.

Boyd, C. O. (1993b). Phenomenology: The method. In P. L. Munhall & C. O. Boyd (Eds.), *Nursing research: A qualitative approach* (2nd ed., pp. 99–132). New York: National League for Nursing.

Boyd, C. O. (1993c). Combining qualitative and quantitative approaches. In P. L. Munhall & C. O. Boyd (Eds.), *Nursing research: A qualitative approach* (2nd ed., pp. 454–475). New York: National League for Nursing.

Breitmayer, B. J., Ayres, L., & Knafl, K. A. (1993). Triangulation in qualitative research: Evaluation of completeness and confirmation purposes. *Image: Journal of Nursing Scholarship, 25*, 237–243.

Burns, N., & Grove, S.K. (1997). *The practice of nursing research: Conduct, critique, and utilization* (2nd ed.). Philadelphia: W. B. Saunders.

Chenitz, W. C., & Swanson, J. M. (1986). *From practice to grounded theory: Qualitative research in nursing.* Menlo Park, CA: Addison-Wesley.

Colaizzi, P. F. (1975). Psychological research as the phenomenologists view it. In R. Valle & M. King (Eds.), *Existential phenomenological alternatives for psychology* (pp. 48–71). New York: Oxford University Press.

Fairman, J. (1992). Watchful vigilance: Nursing care, technology, and the development of intensive care units. *Nursing Research, 41*, 56–60.

Fareed, A. (1996). The experience of reassurance: Patients' perspectives. *Journal of Advanced Nursing, 23*, 272–279.

Fitzpatrick, M. L. (1993). Historical research: The method. In P. L. Munhall & C. O. Boyd (Eds.), *Nursing research: A qualitative perspective* (2nd ed., pp. 359–371). New York: National League for Nursing.

Glaser, B. G., & Strauss, A. L. (1967). *The discovery of grounded theory: Strategies for qualitative research.* New York: Aldine De Gruyter.

Lackey, N. L. (1991). Qualitative research methodologies: An overview, Part 1. *Journal of Post Anesthesia Nursing, 6*, 290–293.

Lincoln, Y. S., & Guba, E. G., (1985). *Naturalistic inquiry.* Beverly Hills, CA: Sage.

Magilvy, J. K., Congdon, J. G., & Martinez, R. (1994). Circles of care: Home care and community support for rural older adults. *Advances in Nursing Science, 16*(3), 22–33.

Miles, M. B., & Huberman, A. M. (1994). *Qualitative data analysis* (2nd ed.). Thousand Oaks, CA: Sage.

Mishel, M. H., & Murdaugh, C. L. (1987). Family adjustment to heart transplantation: Redesigning the dream. *Nursing Research, 36,* 332–338.

Morse, J. M., & Field, P. A. (1995). *Qualitative research methods for health professionals* (2nd ed.). Thousand Oaks, CA: Sage.

Nelson, J. P. (1996). Struggling to gain meaning: Living with the uncertainty of breast cancer. *Advances in Nursing Science, 18*(3), 59–76.

Parse, R. R. (1990). Parse's research methodology with an illustration of the lived experience of hope. *Nursing Science Quarterly, 3,* 9–17.

Paterson, J., & Zderad, L. (1976). *Humanistic nursing.* New York: Wiley.

Ray, M. (1985). A philosophical method to study nursing phenomena. In M. Leininger, *Qualitative research methods in nursing* (pp. 81–92). Orlando, FL: Grune & Stratton.

Ray, M. A. (1991). Caring inquiry: The esthetic process in the way of compassion. In D. Gaut (Ed.), *The compassionate healer* (pp. 181–189). New York: National League for Nursing.

Sandelowski, M. (1986). The problem of rigor in qualitative research. *Advances in Nursing Science, 8*(3), 27–37.

Sandelowski, M. (1997). "To be of use": Enhancing the utility of qualitative research. *Nursing Outlook, 45,* 125–132.

Stern, P. N. (1985). Using grounded theory method in nursing research. In M. M. Leininger (Ed.), *Qualitative research methods in nursing* (pp. 149–160). Orlando, FL: Grune & Stratton.

Stevens, S. Y. (1990). Sale of the century: Images of nursing in the Movietonews during World War II. *Advances in Nursing Science, 12*(4), 44–52.

van Manen, M. (1990). *Researching lived experience: Human science for an action sensitive pedagogy.* Ontario: Althouse Press.

Weitzman, E. A., & Miles, M. B. (1994). *Computer programs for qualitative data analysis.* Newbury Park, CA: Sage.

Wilson, H. S., & Hutchinson, S. A. (1991). Triangulation of qualitative methods: Heideggerian hermeneutics and grounded theory. *Qualitative Health Research, 1,* 263–276.

Chapter 24

Writing the Research Proposal

Geraldine V. Padilla

A research proposal is the plan for a scientific project. The merit of a project is judged on the basis of the clarity, conciseness, and persuasiveness of the proposal. Failure to meet any of these three criteria usually results in some form of rejection. A proposal addresses a number of people such as clinical staff, research assistants, administrators, human subject protection committee members, and scientific reviewers of funding agencies who have the responsibility of approving or implementing scientific projects. Clarity and conciseness in the proposal are achieved through organization, critique, feedback, and revision before submission. A statement about the clinical or scientific significance of the study, which illustrates sound and feasible research methods, generally garners support for the study. This chapter summarizes the procedures for writing a proposal and presents ways of producing clarity, conciseness, and persuasiveness.

The proposal can be used as a first step toward publication. This objective can only be met, however, if the text is well written, explicit, concise, and detailed. Once the researcher accomplishes this, all that remains to complete the final report is to update the literature, explain changes in the original methodology, describe unusual or noteworthy occurrences that happened while implementing the study, and report the findings and their clinical and scientific implications. Final reports must usually be formatted to meet journal specifications.

STRUCTURE

It is common for an investigator to write three or more versions of the same proposal. Proposals must conform to funding agency guidelines, human and animal subjects protection committee requirements, and nursing department forms. Instructions or application kits that outline the proposal requirements should be requested in ad-

Table 24–1

Basic Structure of Proposals

1. *Abstracts* are synopses of the research plan that briefly summarize the study objectives, methods, and expected results.
2. *Business pages* include the following: budget and its justification (Clore, 1985); information on the investigators, consultants, collaborators, and other project staff; sources of research support already obtained by the project staff; resources available for carrying out the project; and signatures of the investigator and administrator.
3. The *research plan* describes what is intended, why the study is significant, what has already been done by the researcher or others, and how the study will be done (US Dept. of Health and Human Services Public Health Services, 1995). Also included are instructions on page limitations, headings, references, personnel qualifications, and human subject consent procedures.
4. *Appendices* include letters of support from consultants and collaborators, detailed descriptions of data collection procedures, and other supporting documents.

vance. If guidelines are not available, the researcher should determine the informational needs of the reader. Although a research project remains the same regardless of who reads the proposal, different audiences require different types and amounts of information. For example, nurses at the study site must know the objectives of the project, the anticipated impact of data collection procedures on patient well-being, and the amount of nursing time required. Scientific terminology should be excluded from proposals aimed at nonresearchers. Federal grant applications undergo rigorous peer review and should therefore include all aspects of scientific method that apply to a project (National Institutes of Health, 1989). The investigator should use the language of the reviewers' discipline to describe design, variables, measurement, procedures, and statistics.

Most proposal guidelines comprise (1) an abstract, (2) business pages, (3) a research plan, and (4) appendices (Table 24–1).

Many aspects of proposal preparation are not under the direct control of the investigator, such as obtaining letters of support, institutional signatures, approval for use of human or animal subjects, consultation, critique, and secretarial support for proposal preparation. The investigator should keep these requirements in mind when determining the time frame for meeting proposal submission deadlines.

When the study involves investigators from different clinical services within an institution or between agencies, collaborative agreements are needed and should be included in the proposal. Collaboration requires ground rules that are clearly understood by all investigators, institutional administrators, and nursing staff involved in the study. This is necessary for the proposal to be completed in a timely manner, for future work to be determined, and for ownership of the research to be understood. A meeting of all collaborators should be held to address proposal writing responsibilities, to determine level of administrative commitment for time, space, and personnel, and to operationalize "ownership" of the study and its results (Waltz, Nelson, & Chambers, 1985). Refer to Chapter 15 for more information on collaboration.

Numerous articles describe the characteristics of poorly written proposals. It is important to keep these characteristics in mind during the proposal development phase (Cuca & McLoughlin, 1987) (Table 24–2).

Table 24–2

Characteristics of Poorly Written Proposals

1. Ill-defined, faulty, diffuse, or unwarranted aims and/or hypotheses
2. Insignificant, unimaginative, unoriginal research problems
3. Inadequate literature review with no analysis or synthesis
4. Weak or inappropriate designs with insufficient sample sizes and inadequate controls
5. Questionable, defective technology
6. Invalid and/or unreliable instrumentation, timing, conditions, or data collection procedures
7. Weak, vague, or inappropriate analyses
8. Inexperienced, unproductive, incompetent investigators as reflected in the preliminary studies or curriculum vitae
9. Inadequate resources (from laboratory facilities to coinvestigator involvement)

ORGANIZATION OF THE RESEARCH PLAN

A well-organized narrative of the research plan weaves the different aspects of the project into a cohesive whole to achieve clarity, conciseness, and persuasiveness. The research plan consists of the following sections:

1. Specific aims
2. Significance
3. Background
4. Preliminary studies
5. Method

From the first sentence of the proposal, the reader should begin to develop a clear picture of the research plan. Every succeeding sentence should add new information that contributes to a reader's understanding of the study. A summary table highlights critical aspects of the study, promoting clarity and helping the reader see the continuity of the research plan (Table 24–3).

Specific Aims

Specific aims of the research plan should be stated in terms of objectives and research questions or hypotheses (predictions). The aims inform the reader about what the investigator hopes to accomplish. Aims are better understood when they are summarized in a model that reflects the major variables and relationships between variables. Such a model helps the reader visualize the conceptual framework (basis) of the study. Development of such a model unfolds as the investigator uses information from scientific reports, expert consultants, and personal clinical and research experience. Figure 24–1 offers a model that shows relationships between research variables.

A hypothetical study examining the impact of decision making (decisional control), exercise, and diet on fatigue in cancer patients is used to portray development of the model. The design includes an experimental group that will participate in decision making (decision-making group) and a control group that will not be participating in decision making (non–decision-making group). The following example is used throughout the chapter.

EXAMPLE

Specific Aim 1. To determine whether patients who participate in decision making on amount of exercise and type of diet report less fatigue during chemotherapy than patients who do not participate in decision making. The researcher believes that type of decisional control (participation in decision making) over exercise and diet (independent variables) influences the fatigue (dependent variable) that patients experience.

Specific Aim 2. To determine whether the magnitude of the impact of decisional control over exercise and diet on reported fatigue during chemotherapy is influenced by the patient's compliance with the optimal exercise and diet program. As noted in Figure 24–1, the degree to

Table 24–3

Example of a Table to Assist in Maintaining the Integrity of the Proposal

SPECIFIC AIMS	OPERATIONAL DEFINITION	WHERE FOUND	RELIABILITY AND VALIDITY	DATA COLLECTION TIMES	DATA ANALYSIS
Experimental subjects report less fatigue than control subjects	Perceived fatigue score = sum of 10-item questionnaire; higher score means more fatigue	Perceived Fatigue Questionnaire (Appendix A)	Internal consistency reliability = .92 Content validity index = .89 Criterion validity = .82	T1 = baseline T2 = after first chemotherapy course, 10-minute patient self-report	*t*-test between means for experimental versus control groups

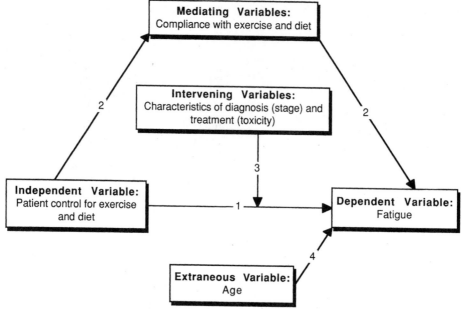

(Numbers 1 through 4 refer to specific aims of the study.)

Figure 24–1
Model of variables and relationships.

which patients comply with exercise and diet (mediating variables) influences the fatigue that patients report experiencing.

Specific Aim 3. To determine whether stage of cancer and toxicity of treatment have an impact on the relationship between type of decisional control and fatigue. The intervening variables (characteristics of diagnosis and treatment) affect the influence of the independent variable (patient control over exercise and diet) on the dependent variable (fatigue).

Specific Aim 4. To determine whether age has a direct impact on fatigue. As seen in Figure 24–1, the researcher anticipates that study results will show that age (extraneous variable) affects fatigue (dependent variable).

Significance

The significance part of the proposal details the importance of the problem under examination. This can be done by including statistics that summarize the scope of the problem in relation to incidence, distribution in different populations, relevance to health, and impact on mortality and morbidity. A statement addressing the expected gains for

nursing and science should also be included. For instance, in the hypothetical study, the researcher might expect to fill the gap in knowledge concerning the importance of patient participation in decision making regarding exercise and diet in preventing extreme fatigue.

Background

The background section of the proposal could be merged with the significance section if page limits are in effect. The background provides literature support for each of the hypothesized relationships and includes information on how the study can be used to fill a knowledge gap in science. Readers find it helpful if the investigator provides a one-paragraph overview of the study at the end of the section.

For the hypothetical study concerning the effects of decision making over exercise and diet on chemotherapy-related fatigue, the background section would include the following:

1. Research on different types of control (the importance of decisional control compared to other types of control in eliciting compliance with self-care prescriptions)

2. A summary of the physiological and psychological theories that link fatigue to type of diet and exercise
3. Influence of disease stage, treatment toxicity, and patient's age on fatigue

Preliminary Studies

The purpose of the preliminary studies section of the proposal is to authenticate that investigators are competent to implement and complete the study. In this section, the preliminary studies that have been done by all researchers associated with the proposed project are listed. These studies are used as building blocks for the hypotheses, design, operational definitions, and procedures of the current study. Pilot studies serve as small, preliminary tests of the project's feasibility. Successful completion of a pilot study could convince others of the viability of the project and of the competence of the investigators.

Nurses in clinical settings often have no previous research experience in proposed areas of study. In that case, the preliminary studies section of the proposal can include descriptions of relevant case studies, quality assurance reviews, nursing care policies, and staff development or patient education projects with which the nurses have been associated. Nurses with little research experience could conduct a pilot study preliminary to a larger project to promote research competence.

Method

The method section is the most essential part of a proposal. Constructing a valid, feasible, cost-effective method for conducting the study is the best way to gain approval from administrators, professionals in nursing and other disciplines, human or animal use committees, and other nurse investigators. The method section includes sample and setting, design, variables, data collection and management procedures, human or animal use protection data, data analyses strategies, and time frames for conducting the study.

SAMPLE AND SETTING

The sample and setting should be described in as much detail as possible. The proposal should include criteria for selecting the setting and subjects.

EXAMPLE

The investigator lists the characteristics of the subjects as

1. Adult males
2. Between the ages of 50 and 80 years
3. With a new diagnosis of squamous cell carcinoma of the lung
4. Embarking on their first course of therapy
5. Not more than 5 pounds underweight
6. Able to maintain a moderate pace on a treadmill

After the subject criteria have been defined, the sampling procedure (for example, convenience, including all eligible patients) should be described, documenting the method used to determine sample size (adequacy of the number of subjects in meeting the study objectives and availability of subjects from the setting in which the study will be conducted). To be competitive, a grant proposal should include a sampling strategy that yields ethnic representation proportional to the population. In some cases, oversampling of an ethnic group is needed.

EXAMPLE

The researcher states that the clinical setting is the outpatient department of a major medical center that annually accrues 200 new patients who fit the criteria. The process for deciding sample size should be addressed in the proposal. Consultation with a statistician is advisable at this time. The following factors are used in determining sample size (Polit & Hungler, 1995):

1. The probability of making a type I error by *rejecting the null hypothesis* (prediction that the mean group scores are the same) *when it is true*, i.e., when it is true that there is actually no significant difference between mean fatigue scores of groups. For example, when developing the proposal, the researcher
   a. Formulates a hypothesis, which is a statement that something is true. The first hypothesis states that patients who participate in decision

making on diet and exercise report less fatigue than patients who do not participate in decision making. The null hypothesis states that there is no difference in fatigue between the two conditions.

b. Randomly assigns 200 patients, 100 to the decision-making group and 100 to the non–decision-making group, so that the fatigue experience in both groups can be compared.

c. Uses a statistical test (*t*-test for independent samples) to find out whether the anticipated data from 200 subjects (100 in each group) will yield a significant difference between the mean fatigue scores. (Considering the number of subjects, the value of the *t* statistic has to be large enough to conclude that there is only a small chance [for example, 5%] of making an error in rejecting the null hypothesis.)

2. *Determination of the anticipated difference between the two groups.* Previous studies or clinical experience can be used as the basis for predicting the difference between the two groups. For example, the investigator might anticipate a difference in weight loss and treadmill capability of about 15% between the decision-making group and the non–decision-making group.

3. The probability of making a type II error by *accepting the null hypothesis when it is false.* For example, the investigator might conclude in the hypothetical example that there is no difference in fatigue between the decision-making and non–decision-making groups when, in fact, there is a difference. One way to reduce the possibility of making a type II error is to set the power of a test high at .80 or greater. This requires a larger number of subjects in the different groups than when power is set at a lower level such as at .50.

DESIGN

The design must fit the specific aims of the study (see Chapter 22). The following discussion addresses the design of the hypothetical example.

The use of a design model helps the reader to visualize the study. The kind of design that fits the aims of the hypothetical study is one that includes grouping (stratification) of subjects. The model in Figure 24–2 shows that subjects are assigned to groups according to age categories (51 to 60, 61 to 70, and 71 to 80 years) and functional status (poor, moderate, good) before random assignment to the experimental (decision-making) or control (non–decision-making) conditions.

Ideally, the proposal specifies the exact number of subjects to be accrued for each predetermined group (age and functional status). When this is not possible, the investigator should provide an estimate of the proportion of subjects in each age and functional status category by using statistics from the setting from which subjects are recruited. The total number of experimental and control subjects should be indicated in the proposal (for example, experimentals = 100 and controls = 100), because that number is predetermined.

Nurses involved in clinical studies should always be concerned about controlling the following variables that tend to affect (confound) results: medical diagnosis, treatment, age, physical and mental status, and gender. In some types of studies, these variables are controlled through sample selection criteria (eligibility criteria such as age) or by statistics. The proposal should clearly describe the methods used to control the variables that are known to influence study results. This is done to ensure that if statistical tests show a significant difference between experimental and control groups, the difference can be attributed to whether the subjects did or did not participate in decision making.

Stratified (grouped) variables can be handled in one of the following two ways:

1. In experimental or quasi-experimental studies, it is useful to control certain variables (such as age and gender) by building them into the design as stratification (grouping) factors. This means that subjects are subdivided into groups according to certain values of the variable that the investigator wants to control. In the example, subjects were subdivided into three

Stratification
Variables

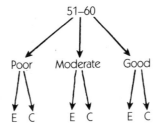

Decision making
YES (Experimental)
NO (Control)

Figure 24–2
Example of experimental design with stratification variables. Subjects accrued under each stratification arm of the design are randomized to the experimental (E) or the control (C) condition.

age groups: 51 to 60, 61 to 70, and 71 to 80 years.

2. A second way to use stratification (grouping) is to ensure that experimental and control groups comprise the same number of participants who are alike in the variables of interest (for example, age, functional status, gender). This strategy does not increase the sample size, because the major comparison is still between the experimental and control conditions. For example, subjects between the ages of 51 and 60 years who have good functional status are assigned to the experimental or control condition in a modified random manner (equal numbers ending up in each condition). The same modified randomization procedure is followed for subjects in the same age category who have poor functional status, and so on for the other two age groups. In other words, the mean ages and the mean functional status scores of subjects in the experimental and control groups will be similar.

When a variable (such as age) is of major interest to the investigator and predictions are made based on the variable, it needs to be taken into consideration when sample size is calculated.

EXAMPLE

Situation 1. If the study includes only an experimental (decision-making) and a control (non–decision-making) condition, fewer subjects are needed because the design consists of only two groups.

Situation 2. Situations in which the investigator is interested in the interaction of decision making with age require that the design include more than just two conditions. Subjects are first categorized into predetermined age groups (51 to 60, 61 to 70, and 71 to 80 years) and are then randomly assigned to either the experimental or the control condition. A total of six groups emerges after subjects are assigned according to age and group. In this case, a much larger sample size is required because of the resulting subgroups. Sample size calculations are per group.

OPERATIONAL DEFINITIONS OF RESEARCH VARIABLES

Each variable in the specific aims requires an operational definition. The definition includes the measurement used to quantify the variable and the validity and reliability of the instrument (Waltz, Strickland, & Lenz, 1991).

In the case of the independent variable (patient participation in decision making), both values of the variable must be defined and adequately described (what constitutes decision making or its absence). The proposal should include the methods used to check the validity of the administration of the intervention (how patient participation in decision making will be carried out) to inform the reviewer of the plans for maintaining the integrity of the intervention. These steps are vital in preventing or minimizing problems in interpretation at the conclusion of the study. If manipulation of the independent variable (assistance in decision making) is not checked for validity and reliability, the investigator might not be able to conclude whether the observed effects are attributable to the treatment or to the omission or incomplete performance of the treatment.

EXAMPLE

An investigator can determine the presence of decisional control for the experimental condition and the absence of decisional control for the control condition by asking subjects to rate degree of perceived decisional control.

1. Administration of the independent variable is judged to be valid if subjects in the experimental decision-making group report greater decisional control than subjects in the control non–decision-making condition.
2. Reliability of the independent variable is determined through checks that show that assistance in decision making was carried out in a consistent manner with each subject.

The proposal should also include a description of "usual" services available to all patients. For example, the proposal might report whether (1) the medical center provides standard written material on exercise and nutrition self-care activities, (2) the clinical setting includes an oncology clinical specialist who sees every patient and writes orders for nursing interventions to prevent extreme fatigue and malnutrition, (3) a dietitian is able to see all patients, and (4) regular patient education programs exist for this type of lung cancer patient.

Operational definitions of the dependent, mediating, intervening, and extraneous variables should also be included in the proposal. It is necessary to report the reliability and validity of each of the measurements, as well as the manner in which the proposed study will reevaluate reliability and validity. The scoring procedure for each measure and the meaning of each score should be included in the proposal.

EXAMPLE

Fatigue can be described as the number of minutes that a subject stays on the treadmill; the greater the time, the more fatigue tolerant the subject. Criterion validity of the treadmill and stopwatch are determined by following the manufacturer's instructions for calibrating the equipment. Reliability is determined by observing the consistency with which treadmill speed is replicated or that a specific rater logs time.

DATA COLLECTION PROCEDURE

A scriptlike description of the procedures used to collect data offers several advantages. It helps the reader to visualize the study in a step-by-step manner, thus facilitating the feasibility of the data collection procedures. The "script" informs the reviewer that the protocol will be consistently implemented during the study.

Of particular importance is the procedure used to obtain human subject consent. It should be clear to the reader that no form of coercion enters into the request for a subject's participation in a study. The proposal should describe how subjects will be identified and approached, what and how information will be provided, and what strategies will be used to revisit potential subjects should they be unavailable or should consent from a family member be necessary.

The time frame for implementing the study should be logical and feasible. It often helps to provide a table that plots the months of the study and the specific activities to be carried out (Table 24–4). The expected subject accrual throughout the study should be included in the time frame. In the case of longitudinal studies, the table needs to show how subject accrual overlaps with repeated data collection from subjects. This gives the reader a good sense of the burden of the study for both the subject and the data collector.

DATA MANAGEMENT

Data management is an often neglected aspect of a proposal. Scientific reviewers want to know how the data will be handled. Questions reviewers ask include the following:

1. Who will be responsible for maintaining confidentiality of subject data?

Table 24–4

Example of 1-Year Timetable

1–2 MONTHS	3–4 MONTHS	5–6 MONTHS	7–8 MONTHS	9–10 MONTHS	11–12 MONTHS
Hire and train staff					
Pilot test					
Instruments					
Procedures					
(10 subjects)					
Collect pretest and posttest data with 10 subjects per week					
Pretest: 10 10 10 10 10 10 10 10 10 10 10 10 10 10 10 10 10 10 10 10					
Posttest: 10 10 10 10 10 10 10 10 10 10 10 10 10 10 10 10 10 10 10 10					
Data Entry - >					
				Data analysis and write-up	

2. Where will raw data be stored? Will it be secured?

3. Who will code or computerize the data? How will data sets be checked for errors in coding or computerizing?

4. How long will raw data be kept? When will it be destroyed?

5. If multiple data collection sites are involved, who will coordinate data collection? Will data be collected in a timely and efficient manner and be kept in a single safe location?

DATA ANALYSIS

An efficient way to write the data analysis section is to provide the reader with an overview of the plan for testing the aims and then to describe the statistical tools used to address each specific aim. In this manner, consistency is promoted throughout the proposal, and the reader has no trouble following the logic of the analysis plan. The sample should be described in general and specific terms with the study design and statistical assumptions in mind. Next, subject dropout and its impact on sample size and power should be addressed. Strategies for testing assumptions of the statistics should also be discussed.

Before addressing the specific aims of a study, analyses are carried out to identify errors in the data set. For example, unusual scores or scores outside of the limits of measurement for specific variables are identified and corrected. This process is sometimes called "data cleaning" and must precede any analysis of a data set.

PROTECTION OF SUBJECTS AND PERSONNEL

To be complete, a proposal must include information on strategies used to protect subjects and research staff from risk. Most health care institutions or agencies are aware of the need to protect human subjects from undue risk, breach of confidentiality, unscrupulous investigators, or trivial studies. To this end, written policies guide the ethical conduct of research with human subjects, administrators enforce these policies, and committees evaluate projects to decide whether studies are ethical and scientific, and whether they have a risk-benefit ratio in favor of the study. Similar safeguards apply to animal subjects and research staff.

CONSULTANTS

Consultants are used because they provide needed expertise in an important area or because objective advice is needed to ensure methodological and theoretical rigor. Sometimes, consultants are used to facilitate entry into a subject pool, to provide balance, or to help with data interpretation. Proposals must describe the objective of having a consultant, must justify the fit of the consultant's background with the objective, and must identify the time frame and cost under which a consultant will be expected to operate. Finally, a proposal should include a letter of agreement from the consultant. Such a letter should clearly list the activities that the consultant has agreed to perform.

Table 24–5

Examples of Funding Agency Internet Addresses and Telephone Numbers

AGENCIES	INTERNET ADDRESS	TELEPHONE
National Institutes of Health	http://www.nih.gov	301-496-4000
NIH Office of Extramural Research—grants	http://www.nih.gov/grants/oer.htm	301-496-1096
National Institute of Nursing Research	http://www.nih.gov/ninr/	
Division of Extramural Research		301-594-6906
Centers for Disease Control and Prevention	http://www.cdc.gov	404-639-3343
American Cancer Society	http://www.cancer.org/	404-329-5734
American Heart Association	http://www.amhrt.org/	214-706-1453
American Diabetes Foundation	http://www.diabetes.org/	703-549-1500
Robert Wood Johnson Foundation	http://www.rwjf.org/main.html	609-452-8701

LITERATURE CITED

Every scientific proposal includes references to support the premise of the study. Proposals need not include bibliographies that encompass all that is known about an area of research. Only the most pertinent references should be used, and the references in the text should match the list of references cited at the end of the proposal.

APPENDIX

The appendix contains material that elaborates on the information provided in the text. For example, investigators might include a few of their own recent publications that are relevant to the study and that were briefly described in the preliminary studies section. Copies of psychometric instruments or descriptions and pictures of physiological measures defined in the text might also appear in appendices. Scripts that detail an education manipulation, consent forms, full-length curriculum vitae, and letters of support or agreement are all appropriate material. Most importantly, information needed to understand a study should be included in the body of a proposal; only supportive information is placed in the appendix. The

Table 24–6

Ten Fatal Flaws of Research Grant Proposals

1. Expecting a research grant to pay for treatment. Example: A project is about delivery of service with research added on.
2. Conducting research in an area where one has minimal expertise. Example: A scientist with expertise in psychological measures adds physiological measures to a study to try to be more comprehensive.
3. Omitting important details of how research tasks will be completed. Example: Assuming that the reviewers can fill in the blanks.
4. Ignoring expert feedback concerning the weaknesses of a proposal. Example: An investigator does not address the flaws in a research grant application identified by a review committee.
5. Starting a project by developing a scale as if that is a minor aspect of the proposed study. Example: Very little information is provided regarding a scale to be developed to measure an important variable in the study.
6. Tacking on a variable or two to a project so that a funding agency will find the study more appealing. Example: Including a "drug abuse" variable to a study, reasoning that the National Institute of Drug Abuse would therefore want to fund a study.
7. Studying a "no-problem" problem. Example: Studying a problem for which the incidence is very low.
8. Making excuses for why a study cannot be done correctly. Example: Failing to provide control conditions in an intervention trial and justifying it by saying that it was not feasible.
9. Using inappropriate tests or measures. Example: Using measures that are not reliable or valid.
10. Failing to write a proposal. Example: Unless an investigator writes a proposal, he or she cannot be funded.

investigator should be selective about the content and length of the appendix.

GRANT APPLICATIONS ON THE INTERNET

Funding priorities and instructions for grant applications involving federal agencies and many private foundations are located on the World Wide Web. Applicants are encouraged to browse through the information on the Internet before calling the agency asking for information about proposal preparation and grant opportunities. Table 24–5 lists a few examples of Internet addresses and agency telephone numbers.

In addition to the aforementioned recommendations for proposal writing, proposals for research grant applications should be wary of 10 mistakes that usually lead to rejection of a research grant application (Oetting, 1986). These mistakes are concerned with the general significance of the research problem, its relevance to the funding agency, and the general rigor of the research plan (Table 24–6).

SUMMARY

A well-written proposal is a precursor to a scientifically sound study and publishable research report. It is used by reviewers to determine the scientific merit and feasibility of a study. A proposal fulfills the valuable role of informing readers about the researcher's ideas. As such, it is vital that the text be well written so that the reader can visualize the plan (how the study will be carried out and data will be analyzed).

Before writing the proposal, the investigator should inquire about institutional or funding agency submission guidelines. This not only facilitates the review process but also promotes a good working relationship between the investigator and the agency.

REFERENCES

US Department of Health and Human Services Public Health Service. Application for a Public Health Service Grant PHS 398. Rev. 5/95, OMB No. 0925–0001, 1995.

Clore, E. R. (1985). Grant budgeting: Preparation and management. *Nursing Economics, 3,* 341–348.

Cuca, J. M., & McLoughlin, W. J. (1987). Why clinical research grant applications fare poorly in review and how to recover. *Cancer Investigation, 5,* 55–58.

National Institutes of Health, Public Health Service, Department of Health and Human Services. (1989). Preparing a research grant application to the National Institutes of Health: Selected articles. Bethesda, MD: Division of Research Grants, Office of Grants Inquiries.

Oetting, E. R. (1986). Ten fatal mistakes in grant writing. *Professional Psychology: Research and Practice, 17,* 570–573.

Polit, D. F., & Hungler, B. P. (1995) *Nursing research: Principles and methods* (5th ed.). Philadelphia: J. B. Lippincott.

Waltz, C. F., Nelson, B., & Chambers, S. B. (1985). Assigning publication credits. *Nursing Outlook, 33,* 233–238.

Waltz, C. F., Strickland, O. L., & Lenz, E. R. (1991). *Measurement in Nursing* (2nd ed.). Philadelphia: F. A. Davis.

Chapter 25

Implementing the Study

Deborah B. McGuire and Katherine A. Yeager

Implementation of a study that has received the necessary institutional approvals, and perhaps even some external grant funding, is one of the most exciting, frightening, and challenging parts of doing clinical research. The researcher has laid the groundwork, cleared a number of hurdles, scrambled around some obstacles, and is ready to go. What comes next? How does an investigator move from planning a study to carrying it out?

The implementation phase of a clinical research project requires a thoughtful, careful, organized, and sequential set of activities rather than an enthusiastic, "gung ho" approach. The reasons for a deliberative approach are many and include the following:

1. Maintenance of sociopolitical equilibrium

2. Assurance of cooperation from coinvestigators and other essential personnel

3. Development of financial and administrative support systems

4. Acquisition of necessary supplies or personnel

5. Management of pilot test procedures

6. Development of data collection, quality control, and data management procedures

Disregard for these areas, or insufficient attention to them, can seriously undermine the success of a clinical study.

In this chapter, an organized and systematic approach to implementing a study is presented. If the study is conducted on a single unit and involves few participants, some of the detail provided in this chapter will not be pertinent. On the other hand, if the study is a clinical trial and involves multiple sites with many personnel, the level of detail may be too general. Researchers with such studies should consult additional resources (Meinert, 1986; Guy, 1991; Melink & Whitacre, 1991). This chapter is divided into five sections: sites for data collection, administrative issues, equipment and supplies, preimplementation, and implementation. Although different investigators do not always adhere to these five areas in the order or depth presented, each area is relevant to any clinical study and must be addressed to some degree. In the following discussions, the term *investigator* is used to mean a single individual or a group of investigators. The chapter is written primarily for the nurse investigator who does not have a clinical nurse researcher available for consultation. It is recognized, however, that clinical nurse researchers working with nurse investigators might well carry out some of the activities described in this chapter.

SITES FOR DATA COLLECTION

There are two key issues related to the sites selected for data collection. The first key issue involves procedures for access to the institutions and to the patients, nurses, and other personnel. It is assumed that the study sites are able to provide the appropriate subjects for the study (see Chapter 13). The second issue addresses actual planning for implementation, including the development of a time frame, orientation of appropriate personnel, adaptation of the study to the system already in place, and considerations with intervention studies.

Procedures for Access

Before implementing a study, the investigator selects a clinical site or sites suitable to the goals and design of the study. This determination should include assessments of subject and professional participation, receptivity toward research, organizational system, economic factors, facilities and resources, and legal or statutory provisions (Varricchio & Mikos, 1987). In addition, researchers need to explore whether competing or overlapping studies are in place and

to discuss with institutional personnel and relevant researchers how to resolve such situations. Persons in the selected clinical sites should have already approved the study, granted access to patients, and generally indicated the nature and depth of the support that they are able to provide. In Chapter 13, Foreman gives guidelines for gaining access to institutions. These guidelines include discussions about organizational politics, making timely and appropriate contacts with key personnel, and gaining interdisciplinary support.

The investigator who wishes to gain access to a site for a study should focus on three important criteria to help ensure successful negotiation (Kirchhoff & McGuire, 1985a). These include the following:

1. *Early negotiation* can occur with the institution even while the proposal is being developed. Such negotiations generally result in proposals that are compatible with the selected sites and, therefore, are more readily approved (Kirchhoff & McGuire, 1985b).
2. *Mutual respect* should be present before, during, and after a study.
3. *Mutual benefit* is the difference between access for the investigator with an "interesting study" versus one whose study will answer an important clinical question for the institution.

Most institutions require that *all* necessary approvals be granted before the beginning of data collection. In any institution receiving federal funds, a Human Subjects Committee or Institutional Review Board (IRB) is in place to protect human subjects. Refer to Chapter 13 for a discussion on IRBs. In many institutions, the nursing departments have a nursing research review process, and there can also be a third review process conducted by a multidisciplinary group. Such review bodies usually examine proposed studies for both clinical feasibility and scientific merit.

Assuming that the necessary approvals have been obtained, the investigator must refamiliarize himself or herself with committees that have approved the study before its actual implementation. For example, if IRB approval was granted some months before, the investigator must make sure that the approval is still valid and that no addendum or modification to the original application is needed. Similarly, if the nursing department approved the study 6 months earlier but requires updates on the status of approved studies every 6 months, then the investigator should notify the department that the study is about to be implemented.

It is extremely important that the investigator check with the nursing department about whether the persons who were initially involved in approving the study are still in place. If not, the study must be explained to new personnel to gain their formal or informal approval and support. The same process must be carried out in medical or other departments germane to the study. Personnel and positions change frequently in clinical settings, sometimes without notice. It is up to the investigator to keep track of such changes, because notifying investigators of staff changes is almost certainly low on the priority list of administrators and clinicians. When these details are addressed in advance, the investigator can feel more comfortable that a social and political environment positive to the study has been achieved (Oda, 1983).

Planning for Implementation

The planning phase can be time-consuming to the investigator, but it is essential to achieve a smooth, logical implementation. Three specific components include devising a time frame, orienting personnel to the study, and ensuring the fit between the study method and procedures at the clinical site. Additionally, there are unique considerations when the study is going to test an intervention.

TIME FRAME

A carefully planned time frame, devised realistically and followed faithfully, goes far toward helping the investigator implement the study as rapidly and smoothly as possible. Devising a time frame for the different activities required in the implementation phase helps keep the researcher on target (Fig. 25–1). The time frame must be both reasonable in its estimation of time needed for different activities and feasible within the existing schedules and activities of the data collection site. For example, an investigator might not want to conduct orientation sessions to the research study during the summer months because many nurses may be on vacation and the remaining nurses bear an increased workload. Many steps of the research process take much longer than anticipated. A good rule of thumb is to estimate the time needed and to double that amount.

Specific activities in the planned time frame can vary from one study to another. If the investigator has external grant funding to support the study, procedures related to setting up accounts, receiving statements, and other fiscal matters must be included in the schedule (these procedures are discussed later). If there is no external funding forthcoming and there are no other hurdles, the time frame should include only those activities related directly to the study implementation, such as orienting personnel, getting necessary data collection tools or equipment in place, and perhaps conducting a pilot study.

ORIENTATION TO THE STUDY

The politically astute investigator makes certain that groups or persons who have a "need to know" about what is going on in the clinical site are informed and their input is solicited, particularly when they control access to patients. The value of advance groundwork in this area has been thoroughly discussed by several authors (McHugh & Johnson, 1980; Oda, 1983; Brooten, 1984; Kirchhoff, 1987).

Personnel who need to know about the study include registered nurses, licensed practical nurses, nursing assistants, unit clerks and secretaries, housekeepers and janitors, pharmacists, social workers, physicians, and many others (Yeager, DeLoney, Crooker, Webster, & McGuire, 1997). In addition, any person or group who might have anything to do with the study is entitled to hear about it. Orientation of staff to the study serves a number of purposes (Table 25–1) and is easily accomplished with some advance planning and selected considerations (Table 25–2). Such orientation to the study can involve speaking with a large number of personnel, and it is unrealistic to expect that this will be accomplished in one or two scheduled meetings at the investigator's convenience. Plans for orientation must therefore be made in concert with the schedules of everyone involved at the clinical site. It is especially important for inves-

TASKS	6/87–9/87	10/87–12/87	1/88–2/88	3/88	4/88–10/89	12/89
Refine research	→					
Question and write proposal	→					
Procure approvals		→				
Submit for funding		→				
Orient and train nursing staff and other personnel			→			
Submit for funding			→			
Preimplementation and revision			→			
Implementation					→	
Monitor data, troubleshoot, and problem solve			→			
Conclusion						→

The study is a randomized experiment in which two different dressing regimens on long-term indwelling central catheters are compared in a population of patients receiving bone marrow transplants.

Figure 25–1
Sample time frame for a clinical nursing study. (From Shivnan, J.C., McGuire, D., Freeman, S., Sharkazy, E., Bosserman, G., Larson, E., & Grouleff, P. [1991]. A comparison of transparent adherent and dry sterile gauze dressings for long-term central catheters in patients undergoing bone marrow transplant. *Oncology Nursing Forum, 18,* 1349–1355.)

tigators to remember staff who work on nondaytime shifts and to make accommodations so that they also can learn about the study.

FIT BETWEEN CLINICAL SITE AND STUDY METHOD

The third area to consider in planning for implementation helps to ensure that the study and its method fit into the system already in place at the clinical site. As noted earlier in this chapter, early negotiations should have already addressed this issue. When the investigator reaches the implementation phase, however, it is necessary to reevaluate the fit between the study methodology and the site.

Table 25–1
Orientation of Staff to the Study

1. Notify personnel that a study is going to be conducted.
2. Inform staff about who and what will be involved.
3. Explain the background, significance, and time frame of the study.
4. Give staff a chance to provide input on various aspects of the study (which can often include important concerns or points overlooked by the investigator).
5. Explain staff responsibilities or degree of participation.
6. Provide the opportunity to clarify questions or misunderstandings before implementing the study.
7. Reinforce the notion that staff input and ideas are welcome.
8. Engender positive feelings about the study and unit participation.
9. Discuss plans for informing staff about progress and further updates.

Before any data collection, the investigator must learn about and observe usual routines in the clinical area (McHugh & Johnson, 1980) and get to know the study culture (Yeager, DeLoney, Crooker, Webster, & McGuire, 1997), because the existing environment can influence the conduct of the study (Rudy, 1991) (Table 25–3). Additionally, the investigator must consider how the study procedures can fit into the routines, practices, and physical layout of the site without disrupting ongoing activities. Potential problems and solutions need to be

Table 25–2
Considerations in Planning for Staff Orientation to the Study

1. Plan to give orientation sessions personally.
2. Identify the persons who need orientation, what vehicles already exist (regularly scheduled staff meetings, departmental rounds, shift change reports), and when the orientation can be scheduled. These strategies help convey to clinical personnel how important they are to the study (Kirchhoff & McGuire, 1985a; Lasoff, 1986).
3. Give clear explanations. For most listeners, everything about the study is new. Explanations should be given in understandable language appropriate for the group being addressed and should briefly highlight the purpose of the study, target sample, informed consent procedures, and data collection plans. Details about background and data analysis can be omitted if not directly pertinent to the audience. For example, for the nursing staff, a study that asks staff nurses to use a particular documentation form might require extensive explanation, teaching, and practice, but for unit clerks, perhaps only a short informational session on the goals, methods, and time frame of the study is sufficient.

Table 25–3

Examples of Clinical Site Practices and Their Influence on Study Methods

1. Are inpatients unavailable because diagnostic tests and procedures are planned for morning hours? Will adjustments in data collection time periods need to be made?
2. When are inpatient medical rounds made and will they interfere with data collection?
3. In a busy outpatient clinic, what is the best time to approach potential patients for participation in a study? Where can interviews be conducted or questionnaires administered?
4. Where are patient charts, medication administration forms, and other essential documents kept? If they are not where they are supposed to be, where else can they be found? Which personnel are critical in helping locate such important material?

identified. Careful observation and analysis of these issues and incorporation of necessary adaptations into the study protocol ensure a smooth fit between the study and the site.

CONSIDERATIONS WITH INTERVENTION STUDIES

Intervention studies require some unique considerations, including the role of the staff, standardization of the intervention, validity issues, and process issues. The involvement and roles of the clinical staff versus the research staff (Nail, 1990) must be delineated. Decisions regarding who will administer the intervention should be decided up front, and the intervention should be standardized as much as possible (Egan, Snyder, & Burns, 1992). Written instructions or a formal protocol for implementation of the intervention serve the study process well (DeLoney, Yeager, Crooker, & McGuire, 1997). Potential confounding factors that may affect internal validity should be identified and mechanisms developed to control or measure them (McGuire et al., in press). Similarly, decisions must be made about what nursing activities can be left to institutional practice versus what can or must be standardized for all study participants (McGuire, Lin, Owen, & Peterson, 1997). Finally, process components of planning and implementing an intervention study (for example, the timing of study events, measurement procedures, and com-

munication mechanisms) must be developed and documented so that the investigator has a permanent record of all decisions and procedures for reference during the course of the study.

ADMINISTRATIVE ISSUES

Two major administrative issues arise when implementing a study. The first relates to finances and costs pertinent to the study and the second involves personnel necessary to the study.

Finances and Costs

The investigator might have already applied for and received external grant funds to support the study or could be relying on internal nonmonetary sources of support. In either case, two important areas related to finances are (1) determining the costs of a study and (2) setting up accounting procedures.

DETERMINING COSTS OF A STUDY

If external funds have been sought, the investigator will have developed a budget for the study with proposed costs categorized (for example, personnel, supplies) and carefully justified in the process of writing a grant application. If a grant application has not been submitted by the investigator, it is important to realize that a study still incurs costs that must be anticipated and identified before implementation. These costs include the expense of personnel, supplies, equipment, technical support (including clerical, secretarial, and statistical), computer costs, possibly travel, and miscellaneous other expenses (for example, telephone charges, Internet subscriptions, duplication).

Table 25–4 lists examples of possible costs that an investigator can encounter in the course of a study. When a grant has been received, many of these costs are covered by the awarded funds. If there are expenses over and above the grant budget or if the investigator does not have a grant to support the research, the investigator must make a careful analysis of project costs and present them to the director of nursing or other relevant administrators to determine

Table 25–4

Examples of Research-Related Costs

1. Will the investigator and one nurse colleague be the only persons who collect data? If so, will it be done on work time and is the nurse manager agreeable to such an arrangement? Or will all nurses in a clinical area be collecting data on work time and is that permissible?
2. Will multiple copies of a lengthy questionnaire be needed to conduct the study? Can the duplication budget of the nursing department cover this expense?
3. Will consultants in research methodology or statistical analysis and interpretation be needed? Who are they, what are their consultation fees, and will the nursing department pay for them?
4. Will secretarial assistance be required to type data collection forms, or will clerical help be needed to schedule outpatients to participate in the study at a special clinic visit?

sources of support. One avenue that should be explored involves the exchange of fees or services with other departments or institutions (McGuire & Harwood, 1989). An additional source of funds, depending on the purpose of the study, may come from manufacturers of products that will be used or tested in the study. For example, in a study that compared complications and side effects, nursing time, and patient satisfaction and comfort between two types of dressings for long-term indwelling catheters, the manufacturer of the experimental dressing provided partial funding for the study as well as dressing materials (Shivnan et al., 1991).

SETTING UP ACCOUNTING PROCEDURES

When grant funds have been obtained, no matter how small or large, accounting procedures must be established. The investigator is responsible to the funding agency for an accurate record of expenditures and can meet this obligation only when a system is devised. Funding agencies often offer the investigator some options for managing the awarded funds. For example, the American Nurses' Foundation (ANF) may allow the investigator to choose whether the full amount of the grant will be sent to the employing institution and be put into an account for the investigator's use or whether the investigator will keep records of expenditures and then apply directly to ANF for reimbursement (up to the amount of the grant that was awarded).

Accounting systems vary among institutions. A hospital generally has a central financial office that manages a variety of fiscal affairs related to institutional operations. Similarly, universities have well-delineated accounting systems. The investigator must determine what accounting system is used within the institution and whom to contact for organizing, setting up, and problem solving. Accounting concerns should be addressed before study implementation, preferably before receipt of grant funds.

Most institutional accounting systems generally release account statements on some predetermined schedule, usually monthly. These statements partition the grant award into the expense categories indicated in the budget. The statements usually reflect how much was spent in each category during the accounting period and how much is unspent. The wise investigator, novice or experienced, makes certain that the reporting system is understandable and examines monthly statements promptly and carefully to keep track of expenditures. This process helps ensure that any accounting errors are detected in a timely fashion. In financial offices handling a large number of grant and contract awards, it is not uncommon for charges to inadvertently be made to the wrong account. Prompt reconciliation of such errors is necessary, because the investigator must ensure that awarded funds are spent appropriately and within the grant funding period. Finally, the investigator should keep copies of all account statements during the funding period because they are needed for the formal financial report prepared for the funding agency at the end of the grant period.

If an investigator does not have access to a formal accounting system or has chosen a reimbursement option (such as that offered by ANF), he or she must devise an individual accounting system. Accurate records of expenditures (such as receipts and bills of sale) must be kept, including date, budget category, specific items, costs, and documentation. Computer software programs that include fiscal or accounting spreadsheets are available to assist with this process.

Personnel

The second major administrative area in implementing a clinical study is that of personnel. Depending on the study, a few or many individuals will be involved representing one or more groups of people (for example, nursing, medicine, clerical). The selection of proper personnel is important not only in designing the study procedures for data collection and analysis but also in seeking financial support for the study and in planning for implementation.

BUILDING AN INTERDISCIPLINARY TEAM

Complex clinical problems often require interdisciplinary teamwork for optimal assessment and management. Similarly, the formal study of such problems may require the knowledge and expertise of an interdisciplinary research team (McGuire, submitted, 1998). In one study of analgesics in oncology outpatients (Hagle et al., 1987; McGuire et al., 1987), personnel included three clinical nurse specialists, six nurse clinicians, two clinical nurse researchers, and one clinical pharmacist. In this study, all personnel "donated" their time to the research, and grant funds supported only a small percentage of a secretarial salary, duplicating costs, supplies, and local travel. In a larger and more complex intervention study in bone marrow transplant/leukemia inpatients (McGuire, submitted, 1998), study personnel included several nurses (both clinicians and researchers), a clinical pharmacist, two dentists (one specializing in oral medicine and the other in oral pathology), a clinical psychologist, a biostatistician, and a hematology/oncology physician (specializing in transplant medicine). In this case, most of the personnel had a portion of their regular salaries supported by the budget on the grant. For any study, when the proposal is first developed, a determination must be made of who will be involved in the research, what their specific roles and responsibilities will be, and how much of their effort (if any) will be supported with an external grant award. As funding agencies increase their emphasis on collaborative, interdisciplinary research, the investigator needs to carefully plan in a logical way the type of personnel needed to study a particular clinical problem (Mayer & Grant, 1987). In many instances, the conceptual framework used to guide a study can also serve to delineate the specific disciplines that should be involved (McGuire, submitted, 1998).

INVOLVING NURSING STAFF

Involvement of nurses at all levels (administrators, unit leaders, advanced practice nurses, and bedside clinicians) in a study can help ensure support and provide information on the culture, personnel, and available resources of a particular setting. The involvement of clinical nurses at the bedside can enhance the study by increasing clinical feasibility, relevance, and credibility. It can also spark nurses' interest in nursing research and provide them with opportunities for personal professional development (Yeager, DeLoney, & Webster, 1997). In some studies, such as unit-based projects in which staff nurses also act as data collectors (Shivnan et al., 1991), involvement can include such tasks as organizing and carrying out orientation and training sessions and making arrangements for the nursing department to receive financial reimbursement for the time nurses spend collecting data. In other studies, when data are collected primarily by grant personnel, the tasks may involve more clinically oriented aspects of the study (Yeager, DeLoney, Crooker, Webster, & McGuire, 1997). In either case, balancing of the staff nurse's research and clinical roles is always necessary (Rempusheski, 1991).

In the unit-based study of dressing regimens for long-term indwelling central catheters mentioned earlier (Shivnan et al., 1991), the investigators needed to give orientation sessions to nursing staff to explain the study, the data collection tools, and their role in the research. Several of the staff nurse coinvestigators who were based on the unit ensured that staff understood the protocol by using a multimedia inservice educational approach, which included posters, demonstrations of dressing techniques, and written handouts. Also among these nurses' study-related responsibilities was repetition of essential information about the study throughout its course whenever needed. In this study, the nursing unit was reimbursed for the time that all staff nurses spent changing dressings as part of the study's experimental protocol. The staff nurse and clinical nurse specialist coinvestigators, however, "donated" their own time in exchange for the opportunity to learn about and be directly involved in research, including dissemination activities such as presentation and publication (Sharkazy & Freedman, 1989; Shivnan et al., 1991).

In a study testing a nurse-implemented psychoeducational intervention for acute oral pain and mucositis (McGuire, submitted, 1998; Yeager, DeLoney, Crooker, Webster, & McGuire, 1997), selected nursing staff were paid out of a grant budget for responsibilities such as unit-based coordination of the study, oversight of their staff nurse colleagues' completion of assessment and documentation of oral pain and mucositis, and collaborative work with the investigators to ensure staff nurse adherence to an oral care standard (Yeager, Clapper, & McGuire, 1996) and pain management algorithm (Webster & von Hohenleiten, 1995). An additional important component of this study was the participation of a clinical nurse specialist who functioned on "donated" time as a consultant to the study by assisting with a variety of study components, ranging from obtaining adequate supplies for oral care to training of staff nurses in using a specific oral assessment tool (Webster, Clark, & Johnson, 1997).

HIRING, TRAINING, AND MANAGING PERSONNEL

An investigator who receives grant funding that includes specific personnel in the budget must hire, orient, and train the staff before implementing the study. Although a large grant can cover a variety of personnel (such as research assistants, secretaries, technicians, clerks, and a project director), it is common in smaller awards for clinical studies to supply funds only for research assistants or data collectors. The following discussion pertains primarily to funded studies that include a budget for hiring personnel.

When the necessary personnel are not already on board, hiring is the first order of business. The investigator must contact the personnel or human resources office of the institution and explore how to develop a formal position description that is within institution guidelines and policies. Then the position must be advertised, applicants must be screened and interviewed, and an individual must be hired for the position. Recruitment can be internal only or internal and external, depending on the needs and desires of the investigator and on the potential for hiring persons from within the site. Additionally, most institutions have clear policies and procedures that govern this

process and are in compliance with federal regulations. Thus, the newly funded investigator should look for expert assistance from appropriate individuals in the personnel or human resources department of the institution.

Once personnel are hired, orientation and training must be carried out. Regardless of the number of staff to be trained, the content and format of the study should be systematically and formally developed for them. The level of content, depth of information, and specific procedures taught depend on the skills and previous experience of the personnel. At a minimum, orientation and training should cover the following:

1. Significance, goals, and methods of the study
2. Clinical phenomenon (or phenomena) under study
3. Policies, procedures, characteristics, and data collection areas of the site
4. Specific roles and responsibilities that personnel are expected to fulfill, as well as the methods with which to fulfill them (including any necessary standardization or interrater reliability procedures)

The newly funded investigator with a budget to hire personnel becomes, in effect, a supervisor of others, regardless of any prior experience in this area. Thus, in addition to hiring and training personnel, the investigator needs to plan for and develop procedures for managing personnel. Important components of this process include knowledge about the process, content, and schedule for performance evaluations at the institution; personnel policies and procedures regarding leave and discipline; potential opportunities and resources for staff development; and mechanisms for communication. The neophyte investigator is advised to seek regular consultation from institutional human resource personnel and other more experienced investigators. One important component of successful personnel management and good research teamwork is the scheduling of regular team meetings. These can be very useful for providing information to study staff and coinvestigators, identifying and solving problems, and enhancing team spirit and cohesiveness (McGuire, submitted, 1998).

EQUIPMENT AND SUPPLIES

Equipment and supplies for a clinical study have already been discussed, but more specific information is needed when the investigator is ready to implement the study. The methodology of a given study dictates what equipment and supplies are required. These could range from expensive diagnostic equipment, such as an electrocardiograph machine (Kirchhoff, Holm, Foreman, & Rebenson-Piano, 1990), to dressing supplies and culture materials (Shivnan et al., 1991), to sophisticated videotapes and playing equipment (McGuire, Owen, & Peterson, 1998). Whenever possible, the investigator should use supplies already available if study-specific supplies are needed; otherwise, supplies must be purchased. Three activities germane to equipment and supplies are ordering, storing, and replenishing.

Ordering Equipment and Supplies

Many institutions where nurse investigators are employed have specific policies and procedures regarding ordering of equipment and supplies (for example, preference for or contracts with certain retailers or vendors, or requirements to purchase from the lowest bidder). Unnecessary delay in acquiring equipment and supplies can be avoided if the investigator knows and adheres to any such policies. Depending on the specific equipment or supplies needed, the investigator may need to request catalogs or visit suppliers to inspect and price the desired materials. In the current climate of managed care and cost containment, institutions may have committees whose task it is to review the usage pattern of supplies and to approve requests for new supply items. Contact with a committee representative may be helpful if changes in usage or additional supplies are needed for the study. Committee representatives can also advise the investigators on whether any additional approval mechanisms are necessary.

Storing Equipment and Supplies

Location of equipment and supplies is extremely important. Materials must be stored in areas that are accessible, logical, and safe (particularly when the materials are expensive). For example, special study dressings should be stored in a clean utility room with other dressings, but they should be specifically marked "for study patients only." Data forms should be stored in the nurses' station with other nursing and patient forms, but they should be placed in a specially labeled folder. Sometimes the use of colors may be helpful in production of new forms specific to a study to alert all staff to a special study form or study-related procedure. In the acute oral pain and mucositis intervention study mentioned earlier, the oral care standard used by all patients (Yeager et al., 1996) was copied onto blue paper, laminated, and mounted in a visible location in patients' rooms. All personnel involved in the study should be told about the location of relevant materials before implementation. Plans to store completed data forms and other materials should be made. Because study forms often contain confidential information, the investigator must obtain a secure storage spot, such as a lockable file cabinet.

Replenishing Equipment and Supplies

Replenishment of equipment and supplies is just as important as storage location. The quantity should be routinely checked to ensure that there is sufficient quantity for projected needs. It is helpful if several persons involved in the study know how and where to obtain additional supplies if needed. Additionally, the study should have designated personnel to check the condition of any equipment and to make sure that any routine or unplanned maintenance occurs in timely fashion.

When the system for ordering, storing, and replenishing equipment and supplies is carefully planned and conscientiously communicated to those involved, a smoother implementation phase results. The actual conduct of the study is also facilitated. In the acute oral pain and mucositis study mentioned previously (McGuire, Owen, & Peterson, 1998), the oral care standard required a specific mouthwash. Major problems occurred when the hospital suppliers ran out of the mouthwash (Yeager et al., 1996). Accurate projections of usage patterns of supplies and communication of this information between clinical personnel and study personnel would have eliminated this problem.

PREIMPLEMENTATION: THE PILOT STUDY

In many instances, the investigator needs to perform a pilot study before implementing the full study. The primary activity in the pilot study is the *testing* of the study procedures and instruments in a small sample that is as similar to the real study sample as possible.

Reasons for a Pilot Study

The major purpose of the pilot study is to identify and correct any problem areas before the study is implemented in its final form. Hagle and colleagues (1987) noted that the advantages of a pilot study included opportunities to evaluate tools, practice collecting data, assess availability of research subjects, and estimate time required for data collection. McHugh and Johnson (1980) further described the pilot phase as

. . . a time for the researcher and the clinical staff to become acquainted and for the researcher to test all the research tools, as well as try out various strategies of performing the research activities so that they are efficient yet . . . cause the least disruption to patient care.

Table 25–5 displays some of the areas that can be addressed. In a pilot study, all procedures should be carried out in the same way as planned for the formal study.

Table 25–5

The Pilot Study: Opportunities for the Researcher

Conducting a pilot study gives the researcher opportunities to:

1. Identify and recruit subjects; obtain informed consent
2. Administer questionnaires or experimental nursing interventions
3. Measure outcomes
4. Use forms to collect and record data from medical records or other sources
5. Assess potential problems in the data collection phase

Table 25–6

Goals of a Pilot Study

1. *Test procedures*—Screening, enrollment, and consent; randomization; adherence to and documentation of use of acute pain and oral care standards; time needed to implement intervention, time needed for patient assessment; collection of all tools and instruments, entry of data, disposition of each patient file.
2. *Test tools*—Determine usability including burden, ease of completion, and time for completion for patients, family members, and study personnel; test paper flow including distribution, collection from patients, staff nurses, and pharmacists, tracking with log-out and log-in systems, procedures for data entry, and filing.
3. *Test intervention*—Evaluate initial intervention session of videotape, written material, one-on-one discussion, and overall patient and family response; evaluate reinforcement visit including discussion and overall patient and family response.
4. *Refine roles of study personnel*—principal investigator and co-investigators, project manager, secretary, unit-based study coordinators, pharmacist, statistician and data manager, dentist, and other (consultant, staff nurses, clinical nurse specialist).
5. *Evaluate overall study timeline*—Realistic maximum amount of patients on study at one time, pattern of accrual per stratum, best time of day to schedule patient visits, daily versus weekly scheduling of data entry, need for and scheduling of full team versus data management personnel meetings.

From McGuire, D. B., Yeager, K. A., Dudley, W. N., Peterson, D. E., Owen, D. C., Lin, L. S., & Wingard, J. R. (in press). Acute oral pain and mucositis in bone marrow transplant and leukemia patients. Data from a pilot study. Cancer Nursing.

With complex intervention studies that use a repeated measures design, a pilot study is especially important. Table 25–6 shows an example of goals developed for a pilot study that the authors conducted before implementing a large, complex, repeated measures intervention study in acutely ill cancer patients (McGuire, Yeager, Dudley, et al., in press). Often during a pilot study, problems surface that the investigator had not anticipated. Solutions can then be devised before implementing the full study. For example, if a study uses a design with randomly assigned treatments, situa-

tions in which two patients randomly assigned to different treatment but sharing
the same room can have important implications for the conduct and the internal validity of the study. Knowing that the clinical
units have two-person rooms ahead of time
allows the investigator to make necessary
adjustments, because it is sometimes undesirable for persons with different interventions to be close to one another (McHugh &
Johnson, 1980); contamination can occur
(inadvertent sharing of information between subjects, one of whom may be a control subject and one an experimental subject). A carefully designed and implemented
pilot study, although time-consuming, is an
extremely important preimplementation activity, because it helps protect the internal
validity of the full study (McGuire, De-
Loney, Yeager, et al., in press).

Workload, Involvement, and Commitment for All Study Participants

The preimplementation phase of the study
is an appropriate time to consider the workload of study personnel, the level of involvement of clinical staff, and the amount of
commitment demanded of subjects through
their participation, especially if they are
acutely ill (Yeager, DeLoney, & McGuire,
1997). In repeated measures designs, issues
of excessive workload for personnel, heavy
staff involvement in a busy clinical environment, and unreasonable commitment
(sometimes called "burden") demanded of
subjects can contribute to high rates of
missing data. Extensive missing data can
jeopardize the investigator's ability to analyze the results and draw meaningful conclusions. Thus, successful completion of a
study is achieved, in part, when the rate of
missing data is low or zero. The pilot study
is therefore also extremely important as a
mechanism for carefully examining issues
that can contribute to missing data and
helping to devise a realistic data collection
plan to maximize the chances for complete
data and to preserve study validity (Mc-
Guire, DeLoney, Yeager, et al., in press). For
example, after completion of the pilot study
referred to in Table 25–6, the investigators
made major changes in the administration
schedule of tools because of difficulties and
burden encountered in the pilot study while
collecting large amounts of information

from acutely ill patients who were experiencing pain and were sometimes cognitively
impaired as a result of sedative medications
and other factors (McGuire, DeLoney, Yeager, et al., submitted, 1998).

IMPLEMENTATION

The investigator should be ready to implement the project following the pilot study
and to implement any changes that result
from the pilot. Although there are many
aspects to implementation, only six areas—
informed consent, study protocols, collection
of data, monitoring data, troubleshooting
and problem solving, and progress and final
reports—are addressed in this chapter.
These areas are essential to any clinical
nursing study. Knowledge about them is
critical to the nurse who wishes to conduct
a successful study.

Informed Consent

The investigator who implements a study
may be the person to obtain informed consent from study subjects or may supervise
others in this process. In either case, it is
imperative that proper procedures be followed when obtaining consent. Investigators must make certain that they have the
knowledge and experience to explain and
conduct their studies (Cassidy & Oddi,
1986). They must be able to use research
procedures safely and protect their patients'
well-being. Informed consent documents
and procedures (including the treatment or
study goals, risks, benefits, and the rights
of the participants) must be fully explained
to potential participants (Chamorro & Appelbaum, 1988). Educational level and other
pertinent factors related to patients' informational needs must be addressed in this
process (Larson & McGuire, 1990). See
Chapter 13 for a more in-depth discussion
of informed consent.

Study Protocols

Development of a study protocol to guide
and document important study procedures
serves many purposes. First, it is a necessary step to standardize study procedures if
more than one person will be working on

the study. These procedures should include instructions for obtaining informed consent, randomly assigning patients to treatments (in intervention studies), interviewing subjects, and completing instruments, including the sequence of instrument completion if multiple instruments are used (Meinert, 1986). Second, a study protocol can assist in providing the history of a study and documenting when and why specific decisions were made; this record is often helpful when problems are repetitive. Third, the study protocol can serve as a central source of essential study information such as instructions and explanations about how to assign study identification numbers or develop copies of study rosters and instruments. The ideal tactic, if resources allow, is to compile all study protocols into a notebook, which is then duplicated and distributed to all team members.

Collection of Data

Burns and Grove (1997) wrote, "The initiation of data collection is one of the most exciting parts of research" (p. 383). The investigator is *finally* getting started and gathering data that answer the research question. This phase of implementation is always a step into the unknown for any researcher, novice or experienced. Implementation of the study depends on the data collection plan, which should be developed carefully and in concert with results from the pilot study if appropriate (Burns & Grove, 1997). During implementation, the investigator finds out whether data collection will proceed as designed, whether the planned procedures will really work, and whether other expectations are met.

Burns and Grove (1997) delineated four categories of problems that can occur during data collection. First, people problems can be manifested through lack of available sample, unanticipated (and undesired) external influences on the study subject (for example, influence of family or friends), poor interactions between researcher and subject, and passive interference with the study by staff or other personnel. Second, researcher problems can develop, including interactions with subjects and others who interfere with timely completion of study instruments, lack of skill in using specific types of data collection instruments or pro-

cedures, development of researcher versus clinician role conflict (which may be especially prominent when staff nurses are functioning as data collectors), and trouble maintaining objectivity and perspective. Third, institutional problems can occur, for example, institutional personnel may change, study units may be moved or reorganized, or patient record systems may be overhauled. Even more importantly, changes in referral and practice patterns can occur that affect the availability of potentially eligible subjects (McGuire et al., 1997). Finally, a variety of random events may occur that cause frustration and interference with data collection, for example, research tools are lost in the mail, the copying machine fails just when more instruments are needed, data forms get "lost in space," and so on. In planning for, and implementing, the data collection phase of the study, the investigator needs to anticipate every sort of problem and have possible solutions in mind if they occur. When unforeseen problems do occur, the investigator should try to be flexible and creative, and call on the collective wisdom of the research team members or researchers with more experience.

Monitoring of Data

During the data collection process, the investigator must examine carefully all the end products, that is, all instruments, forms, and reports. This process is called monitoring, and it is essential for adequate quality control in any study (Table 25–7). There is always a possibility that tools were improperly or incompletely filled in, cultures were not obtained correctly, instructions were misunderstood by data collectors, or calculations of scores were inaccurate. The best policy, if possible, is for the investigator to examine each set of data as it is collected. Any potential problems can be detected immediately and corrected, before too much incorrect data information is accrued or it is too late to go back and collect accurate data. If the investigator is unable to review each set of data, a team member should be assigned to check (that is, edit) all forms for accuracy and completeness within a specific time period so that corrections can be made in the data or other adjustments made as necessary. For the sake

Table 25–7

Monitoring of Data

Continuous monitoring of data collection helps to:

1. Keep the investigator on top of the research as it is progressing, giving an idea of the general findings and how many patients have participated in the study
2. Control the quality of the data and ensure that they are being collected in the most appropriate and methodologically rigorous way possible
3. Ensure that when the desired number of subjects for the study has been attained, the data are ready for entry into a computer or ready for analysis

of objectivity, this person should not be the same individual who collected the data originally. A specific method for documenting this editing step, such as a sign-off mechanism, can be helpful for accountability. Such a monitoring system is vital to a successful project.

Troubleshooting and Problem Solving

Tracking the entire process of data collection is important so that if problems arise, they will be recognized early. Some problems can become recurrent, or they can mushroom into larger and more severe problems that affect the success of the study. If problems are identified, the investigator must take action. Unforeseen problems that arise in clinical research are varied and caused by many factors, including the research question, procedures, institutional variables, patient variables, data collector variables, and other factors. Examples of problems and solutions are displayed in Table 25–8.

With the many and varied types of research questions and hypotheses that investigators can study in clinical research, the potential number and nature of problems expands exponentially. The important things for the investigator to keep in mind are the following questions: What am I studying? How am I collecting the data? How do I expect the data to be generated? What problems have I already solved? What other problems could arise?

If the investigator continually asks these questions, monitors the data, and communicates with all personnel involved in the study—both formally and informally—the process of troubleshooting and problem solving should be simplified. The study should continue from implementation to completion without major difficulties or disasters.

Table 25–8

Examples of Problems and Solutions

Situation 1
Problem: In an oncology outpatient study (Hagle et al., 1987; McGuire et al., 1987), the number of eligible subjects was less than expected.
Solution: An additional site for data collection was added, and patient accrual increased.

Situation 2
Problem: Staff nurses collecting data obtained catheter cultures on nonscheduled days if they had missed the culture on its scheduled day (Sharkazy & Freedman, 1989).
Solution: The missed culture was considered "missing data," and the nurses simply obtained the culture on the next scheduled date, thus allowing appropriate data entry and analysis.

Situation 3
Problem: Randomizations to dressing regimens were made when patients were admitted to a bone marrow transplant unit (Sharkazy & Freedman, 1989). Although this procedure generally worked well, there were some patients who were randomized, began the study, and then were discharged because they did not meet medical criteria for transplantation.
Solution: Patients were randomized to their dressing regimens as late as possible once it was clear that they were to receive a transplant, and attrition decreased almost completely.

Situation 4
Problem: Changing referral and treatment patterns caused major changes in the characteristics of potentially eligible patients for an intervention study using a stratification schema based on treatment (McGuire et al., 1997).
Solution: The stratification schema was collapsed so that only two major strata remained, thus allowing accrual of a wide range of patients who could be categorized by more specific treatment regimens ex post facto.

Progress and Final Reports

As the investigator moves through the implementation and completion of a study, there are two different types of reports that need to be made. While the study is ongoing, progress reports on the status of the study may be given to interested parties such as staff, administrators, or representatives of the funding agency if a grant has been received. These reports usually focus on the status of the study, for example, how many subjects have been entered or what kinds of problems have been encountered and how they were solved. When the study is completed, the investigator prepares one or more final reports, which are submitted to various places and persons, for example, to the funding agency, administrators of the institution in which the study was conducted, or the nurses on the study units. With both progress and final reports, formats can be informal or formal.

INFORMAL REPORTS

The informal report is usually used internally, because it is a good way to give regular progress reports to the research team, nursing staff, or other personnel directly involved in or supportive of the study. The investigator can easily give informal reports by making arrangements with unit administrators to meet with staff at a regularly scheduled or specially called meeting. The environment and tone should be casual, and the meeting brief and to the point, although time should be allowed for questions and discussion. Food is usually a welcome addition to such meetings. This process keeps staff up-to-date, helps maintain their interest and cooperation, allows for detection and discussion of problems or concerns, and increases their investment in the study. In addition, the investigator might want to provide similar progress reports to nursing administrators, physicians, and other key persons who support the study. These informal progress reports demonstrate that the investigator is capable of carrying out the study and fulfilling the requirements of clinical research. At the completion of the study, the same type of informal report mechanism can also be used to share findings and implications with staff, administrators, and others. The investigator's willingness to meet informally with staff and others not only demonstrates awareness of the need for regular communication between study personnel and institutional personnel but also affirms the important contributions they make to the study.

FORMAL REPORTS

Agencies or foundations awarding external grant funds often request formal progress reports annually, halfway through the funded period, or at the end of the funded period. These agencies usually provide the investigator with specific information about the content of the report, special forms on which to write it, and the name and address of the person to whom it should be submitted. Careful preparation of accurate and informative formal progress reports is important because it provides the investigator with a mechanism to demonstrate to the funding agency that the study is going well and that the funds are being used as intended. In some instances, continuation of funding for the second or subsequent years of a study may be contingent on satisfactory progress reports.

At the completion of the study, the investigator usually prepares a formal final progress report. If this report is for the funding agency, there will be a specific format and length, as with the progress report. Prompt, accurate preparation and submission of the report is recommended. If the formal final report is for internal use only, it is a good idea is to use a standard research report format, such as that found in research journals such as *Nursing Research* or *Research in Nursing and Health*. In preparing such reports, the inclusion of a brief but comprehensive abstract that clearly indicates the major findings of the study is useful for many purposes, and it is certainly appreciated by busy administrators who may have competing demands on their time. In preparing any formal report, the inexperienced writer should seek consultation and assistance from others who are more experienced (refer to Chapter 27).

SUMMARY

The purpose of the implementation phase is to put the research plan into action. Close attention to clinical sites, administrative issues such as finances and personnel, man-

agement of equipment and supplies, a carefully conducted pilot study, and systematic implementation of the full study should ensure a well-executed study and successful outcome for the investigator.

REFERENCES

Brooten, D. E. (1984). Making it in paradise [Editorial]. *Nursing Research, 33*, 318.

Burns, N., & Grove, S. K. (1997). *The practice of nursing research: Conduct, critique, & utilization* (3rd ed.). Philadelphia: W. B. Saunders.

Cassidy, V. R., & Oddi, L. F. (1986). Legal and ethical aspects of informed consent: A nursing research perspective. *Journal of Professional Nursing, 2,* 343–349.

Chamorro, T., & Appelbaum, J. (1988). Informed consent: Nursing issues and ethical dilemmas. *Oncology Nursing Forum, 15*, 803–808.

DeLoney, V., Yeager, K., Crooker, S., & McGuire, D. (1997). Clinical issues in implementing non-pharmacologic interventions [Abstract]. *Proceedings of the American Cancer Society 4th National Conference on Cancer Nursing Research,* 100.

Egan, E. C., Synder, M., & Burns, K. R. (1992). Intervention studies in nursing: Is the effect due to the independent variable? *Nursing Outlook, 40*, 187–190.

Guy, J. L. (1991). New challenges for nurses in clinical trials. *Seminars in Oncology Nursing, 7,* 297–303.

Hagle, M. E., Barbour, L., Flynn, B., Kelley, C., Trippon, M., Braun, D., Beschorner, J., Boxler, J., Hange, P. A., McGuire, D. B., Bressler, L.R., & Kirchhoff, K. T. (1987). Research collaboration among nurse clinicians. *Oncology Nursing Forum, 14,* 55–59.

Kirchhoff, K. T. (1987). Nurses and physicians must interact for valid clinical research. *Research in Nursing and Health, 10,* 149–154.

Kirchhoff, K. T., Holm, K., Foreman, M. D., & Rebenson-Piano, M. (1990). Electrocardiographic response to ice water ingestion. *Heart & Lung, 19,* 41–48.

Kirchhoff, K. T., & McGuire, D. B. (1985a). Gaining access to a clinical setting for research. *Nurse Educator, 10*(5), 2–26.

Kirchhoff, K. T., & McGuire, D. B. (1985b). The nursing research review process in a clinical setting. *Journal of Professional Nursing, 1,* 311–314.

Larson, E. L., & McGuire, D. B. (1990). Patient experiences with research in a tertiary care setting. *Nursing Research, 39,* 168–171.

Lasoff, E. M. (1986). Improving nurses' cooperation with clinical research. *Journal of Nursing Administration, 16*(9), 6–7.

Mayer, D. K., & Grant, M. (1987). Identifying and utilizing key personnel for cancer nursing research. *Oncology Nursing Forum, 14,* 91–93.

McGuire, D. B. Manuscript submitted. Using a conceptual framework to develop an interdisciplinary research team. *Nursing Outlook.*

McGuire, D. B., Barbour, L., Boxler, J., Braun, D., Flynn, B., Hagle, M., Hange, P., Kelly, C., Trippon, M., Bressler, L., & Kirchhoff, K. T. (1987). Fixed-interval versus as-needed analgesics in cancer outpatients. *Journal of Pain and Symptom Management, 2,* 199–205.

McGuire, D. B., DeLoney, V. G., Yeager, K. A., Owen, D. C., Peterson, D. E., Lin, L., & Webster, J. Submitted, 1998. Maintaining study validity in a changing clinical environment. *Nursing Research.*

McGuire, D. B., & Harwood, K. V. (1989). The CNS as researcher. In A. B. Hamric & J. A. Spross (Eds.), *The clinical nurse specialist in theory and practice* (2nd ed., pp. 169–203). Philadelphia: W. B. Saunders.

McGuire, D. B., Lin, L., Owen, D., & Peterson, D. (1997). Methodologic decisions: Reality and compromise [Abstract]. *Proceedings of American Cancer Society 4th National Conference on Cancer Nursing Research,* 99.

McGuire, D. B., Owen, D. C., & Peterson, D. E. (1998). Nursing interventions for acute oral pain and mucositis [Abstract]. *Oncology Nursing Forum, 25,* 341.

McGuire, D. B., Yeager, K. A., Dudley, W. N., Peterson, D. E., Owen, D. C., Lin, L. S., & Wingard, J. R. (in press). Acute oral pain and mucositis in bone marrow transplant and leukemia patients: Data from a pilot study. *Cancer Nursing.*

McHugh, N. G., & Johnson, J. E. (1980). Clinical nursing research: Beyond the methods books. *Nursing Outlook, 28,* 352–356.

Meinert, C. L. (1986). *Clinical trials: Design, conduct, and analysis.* New York: Oxford.

Melink, T. J., & Whitacre, M. Y. (1991). Planning and implementing clinical trials. *Seminars in Oncology Nursing, 7,* 243–251.

Nail, L. M. (1990). Involving clinicians in nursing research. *Oncology Nursing Forum, 17,* 621–623.

Oda, D. S. (1983). Social and political facilitation of research. *Advances in Nursing Science, 5*(2), 9–15.

Rempusheski, V. F. (1991). Incorporating research role and practice role. *Applied Nursing Research, 4*(1), 46–48.

Rudy, E. B. (1991) Facilitating clinical research: Nurse to nurse support [Editorial]. *Applied Nursing Research, 4*(2), 49.

Sharkazy, E., & Freedman, S. E. (1989). Implementing nursing research on an inpatient unit [Abstract]. *Oncology Nursing Forum, 16*(Suppl.), 209.

Shivnan, J. C., McGuire, D., Freedman, S., Sharkazy, E., Bosserman, G., Larson, E., & Grouleff, P. (1991). A comparison of transparent adherent and dry sterile gauze dressings for long-term central catheters in patients undergoing bone marrow transplant. *Oncology Nursing Forum, 18,* 1349–1355.

Varricchio, C., & Mikos, K. (1987). Research: Determining feasibility in a clinical setting. *Oncology Nursing Forum, 14,* 89–90.

Webster, J., Clark, J., & Johnson, P. (1997). Incorporation of a standardized oral assessment guide in the bone marrow transplant setting. Poster presentation at the Seattle Marrow Transplant Nursing Consortium's Sixth International Conference, Seattle, WA, October.

Webster, J. S., & von Hohenleiten, C. (1995). Development and implementation of an oral pain algorithm in bone marrow transplant patients [Abstract]. *Oncology Nursing Forum, 22,* 383.

Yeager, K. A., Clapper, L., & McGuire, D. B. (1996). Challenges in developing and implementing an oral care standard for hematology and bone marrow transplant patients: Working toward 100% acceptability [Abstract]. *Oncology Nursing Forum, 23,* 311.

Yeager, K., DeLoney, V., Crooker, S., Webster, J., & McGuire, D. (1997). Integrating intervention research into the clinical setting [Abstract]. *Proceed-*

ings of American Cancer Society 4th National Conference on Cancer Nursing Research, 101.

Yeager, K., DeLoney, V., & McGuire, D. (1997). Challenges in studying bone marrow transplant patients. Poster presentation at the Seattle Marrow Transplant Nursing Consortium's Sixth International Conference, Seattle, WA, October.

Yeager, K., DeLoney, V., & Webster, J. (1997). Nursing research in the clinical setting: keys to success [Abstract]. *Oncology Nursing Forum, 24,* 282.

Data Analysis

Mary R. Lynn

In any quantitative study, the data must be reduced in scope for it to be meaningfully interpreted. It is here that statistical methods come into play, because they facilitate the ability to make sense out of great quantities of data. Statistical methods range from techniques as simple as determining the mean of a set of numbers to the complex use of structural equation modeling to test elaborate conceptual and measurement models. This chapter discusses concepts and issues related to the analysis of data. For details on the use or applicability of any particular statistical method, refer to a statistics text, several of which are of particular value to health care professionals in the analysis of data (for example, Knapp, 1985; Munro, 1997).

PURPOSE OF STATISTICS

Statistical methods are used in the analysis of data for two reasons—to describe the important *variables** in a study (descriptive

statistics) and, when relevant, to make inferences about a population based on information contained in a sample (inferential statistics). It is the inferential use of statistical methods that is commonly thought of as the purpose of statistics, although the descriptive uses are just as important.

LEVEL OF MEASUREMENT

One of the common issues in statistical analysis is the level of measurement of the involved variables. The four levels of measurement, introduced by Stevens (1946), are nominal, ordinal, interval, and ratio. *Nominal* measures, from the Latin "of or belonging to a name," are measures in name only. In other words, variables that are measured on a nominal scale have numbers assigned to them for convenience only; the numbers have no mathematical meaning. In a nominal scale, a "1" is simply different from a "2" and is not seen as less than or half of the number 2. Typical nominal measures are classification variables such as gender ("Select 1 if you are female and 2 if you are male) or occupational status (1 = full-time, 2 = part-time). Nominal measures are discrete in that each value is mutually exclu-

---

Variable refers to a finding or characteristic that can change (for example, weight) or can be expressed as more than one value within a category (for example, gender).

sive and there is no measurable interval between the values.

Ordinal measures are ranked in some manner. Like nominal measures, they are also discrete because the numbers are in order but there is no consistent or measurable interval between the rankings. Using ordinal measures, distinctions between higher and lower, bigger and smaller, or even faster and slower can be made but no other direct comparisons can be made. Questionnaire item response formats that range from "Strongly disagree" to "Strongly agree" or from "Unimportant" to "Extremely important" are examples of ordinal measures; it is known that "Extremely important" is more highly rated than "Important," but the distance between the two response points is not known.

Interval and ratio measures are ordered and continuous, that is, the interval between points on the scale can be measured, but differ in the meaning of zero. In interval measures, zero is an arbitrary point. Ratio measures are distinguished by having an absolute zero: zero means "none of." Temperature has both interval and ratio measures; Fahrenheit or centigrade are interval measures because zero is an arbitrary point in that values below zero are both common and expected. However, the Kelvin scale is ratio measure because zero (0°K) is absolute zero, the coldest theoretical temperature at which the energy of motion of molecules is zero. (If the motion of molecules is zero, however, a thermometer would fall apart; nonetheless, zero in the Kelvin scale does mean "none of.") Most physiological measures are at the ratio level of measurement. The importance of the distinction between interval and ratio measures is that only with ratio level measures can comparative statements of proportion or ratio be made. To say a blood sugar of 100 is twice as high as a 50 blood sugar is accurate; to say that 100°F is twice as hot as 50°F is not, because Fahrenheit temperatures exist below zero. However, interval and ratio measures are usually treated the same in statistical analysis.

The importance of the level of measurement is that it is thought to dictate which statistics are to be used when describing variables and, to a great extent, which ones are used in statistical inference. There is considerable controversy about how stringently the level of measurement does, in fact, prescribe which statistical test is used. This question most often arises when a researcher wants to use parametric statistics, those statistics that are based on the assumption that the data are normally distributed and at least interval level, in the analysis of data derived from questionnaires based on the Likert response format. The argument is that even though the Likert response format for the items is ordinal, when the items are summed for analysis, they "approach" the interval level. Purists say the tie between level of measurement of a variable and the statistics to be used is unequivocal (for example, Stevens, 1946). Others (for example, Armstrong, 1981; Knapp, 1990) suggest that it is not so clear; when the researcher has items with a number of response options that are summed to create total scores for which zero is a possibility and the meaningfulness of an instrument is inferred to be interval, then the resulting data are supposed to be appropriately amenable to being analyzed using parametric statistics.

DESCRIPTIVE VERSUS INFERENTIAL STATISTICS

Descriptive statistics are used to organize and summarize the information on specific variables. Most often these statistics are used to describe the *central tendency* (where distribution of that particular variable is centered, or the typical score) and *dispersion* (how the scores are distributed around the measure of central tendency) of variables. Because there are several methods for determining the "average" and the dispersion, knowing the level of measurement of the variable is essential in determining which measures are to be used. Table 26–1 identifies the appropriate measure of central tendency (the "average"), dispersion (variability), and correlation (relationship between two variables) for each level of measurement.

Frequency distributions are an additional means of describing the dispersion of a set of data. Generally data in a frequency distribution are grouped into mutually exclusive categories with the count of observations that exist in that category shown either on a table or in a graphic description such as a histogram or line graph. Occasionally, the bivariate relationship or correlation

Table 26–1

Appropriate Measures of Central Tendency, Dispersion, and Correlation for Variables at the Four Levels of Measurement*

MEASURE OF CENTRAL TENDENCY,† DISPERSION, CORRELATION	LEVEL OF MEASUREMENT			
	Nominal	**Ordinal**	**Interval**	**Ratio**
Mode Range Chi-square	**X**	X	X	X
Median Semi-interquartile range (SIQR) Kendall's tau, Spearman rank order		**X**	X	X
Mean Standard deviation Pearson product-moment (PPM)			**X**	**X**

Ideal combination is boldface. However, when interval or ratio data are skewed, the median and semi-interquartile range should be used instead; the Pearson product-moment correlation is still appropriate.

†*Below each "average" or measure of central tendency for which there are specific measures of variability (dispersion) and the relationship between two or more variables.*

between variables is explored when describing the variables in a data set. Depending on the level of measurement of these variables, different techniques are used (see Table 26–1). When correlation or association statistics are applied for descriptive uses, the results cannot be used to make any statements or inferences about subjects other than those studied. Assertions of the existence of a relationship between these variables in the population cannot be made without assessing the significance of the correlation.

Inferential statistics are used when the intention is to generalize the findings from a sample to the population from which the sample was drawn. Most inferential statistics have certain assumptions that must be met for their use, such as the extent to which the data reflect a normal distribution, the level of measurement of the data to be analyzed, and the method for obtaining the sample. The two major types of inferential statistics, *parametric* and *nonparametric* statistics, differ in the extent to which the data should reflect a normal distribution (parametric) or are distribution-free statistics (nonparametric) and the need for specific levels of measurement for variables being analyzed—interval or ratio data (parametric) and nominal or ordinal data (nonparametric). However, they do not differ in the assumption that all data are ob-

tained from subjects selected according to some chance (random) mechanism.

STATISTICAL INFERENCE

Statistical inference, a formal method for drawing conclusions about populations from information obtained in samples, is based in hypothesis testing and probability theory. Whether overtly stated or noted, any inferential statistical analysis is testing one or more hypotheses or questions about a population. The purest form of hypothesis is the *null hypothesis*, a statement that the researcher hopes to refute. For example, if a nurse is interested in comparing the self-care skills of patients in a new outpatient education program to those of patients not in the program, the null hypothesis might be "There is no difference in the self-care skills of patients in the outpatient education program when compared to patients who are not in the outpatient program."

The convention of using a statement or hypothesis about what is hoped to be rejected rather than what is intended to occur is where probability theory comes into play. In research, and therefore statistical analysis, nothing can be *proved*. Why? Because the researcher is not studying all persons who might fit the classifications or groupings, and the researcher is doing so with perfect tools or measures. Although statements about populations can be refuted because a sample may provide overwhelming evidence to the contrary (rejecting the null), that same contrary position cannot be "proved." So, in inferential statistics, the options are to reject a null hypothesis or to fail to reject it. To state that a null hypothesis, or any other hypothesis, has been "accepted" or supported is statistically incorrect.

A null hypothesis can be either true or false, and the conclusion reached from the interpretation of the data analysis either agrees or disagrees with this underlying true state of the population. Accordingly, when hypotheses are tested, there are four possible outcomes (Table 26–2). In Table 26–2, no error occurred in the conclusion reached in the first and fourth outcomes, because the conclusion reached matched the true state of the hypothesis. Although no error was committed in the first outcome, this outcome results in a weak statement about the hypothesis tested, because inferential statistics are used to make statements about rejection rather than support of a null hypothesis. The fourth outcome is the desired outcome because a false hypothesis was rejected.

Errors occurred in both the second and third outcomes because the conclusion did not agree with the true state of the population as described in the null hypothesis. Because samples rather than populations are being studied, these errors have some likelihood of occurring. It is possible that a decision based on a sample of subjects may not represent the true nature of events; the *significance level (p)* tells how probable it was that an incorrect conclusion was reached.

Alpha (α) is the probability that the second outcome (a true null hypothesis is rejected) might occur, and *beta* (β) is the probability that the third outcome (not rejecting a false hypothesis) might occur.

The probability of making a *type I error* is established by the researcher based on the researcher's willingness to make such an error. Traditionally, alpha is set at .05, meaning that the researcher is willing to conclude that a hypothesis is false only when it is, in fact, true no more than 5 of 100 times. Stated otherwise, even when a null hypothesis is true, there is a chance (α) that it could be concluded to be false. When concern over making such a mistake is high, such as when human life is at risk, alpha is set even more conservatively by choosing .01, .001, or an even more conservative value. The need to have the level of confidence in the conclusion reached to be as high as 99.9% is reserved for research with tremendous implications for the eventual recipients of the results of the research. An example is testing the tumor reduction capacity of a new oncologic agent or the ability of a medication to increase immune function in a patient population whose function has been compromised. The researcher chooses such a conservative level of significance because it is necessary to be unwilling to conclude the medication has a positive effect unless it is impossible to conclude otherwise.

Occasionally, the level of significance is set as $\alpha = .10$ when the research is exploratory and non–life-threatening, that is, research is being done to get a preliminary idea of the structure of events or whether variables are promising to include in future research.

Table 26–2

Possible Outcomes from Statistical Testing of Hypotheses

OUTCOME	HYPOTHESIS (HO) TRUE STATE*	CONCLUSION REACHED AFTER ANALYSIS	REJECTION DECISION	TYPE OF ERROR
1	Ho True	Ho True	Do not reject Ho	None
2	Ho True	Ho False	Reject Ho	Type I error
3	Ho False	Ho True	Do not reject Ho	Type II error
4	Ho False	Ho False	Reject Ho	None

This is a hypothetical situation, as the "truth" about the hypothesis is never known; otherwise the research would be unnecessary.

STATISTICAL SIGNIFICANCE

The result of a statistical test is deemed "significant" if the attained level of significance *(p)* is less than or equal to the a priori level of significance (α) established for the study. *Statistical significance* provides the researcher with the opportunity to say that data from the sample provide convincing evidence that what was found in the study would occur for the whole population, if studied, at $1 - \text{alpha}$* level of confidence. Stated differently, a significant finding is one unlikely to have occurred by chance alone. For example, when two or more groups are being compared and found to be "significantly different ($p < .05$)," the difference found between the groups is sufficient to warrant a conclusion that the samples come from "different populations" with 95% confidence. This is often confusing to persons learning about statistical inference who may wonder how this can occur when a single group was divided into two groups, one that received treatment and one that did not. The reason is that although the groups were similar at the outset, at the end of the study the impact of the intervention was such that the treatment group was no longer in the same population as the untreated group *with respect to the variable upon which they were found to significantly differ.* Similarly, when two variables are found to have a "significant correlation of .42 ($p < .05$)," they are said to relate to each other in a moderately positive manner such that as variable *A* increases, variable *B* tends to also increase. The fact that the variables related at $r = .42$ in the sample suggests that there will also be a systematic (nonchance) positive relationship between the variables.

Conversely, when groups being compared are found to not differ significantly, the interpretation is that whatever differences do exist are chance differences and are not large enough to conclude that they are systematically or genuinely distinct. Two variables found to correlate at the level of .54 ($p > .05$) are not significantly related to each other, so the correlation between those two variables in the population correlation should be seen as zero.

One of the most common mistakes subse-

quent to significance testing, in which some tests resulted in significant results and some did not, is for the researcher to treat all aspects of the analysis as meaningful, when they are not. This most commonly occurs with correlation coefficients. When a correlation between two variables is found to be not statistically significant, *regardless of the magnitude of the correlation,* the correlation between these same variables in the population is inferred to be zero, assuming the null hypothesis was that the population correlation was equal to zero. Regardless of any statistical testing, the results found for a sample do apply to the subjects or variables included in the study but, in the face of nonsignificant findings, these same results have no application to the population from whom the sample was drawn.

CLINICAL VERSUS STATISTICAL SIGNIFICANCE

Statistical significance does not connote practical significance and vice versa. To illustrate, consider the following two situations. In the first situation, a study is done comparing the effectiveness of iodine-based solution A to iodine-based solution B in reducing skin bacteria preoperatively. After a tightly controlled study, solution B was found to significantly reduce bacteria ($p < .05$), with the average reduction being 1000 colonies of usual skin flora X. In the second situation, a study of tube feeding administration is conducted with 100 subjects to determine whether there is any increase in distress when tube feeding is administered directly from the refrigerator versus being warmed to room temperature. After intensive study, it was determined that there was no significant difference in distress between the tube feeding trials.

In the first case, there is statistical significance without any real clinical significance. A reduction of 1000 colonies is of no particular clinical value because colonies are measured in the millions. Whereas in the second situation, there is clinical significance without any statistical significance. The lack of a significant difference in distress in a solid study of temperature of administrations suggests that the age-old tradition of warming tube feedings may not be necessary.

---

*1 (100% confidence in results) minus alpha (probability of a type I error).

SELECTION OF AN ANALYSIS PROGRAM

Until recently, statistical analysis was relegated to large mainframe systems; currently, a desktop personal computer can manage the analysis of most research data with one of the many analytical software programs available. Most of the commonly used programs (for example, SPSS, SAS [1988], SYSTAT) offer similar arrays of procedures, although they are available at different costs and require different skills or tolerances to use. Students tend to use the program used at their schools, but clinicians have fewer at-hand options. Table 26–3 provides summary information on the aforementioned commonly used programs as well as on Epi Info (Dean et al., 1994), the computer program mentioned in the next section. Another source of analysis is the spreadsheet program. For example, Microsoft Excel can perform most basic statistics (measures of central tendency and dispersion, t-test, correlation, regression) and is available on many PC-based systems.

PREPARATION OF DATA FOR ANALYSIS

Preparation of data for analysis usually proceeds from transforming the data from its raw form to an analyzable form. The steps involved in the data preparation include data entry, data verification, and data cleaning. Precision in the execution of each of these steps helps ensure having a data set that is as accurate as possible.

Data Entry

It is rare that the data from any study are analyzed without some form of computer interface. To conduct this analysis, the data most be converted to a data set amenable to analysis by the particular software program to be used. Data entry can be conducted by manual or electronic means. Manual data entry usually includes direct entry into the analysis program or indirect entry by first entering the data into a database, a spreadsheet or even a word processing program, and then exporting the data file to the analysis program. The data from most small-scale projects are entered directly into the statistical program to be used in the analysis although the method of data entry varies from one program to another. For example, SPSS (Norusis, 1993) has a data entry screen that emulates a traditional spreadsheet, with the columns being the variables to be entered and the rows being the study participants. Data from each participant is entered on a single line with data entry continuing from the first to the last relevant variable for that person.

Direct data entry or importing a data set created outside the analysis program requires that each variable be named and the magnitude of the data to be entered for that variable be known so that sufficient space is allocated to that variable. Specification of that space can become a very detailed process for imported data, depending on the format of those data. If the data for each subject are delimited, that is, a common delimiter (space, comma, or other character) is placed between each variable and each record, then importing data is relatively straightforward and the program allocates the appropriate amount of space needed for each variable. On the other hand, if data are not delimited or are incomplete, the process of importing the data can be complicated. The program then needs to be directed to the precise location and size of each variable (in terms of both number of digits and number of digits after the decimal point if decimals are not included in the data set) and the convention used for missing data. Details on conversion of such data sets are contained in the instruction manuals that accompany the specific analysis program.

Electronic data entry is usually done by means of optical mark readers (OMR), or "scanners," which are popular because they circumvent the human element in data entry errors. This method is generally limited to data collected in a multiple-choice format because the scannable sheets are usually the familiar "bubble sheets" upon which study participants record their responses. Software programs do exist that can read and directly enter text and handwritten responses, but these programs are prohibitively expensive for most researchers. The expense of an OMR machine and its accompanying software can also be prohibitive. In addition, the issue of multiple responses, partially darkened responses, and the propensity for people to get "off track" (for example, putting the answer to question 3 in the slot corresponding to question 4) when

Table 26-3

Features and Purchase Information for Commonly Used PC-Based Statistical Analysis Programs

PROGRAM	DATA ENTRY	DATA VERIFICATION	UNIVARIATE STATISTICS	MULTIVARIATE STATISTICS	MEASUREMENT/ SCALE CONSTRUCTION	CFA/SEM*	GRAPHICS	EASE OF USE	PLATFORM	PRICE
SPSS SPSS, Inc. 444 N. Michigan Ave. Chicago, IL 60611 1-800-543-2185	Y	N	Y	Y	Y	N†	Y	Easy	PC, Mac, mainframe	$150–$200 (students); $1400 (nonstudents)
SAS SAS Institute, Inc. SAS Circle Box 8000 Cary, NC 27512 1-919-677-8000	Y	Y	Y	Y	Y	Y	Y	Difficult	PC, Mac, mainframe	$35 plus $60 per year licensing fee
SYSTAT SPSS, Inc. 444 N. Michigan Ave. Chicago, IL 60611 1-800-543-2185	Y	N	Y	Y	Y	N	Y	Moderate	PC, Mac	$150–$200 (students); $995 (nonstudents)
EPI INFO Division of Surveillance and Epidemiology Epidemiology Program Office Centers for Disease Control Atlanta, GA 30333 1-404-728-0545	Y	Y	Y	Some	N	N	Y	Difficult	PC	Free

*Confirmatory factor analysis (CFA)/structural equation modeling (SEM) included in the program.
†SPSS produces a variety of stand-alone programs for specific applications such as SEM which can be purchased separately.

marking responses on the sheets cannot be remedied by the software that converts input data from the sheets into a data file. Some corrections will, in all likelihood, still have to be made by hand-editing the data file once it is created.

Data Verification

Independent of the means of data entry, the activity of data entry is fraught with opportunities for errors to occur. Accordingly, the data must be assessed for accuracy, which is referred to as *data verification*. The traditional means of data verification is to print the data file and compare it number by number with the original data source. Although this procedure is simple, it is impractical in the presence of numerous subjects, variables, or both. Additionally, even for a relatively small data set, this approach is tedious, optimally done with two people participating—one reading the values in the data file while the other checks those values against the original protocols—and is not an assurance of "clean" data. More technologically advanced methods of data verification exist, which, although not necessarily easier than the "hands on" method, do provide alternative means for ensuring the reasonable accuracy of the data set.

Many analysis programs have means of data verification: SAS and Epi Info are two programs commonly used for this purpose. Both programs require the user to enter all of the data twice in two separate files, which are then compared for discrepancies. In SAS, the PROC COMPARE procedure can be used to check the contents of two supposedly identical data files. After the data have been entered independently into two separate SAS data files, the COMPARE procedure compares the contents of each file, datum by datum, and produces a printout that identifies the discrepancies between the two files. The user must then consult the original data protocol to determine, for each identified mismatch, which of the two entries is the correct one. Then the proper changes are made to one of the original data files and the other file is discarded. The major requirement for running this procedure is that each file must contain an identification variable that uniquely identifies each record in the file, necessary because this unique record identifier is the mecha-

nism by which the program matches the records in the two files.

Epi Info uses a different method to verify data. In this approach, data are entered once in their entirety. Then, the data are entered a second time, with the first file serving as a template for the second entry. This allows each piece of data entered in the second file to be compared to its counterpart in the first file at the *exact moment* it is being entered. In the event of an inconsistency between the previously entered data and the data being entered, a signal prompts the user about the inconsistency. The advantage of this real-time feedback approach to data verification is that the user can compare his or her entry to that on the data protocol immediately to determine the proper value. If the value being entered in the current data file is incorrect, then it can be remedied immediately. However, if the error lies in the underlying template file, that file must be opened and edited before the second data entry session can be continued.

These methods represent computer-based approaches to ensuring accurate data entry, but they have some limitations. First, all of the data to be analyzed must be entered twice, which can be time-consuming. Also, there is no protection against the case in which the same datum is incorrectly entered twice.

Another means to increase the accuracy of a data file is an alert that can be programmed to reject data entry errors in a database program. Microsoft Access allows the creator of the database to set parameters or boundaries on the range of data that can be entered in a given field, therefore eliminating out-of-range values. For example, if a user enters a 5 in a field that is set up to accept only values between 1 and 2, the user is notified immediately of the error and prompted to enter a number within the proper range for that field. This has no effect on errors that are within the proper range of values for any field, however.

Data Cleaning

The final step before the actual analysis begins is to "clean" the data set by eliminating errors not picked up in the data entry and verification (Barhyte & Bacon, 1985; Suter, 1987). This cleaning is an essential, but often forgotten, step in preparing data for analysis. One easy method used to clean data is to print the data file and examine it for obvious errors in placement of data and numbers that appear to be unusual for the variables included. Such a strategy aids in the identification of values that are out of range for the variables entered, but it does not reveal entry errors in the data if they are within range. Out-of-range values are more easily seen from frequency distributions for each variable, which are easily obtained from any statistical analysis program. Another method of data cleaning is to run cross tabulations on variables that have combinations that are not reasonable, such as opposing gender and diagnosis to be sure only women have hysterectomies and only men have transurethral resections. Not all data sets have such illogical combinations, so this procedure might be of limited value in such circumstances.

Outliers

Outliers in a data set are those observations that do not seem to belong to the same set as the others. Suppose the age of five participants was 24, 27, 22, 48, and 25 years. The participant with the age of 48 years would seem out of place with the other subjects who are more than 20 years younger and have similar ages. Determining when an outlier exists and what should be done with it is not completely clear. Outliers tend to be classified as observations more than 3 or 3.5 standard deviations from the mean. When one or more outliers are identified, the options are to ignore the situation, drop the observations, transform the observations in some way, or analyze the data with and without the outliers to determine whether they really do have some impact on the results. The last option is probably the most legitimate because it acknowledges the existence of the outliers but does not artificially delete or alter them in order to conduct the analysis.

For example, a master's student was conducting her thesis research by assessing the effect of touch on the self-perceptions of patients undergoing ostomy surgery for the first time. In this study, she assessed the self-perceptions of nine control subjects before surgery and at discharge. Following collection of the control group data, she implemented her intervention of deliberate, appropriate touch as a part of routine postoperative care to nine treatment subjects who were also assessed for self-perception before surgery and at discharge. Unknown to her, the wife of one of the nine treatment subjects filed for divorce immediately after his surgery. His at-discharge self-perception score was several standard deviations below his preoperative score and that of the other treatment participants. When the self-perception scores of the nine control and nine treatment subjects were compared, there were no significant differences in their self-perception scores. However, when the treatment group was reduced to eight subjects by eliminating the data from the affected patient and their average scores were compared to those of the nine control subjects, the treatment group had a significant increase in their average self-perception scores. Although it would be a misrepresentation of the results of the study to report only the latter result, presenting both sets of results provides the only truly accurate view of the research situation.

This example also points out the relationship between sample size and the influence of outliers. The inclusion of this patient in the treatment group had a profound effect on the results of the study, because the sample size was so small. Had the treatment group had 50 or 100 participants, it is unlikely that his inclusion would have made much of a difference in the results. Small samples are always more sensitive to the effect of the "deviant" participant.

SELECTING THE STATISTICAL TEST

Selection of the appropriate statistical test is based on several considerations, among them the hypotheses being tested and the level of measurement of the variables. Table 26–4 provides an overview of selected common statistical tests that are appropriate for independent and dependent variables of varying levels of measurement for each of several types of research questions. What is not apparent from the table is that there are alternative statistical means by which many data sets can be analyzed. This occurs when, despite the original level of measurement, the data are reclassified into a different level of measurement. For example, if the goal of a researcher is to assess the

Table 26–4

Level of Measurement and Focus of the Research Hypothesis/Question for Selected Statistical Tests

STATISTICAL TEST	VARIABLE		FOCUS OF HYPOTHESIS/QUESTION		
	Independent	Dependent	Association	Difference	Correlation
Chi-square	N*	N	X		
	N	N	X		
	O	N	X		
	O	O	X		
Kendall's tau and Spearman rank order	O	O			X
	O	I			X
	I	O			X
Pearson product-moment	I/R	I/R			X
Regression	I/R	I/R			X (and prediction)
Z or t single group comparison	n/a	I/R		X	
Mann-Whitney U	N	O		X	
	O	N		X	
t-Test (two groups only)	N	I/R		X	
	O	I/R		X	
ANOVA (2 or more groups)	N	I/R		X	
	O	I/R		X	

Level of measurement of the variables is indicated by N = nominal, O = ordinal, and I/R = interval/ratio.

relationship between the age of the subjects and their ability to cope with their diagnosis, a Pearson correlation might be calculated, because both variables are at least interval in nature. However, upon finding a positive relationship between age and coping, the question of whether older participants differ from younger subjects might arise. To perform this analysis, it would be necessary to categorize the participants into older and younger groups (often done by ordering the subjects by age, dividing them into thirds, eliminating the middle third, thereby creating an older and younger group), making it an ordinal variable, and then performing a t-test. The ability to manipulate the data by transforming it into other configurations is a convenient feature offered in most data analysis programs.

INTERPRETATION AND PRESENTATION OF THE RESULTS

While the presentation of the results of the statistical analysis is fairly clear, it is never as simple as it seems. The text must describe what was done and what was found using supporting tables and illustrations of the results. Texts and tables are mutually exclusive presentations, in that what is presented in one is not presented in the other. It takes some experience to learn what to present in which venue, but with time and practice it becomes fairly straightforward.

The text portion of the presentation describes the process of getting to the results; the details about the demographic variables and most of the final statistics from the inferential tests are usually presented in tables. When there are only a few results of either type, a table may or may not be necessary.

Some researchers have a tendency to present "glitz" in their results, to make the analysis *seem* sophisticated and elaborate. Rarely does this approach succeed; instead, this approach is usually interpreted as being convoluted and unnecessarily cumbersome. An analysis *is* sophisticated and elaborate if the hypotheses are fully tested, the results are presented in the most direct and comprehensible manner, and all is done in a simple, straightforward manner.

Construction of tables also takes practice and is best learned by examining the tables presented in journals such as *Nursing Research* or *Image* or in a publication manual (for example, American Psychological Association, 1994). Although the construction of a table is somewhat dependent on the purpose of the report, there are a few points to consider in all tables.

1. The title should identify all the major components of the table in terms of type of variables, subjects, and statistics presented. Generally, variables are listed in the first column with subsequent columns devoted to statistics being reported.

2. Any single column should contain only one statistic, for example, percentage, median, or *t*-test value. An exception is in the presentation of means and standard deviations in the same column, which can be handled by labeling the column for both (Mean [SD]) and then reporting the data in that same manner (for example, 45.43 [5.2]). This approach saves considerably on the space needed for the table as well as on the effort it takes to understand it.

3. All variables presented in the results section of a report, whether they are descriptive or inferential, need to have the appropriate measures of central tendency (typical value) and dispersion (variation) also presented. Demographic variables are described by a mixture of these measures, because they usually vary considerably in their levels of measurement. For example, the most common demographic variables are gender, ethnicity, marital status, socioeconomic status, age, and years of education, and, in a clinical study, often there are diagnostic variables. Gender, ethnicity, marital status, and diagnosis are nominal variables, socioeconomic status is ordinal, with age and years of education being ratio level. Using Table 26–1, the appropriate measures would be used depending on the variable being described.

A note about how demographic variables are collected pertains to their eventual analysis. It is *never* in the best interest of the analysis to collect demographic variables that are otherwise interval or ratio variables by reducing them to nominal or ordinal measures. For example, the subject should be able to give his or her age rather than giving the subject age categories to choose from. The need for precision in reporting these variables is lost when they are unnecessarily categorized. The exception to this caution pertains to income, which probably needs to be categorized to encourage participants responding to the question. But that is probably the *only* exception.

Variables used in the inferential analysis also need to have their central tendency and dispersion described along with the presentation of the outcome of the analysis or the final statistics. These statistics are not, however, necessarily presented in the same place within the report. For example, if several *t*-tests (statistical comparisons between the means of two groups testing the hypothesis that the groups are not different) are presented, then the researcher might find any of several presentation configurations: (1) a table with means and standard deviations presented in columns with the *t*-test being the final column of the table, (2) a table of means and standard deviations and a separate table of *t*-test values, or (3) a table of means and standard deviations with the *t*-test results presented in the text. The level of significance attained (*p*) for significant comparisons is usually indicated by means of an asterisk placed next to the *t*-test value, with the actual *p*-level noted at the base of the table. Although it has become convention to present a variety of *p*-values at the base of the table, this seems to suggest that reviewers of the findings will see some results as "more significant" than others. This is not true. The level of significance is an a priori decision for any study and that level is the only level against which all statistical results should be assessed. To place a single *p*-value (for example, $*p < .05$) at the base of a table to correspond to all statistical values noted with an asterisk (*) should convey exactly the same thing that has become this common orchestra of *p*-values, and it does so with much less clutter and "noise."

SUMMARY

Statistical analysis is a complicated subject, one that is not as "black and white" as some statistics professors or consultants would suggest. In any situation, there are likely to be several different analytical techniques that could be applied to achieve the same or similar end. The ability to choose among techniques requires considerable experience with the techniques themselves as well as with the data manipulations that are often required. Because statistical analysis can be complicated, it is often advisable for the researcher to consult a statistician, one with whom the researcher is comfortable and who can communicate effectively as well as "speaking statistics." Few people can manage all the analysis of even a simple study without some form of assistance, and several consultants may assist with the many analysis decisions of complicated studies.

A person in charge of a study does not necessarily know all about the analysis issues and statistics being applied, but such expertise must be available to assist in understanding the data and making sense of the results. Even persons who have had statistical coursework do not necessarily recall it; however, the researcher must be willing to learn about the statistics used and to know where or from whom to get help.

REFERENCES

American Psychological Association (1994). *Publication manual of the American Psychological Association.* (4th ed.). Washington, DC: American Psychological Association.

Armstrong, G. D. (1981). Parametric statistics and ordinal data: A pervasive misconception. *Nursing Research, 30,* 60–62.

Barhyte, D. Y., & Bacon, L. D. (1985). Approaches to cleaning data sets: A technical comment. *Nursing Research, 34,* 62–64.

Dean, A. G., Dean, J. A., Coulombier, D., Brendel, K. A., Smith, D. C., Burton, A. H., Dicker, R. C., Sullivan, K., Fagan, R. F., Arner, T. G. (1994). Epi Info, version 6: A word processing, database, and statistics program for epidemiology on microcomputers. Atlanta: Centers for Disease Control and Prevention.

Knapp, R. (1985). Basic statistics for nurses. (2nd ed.). Albany, NY: Delmar.

Knapp, T. R. (1990). Treating ordinal statistics as interval scales: An attempt to resolve the controversy. *Nursing Research, 39,* 121–123.

Munro, B. H. (1997). *Statistical methods for health care research* (3rd ed.). Philadelphia: J. B. Lippincott.

Norusis, M. J. (1993). SPSS for Windows base system user's guide. Chicago: SPSS.

SAS Institute, Inc. (1988). SAS procedures guide, release 6.03 edition. Cary, NC: SAS Institute, Inc.

Stevens, S. S. (1946). On the theory of scales of measurement. *Science, 103,* 677–680.

Suter, W. N. (1987). Approaches to avoiding errors in data sets: A technical note. *Nursing Research, 36,* 262–263.

SUGGESTED READINGS FOR STATISTICS

Goodwin, L. D. (1984a). The use of power estimation in nursing research. *Nursing Research, 33,* 118–120.

Goodwin, L. D. (1984b). Increasing efficiency and precision of data analysis: Multivariate vs. univariate statistical techniques. *Nursing Research, 33,* 247–249.

Hays, W. L. (1988). *Statistics.* (4th ed.). Philadelphia: Holt, Rinehart & Winston.

Jackson, N. E. (1982). Choosing and using a statistical consultant. *Nursing Research, 31,* 248–250.

Jacobsen, B. S. (1981). Know thy data. *Nursing Research, 30,* 254–255.

Jaeger, R. M. (1990). *Statistics: A spectator sport.* (2nd ed.). Newbury Park, CA: Sage.

Knapp, T. R., & Campbell-Heider, N. (1989). Numbers of observations and variables in multivariate analyses. *Western Journal of Nursing Research, 11,* 634–641.

Knapp, T. R. (1995). Regression analysis: What to report. *Nursing Research, 44,* 58–59.

Knapp, T. R. (1996). The overemphasis on power analysis. *Nursing Research, 45,* 379–381.

Lynn, M. R. (1990). Don't be fooled by statistical significance. *Journal of Pediatric Nursing, 5,* 350–351.

Lynn, M. R. (1990). Choosing (and sticking with) a level of significance. *Journal of Pediatric Nursing, 5,* 401-4–3.

Munro, B. H. (1997). *Statistical methods for health care research.* (3rd ed.). Philadelphia: J. B. Lippincott.

Reid, B. J. (1983). Potential sources of type I error and possible solutions to avoid a "galloping" alpha rate. *Nursing Research, 32,* 190–191.

Rose, D., & Sullivan, O. (1993). *Introducing data analysis for social scientists.* Suffolk, England: St. Edmundsbury Press.

Shavelson, R. J. (1996). *Statistical reasoning for the behavioral sciences.* (3rd ed.). Boston: Allyn and Bacon.

Vogt, W. P. (1993). *Dictionary of statistics and methodology: A nontechnical guide.* Newbury Park, CA: Sage.

Yaremko, R. M., Harari, H., Harrison, R. C., & Lynn, E. (1982). *Reference handbook of research and statistical methods in psychology: For students and professionals.* New York: Harper.

Chapter 27

Writing the Research Report

Susan L. MacLean

WHY WRITE THE RESEARCH REPORT?

The nurse clinician is an important contributor to the development of knowledge for nurses and for solving modern health care problems. Yet, clinicians are often not prepared for roles as researchers and authors. Preparation of the scientific paper may seem overwhelming with all the traditions, rules, and guidelines. However, an author with a logical and systematic mind, perse-

verance, a robust ego, and a willingness to rework and rewrite can be a very successful and important contributor to the scientific literature.

There are many important reasons to write and publish the research report: to contribute to the development of a foundation for practice, to provide visionary leadership, and to achieve personal satisfaction. This chapter is intended to help authors, particularly inexperienced authors, acquire writing skills for successful publication of their research. Throughout the chapter, rules, guidelines, helpful hints, and additional writing resources are mentioned.

Foundation for Practice

The most important reason for publishing research is to provide a foundation for practice. Just about every nursing textbook mentions the need for research-based practice, and every research article concludes with a discussion on the implications of the research for practice. Yet, in the enormous volume of nursing practice literature, there is little practice that is truly based on research. The bottom line is that more research must be conducted and published.

Visionary Leadership

There is an urgent need for information in the modern health care environment. The clinician is faced with changing economic and administrative policies, new care providers and delivery systems, rapidly emerging technologies and health interventions, and serious ethical issues related to accessing quality health care. Research data are critically needed to establish the efficacy of these changes and innovations. Nurses need to be visible in solving these problems by conducting research and publishing the findings. Visionary leadership by nurses requires that they have strong communication skills so their message is heard.

Personal Satisfaction

Personal satisfaction carries most individuals through the very hard work of writing the research report. Seeing a research article published in a scientific journal for the first time is thrilling. The pleasure of completing a research study and publishing the results continues to excite even after multiple publishing experiences.

WHAT IS A SCIENTIFIC PAPER?

The scientific paper is most often a formal report of an empirical study. Writing the empirical report is the primary focus of this chapter. Other types of papers also are considered scientific, for example, critical reviews of published material, papers that examine theoretical or methodological perspectives, research briefs, monographs, case histories, clinical application papers, and papers describing issues in practice, education, administration, and research. Each of these papers is considered a scientific report when it is based on research. While the preparation of these various papers is not specifically addressed, the material in this chapter on writing is valuable to authors writing all types of scientific papers.

PREPARATION FOR WRITING

Careful planning and preparation are essential for producing a publishable research report. The report should reflect the same clear, concise, and organized thinking that went into the study. Before one starts to write, decisions must be made on whether the research merits publication, what is the appropriate audience, what is the best publication medium, and what are the resources needed to produce the manuscript.

Merit

One of the first questions that must be answered is whether the research is worth publishing. No amount of commitment and writing skill can get a poorly designed research study published. Editors can fix flawed writing, but there is little they can do with flawed research.

CHARACTERISTICS OF MERIT

Answering several questions can help determine whether the research is worth writing about and publishing (see box).

RESEARCH LIMITATIONS

Research is often characterized by tradeoffs. For example, to gain control over many demographic variables, some subjects with certain characteristics might be eliminated from the study. This decision, however, will decrease the generalizability of the findings. Most studies also have some unanticipated methodological problems. These problems may cause unexpected results. The results

➤ Questions for Determining the Worth of Writing and Publishing Your Research Report

1. Was the study conducted in a systematic, reliable, and valid manner?
2. Was the research question important, timely, and provocative?
3. Did the research build or expand knowledge on the study topic?
4. Did the research observe ethical standards?
5. Can the results be generalized to a broad population?

also might contradict the results reported by other investigators. Each problem should be examined for any limitations it might cause when interpreting the results of the study. It is possible that the publication of a research report might be premature and require further study. On the other hand, if the research was conducted in a valid and reliable manner, then problems such as conflicting and unexpected results may provide valuable new insights when reported.

RESOURCES ON MERIT

There are several resources that can help authors evaluate the scientific merit and quality of their research studies. Many research textbooks, such as the one by Polit and Hungler (1995), provide guidelines for evaluating research. The *Publication manual of the American Psychological Association* (American Psychological Association [APA], 1995) also provides information on evaluating the merit of the study. The advice of experienced researchers and authors also is helpful. Authors, particularly those who have not been reviewers, should talk with editors and reviewers about the criteria they use to evaluate merit in submitted research manuscripts.

Research Audience and Media

Once the author decides that the research merits publication, the type of publication is

selected. Important decisions must be made concerning the desired audience and the medium to best reach that audience. This information determines the type of manuscript to be written.

RESEARCH AUDIENCE

The research report may be included in a journal devoted only to research articles or it may be included in general or specialty journals that publish other types of articles as well. In either case, the tone of a research article is generally more formal. The format of the report usually adheres to the traditional style of research reports discussed later in this chapter. However, the audience that reads the research article may vary depending on their underlying interest in the publication. Pure research journals have large audiences of researchers whose interests often lie with the theoretical, methodological, and statistical aspects of the study. In contrast, the readers of a journal that publishes some research articles may be more interested in learning about the research problem, the findings, and the application of the findings to practice.

PUBLICATION MEDIA

Once the emphasis of the article and the appropriate audience are determined, the next step is to identify the best publication medium. Journals are the most common medium for publishing research reports. Several articles are available to help authors select an appropriate journal (McElmurry et al., 1981; Johnson, 1982; Swanson, McCloskey, & Bodensteiner, 1991). A detailed discussion of the journal selection process is presented in Chapter 28.

Research also is published in books, films, videos, and electronic media. Electronic publishing is a rapidly growing business. Desktop publishing systems, CD-ROM, electronic libraries, and online journals are expected to rapidly increase dissemination of information and to increase the dissemination of research to a wider audience (Parse, 1991; Killion, 1994). Many editors require manuscripts to be submitted on disk, and some have online submission mechanisms.

AUTHOR GUIDELINES

After selecting the desired publication medium, the author should obtain a copy of the author guidelines. Authors must develop the research article according to the specific rules for content and format. Not following the author guidelines is one of the most common reasons for instant rejection of a manuscript. The author also should review the latest issues of the publication to learn how similar articles were written.

Time, Energy, and Motivation

Finding the time and energy to write the research report is one of the most discouraging aspects of writing. Clinicians have multiple responsibilities and interruptions during their workday, and neither are conducive to productive writing. Too often the research report is delayed or never produced because the author just did not have the time to write. The following are some techniques that writers use to create the time, energy, and motivation for writing:

1. Before getting into the serious writing mode, the writer should take time to get prepared. This is the time to update the literature; identify the audience and desirable publishers; review journals, articles, and publishing guidelines; write letters of inquiry to editors to determine their interest in the manuscript; gather writing tools and reference books; arrange for equipment and a place to write; and make plans for managing both professional and personal obligations that may interfere with the writing timetable.
2. When ready to write, the writer should schedule blocks of time when energy and creativity are high, such as early in the day or once the children have gone to bed. About halfway through the writing project, the motivation to write is much stronger and the writer is able to write even when the sun is shining or the in-box is piled high.
3. The writer should schedule his or her time, adhere to the schedule, and control the urge to become distracted. The urge to clean the office or home is the greatest while trying to write.
4. Writers should make arrangements for a private place to work, close the door, have their calls screened or use an answering machine, and discourage unannounced visitors. The closed door is the best strategy for discouraging interruptions; it says "something important is going on here."
5. Writers should never feel guilty or defensive about using time for scientific writing; guilt uses up too much energy. They should remember, instead, the reasons why they are writing.
6. Writers should never feel anxious or lack confidence about writing, which also uses up energy. They should remember, instead, all of their accomplishments such as conducting the research study in the first place.
7. Writing is hard work, even for experienced authors. Writers often set productivity goals such as writing so many pages or words per day. To help keep the momentum going, writers can set a daily writing goal even if it is just writing a sentence or paragraph. The biggest time waster is the time that is spent getting back into writing after it has been put aside for a few days or weeks.
8. When all else fails and the time and energy are just not there, a colleague or student can be asked to help with the manuscript. Collaboration can be both a motivator and a time saver, and it might just be something that the other person needs to do or learn. (See box for helpful tips for productive writing.)

> ## Helpful Tips for Productive Writing

- Take time to prepare before writing.
- Schedule blocks of time to write when energy and creativity are high.
- Adhere to a schedule for writing.
- Work in a private place.
- Avoid feeling guilty about using time to write.
- Develop confidence about writing.
- Set incremental goals for productivity, for example, number of pages per writing session.
- Invite a colleague to help with the manuscript.

WRITING STYLE

Once the author begins to write the research report, there are new hurdles to overcome. Research articles are often perceived as dull, tedious, ambiguous, or pretentious. Reviewers are inclined to postpone review of difficult-to-read manuscripts, and many nurses will not read a tedious, time-consuming article. Although the scientific paper is not written with the flair of a literary publication, the writing still should be interesting and provocative. The research report is, after all, a story of a problem, a solution, and the consequences. When asked what makes readers care, an experienced author wrote, "They care when the writer suspends them between a question and an answer . . . between a contradiction and its resolution" (Kress, 1993).

Expression of Ideas

ORGANIZATION OF CONTENT

Organizing the content of a research report is fairly straightforward. The topics follow in a standardized and logical order (introduction, literature review, purpose, and so forth). The use of topical headings helps to lead the reader through the report. The organization of ideas, however, is more difficult to achieve.

ORGANIZATION OF THINKING

A common problem in writing is the lack of simple, clear, smooth expression of ideas (APA, 1995). Nursing is not the only profession to wrestle with "plain English." In the book *Plain English for Lawyers*, Wydick (1985) stated, "We lawyers cannot write plain English. We use eight words to say what could be said in two. We use arcane phrases to express commonplace ideas. Seeking to be precise, we become redundant. Our sentences twist on, phrase within clause within clause, glazing the eyes and numbing the minds of our readers" (p. 3). Wydick could easily have been speaking about writing by nurses.

Although scientific papers are scholarly, long complex sentences, wordiness, and long pompous words are unnecessary. Common errors such as short choppy sentences; overly long sentences and paragraphs; lack of continuity in sentences, themes, and ideas; lack of transitions, with poor introductory and summary sentences; misspelled words; and verbosity make it difficult for the reader to follow and understand the report (APA, 1995; Polit & Hungler, 1995). *A Rulebook for Arguments* (Weston, 1992) is a resource that can help an author develop a logical presentation of ideas.

Several strategies can help improve the expression of ideas:

1. Be frugal with words, especially adjectives and adverbs. Cross out all words that are not needed for sensible, complete sentences.
2. Vary the length of sentences and paragraphs.
3. Focus on one point per paragraph; several different points confuse the reader and obscure the importance. A writing teacher described the problem as a tossed salad with very little dressing—lots of ideas with little holding the paragraph together.
4. Use transitional words and phrases to relate new ideas to previous ideas. Developing ideas systematically helps the reader follow the direction of the author's thoughts.
5. Use consistent terms. This is especially important for linking ideas.
6. Use consistent verb tenses. Consistent use of verb tense helps the reader to differentiate past activities from current thinking. For example, use the past tense for the literature review, for the methods section, and for reporting procedures, interventions, and statistical tests in the results section. Use the present tense to describe interpretations of statistical tests in the results section and for the conclusions and implications in the discussion section.
7. Read the paper aloud to identify problem areas in expression, rhythm, and organization. Abrupt transitions, ambiguous sentences, and gaps in organization are more obvious when spoken.
8. Ask colleagues to read the paper and identify confusing and weak areas.

OBJECTIVITY

Scientific papers are objective reports. Opinions, subjective statements, exaggerations, sexist language, stereotypes, and emotionally laden words should be avoided. In the discussion section of a research report, the author provides interpretations, conclusions, and recommendations. These are subjective statements; they differ, however, from opinion, because they are based on the study data.

Word Selection, Grammar, Sentence Construction, and Spelling

Many communication problems are caused by the incorrect selection of words, spelling errors, and poor grammar. Each error causes the reader to question the author's qualifications to conduct a reliable and valid study.

WORD SELECTION

Several types of words make it difficult for the reader to understand the author's ideas. Words that are easily confused, colloquialisms, and jargon should be eliminated from the manuscript. For example, commonly confused words include those that look alike (all ready and already), sound alike (it's and its), and have slight differences in meaning (affect and effect). Colloquial words are those used in conversation but not in formal English. Some examples are "irregardless," "humanness," and "the reason being that." Jargon is technical vocabulary. Jargon is not easily understood by readers outside the profession, and the words are often inflated, polysyllabic, and obscure.

GRAMMAR AND SENTENCE CONSTRUCTION

Correct grammar and sentence construction are important for clarity in expressing ideas. Mistakes in punctuation frequently occur with colons, semicolons, hyphens, commas, and dashes. Problems with noun and verb agreement also are common (APA, 1995). Certain types of nouns are difficult to work with because they sound plural but are singular (news and pediatrics), and other nouns sound singular but are plural (data, hypotheses, alumni, sequelae). There are many resources available in bookstores to help authors with basic grammar and sentence construction. Several manuals also include information that may be helpful for

research writing such as the APA manual (APA, 1995), Gibaldi and Achtert (1988), and Strunk and White (1979).

SPELLING

Correct spelling is essential for both common words and technical language. Errors are most often missed in the last revision of the paper. The writer should persevere, reading the paper one last time before sending it to the editor or returning the page proofs.

Editorial Style

Editorial style refers to the rules or guidelines used by publishing houses to ensure a consistent presentation of materials by the authors. The rules cover topics such as the correct way to cite references; design tables, graphs, and figures; set margins; use punctuation; or capitalize words (APA, 1995). Adherence to a specified editorial style is mandatory, and manuscripts not conforming to the style often are returned to the author unread.

Most publishers describe their required editorial style in one or more issues of their publication in a section called "Information for Authors." Some publishers, particularly for books, send a copy on an abbreviated style manual to the author. Authors should obtain a copy of the required style manual before starting to write. If questions occur that are not addressed in the manual, the best source of information is the editor or editorial staff.

Concluding the Preparation Phase

Before beginning to write the research report, the writer should pause to review the preparation phase: the overall goal for writing the scientific paper was identified; techniques for determining the merit of the research and for mobilizing time, energy, and motivation were considered; the manuscript audience, medium, and focus were selected; finally, strategies for improving writing style and the expression of ideas were identified. Keeping sight of the writing process from the beginning to the end helps keep the project on track and make it a more pleasurable experience for the writer. Each accomplishment is a step closer to completing the exciting but hard work of writing the research report.

WRITING THE RESEARCH REPORT

Although many types of articles can be written concerning the research study, the research report is the best source of information for all manuscripts. For example, a clinical article could be written about the practice implications of the research findings. This information could be extracted from the research report and further developed for the clinical article. Also, the clinical article could refer readers to the published research report for details concerning the study methodology. This reference to the published report decreases repetition of material and saves valuable space that can be used for the clinical content. The reference within the article also decreases copyright issues. Thus, the most practical method for broadly disseminating the results of a study is to first prepare the research report.

The organization of the research report usually follows a traditional publication format (APA, 1995). Authors often find the "cookbook" type of structure helpful during their early efforts with writing research reports. For additional guidance on the content and construction of the research report, refer to the APA manual (1995) and Polit and Hungler (1995).

The content of the research report is organized in the following manuscript sections: Introduction, Methods, Results, and Discussion (APA, 1995). Also included is an abstract and the title page. Space limits the amount of information and the depth of discussion in each section of the research report. In most research reports, the emphasis is usually on the findings and discussion, with less emphasis on introductory sections. Twelve to 15 double-spaced, typed manuscript pages are usually allotted to convey what Tornquist (1983) succinctly summarized as "Why I did it (introduction, rationale, background, problem, and literature review); what I did (methods); what happened (findings); and what it means (discussion, implications, conclusions)."

Introduction

Introductory sections of the research report include information about the nature and significance of the problem, the study purpose, the research variables, the literature review, and the research questions or hypotheses. Most of the material for the introduction comes from the original research proposal. Because of space limitations in the published report, only information relevant to the report topic is included.

PROBLEM AND SIGNIFICANCE

Within the first few introductory sentences, the reader should have a clear understanding of why the research was done. Authors mistakenly write paragraphs, sometimes pages, without making a clear statement of the problem and study purpose. Meanwhile, the reader is floundering in a sea of words, trying to appreciate the significance, without knowing what the problem is. Few readers have the time or patience to figure out why they should read the article. So, the writer should begin the research report with a clear statement of the problem and purpose, providing the details in subsequent paragraphs.

LITERATURE REVIEW

During the proposal writing phase of the research, the investigator diligently works to identify the study problem and document its nature and significance. The challenge in the report writing phase is to reduce the proposal material into a few paragraphs.

Identifying the conceptual framework for the study is a good way to introduce the literature because the framework identifies the variables and relationships that are relevant to the research study. A brief review of the literature identifies supporting and contradicting studies and gaps in existing knowledge. It may be important to update the literature from the earlier written proposal and add new findings to the research report. Tangential studies and lengthy literature discussions from the proposal are not included in the written report.

STUDY PURPOSE, VARIABLES, QUESTIONS, AND HYPOTHESES

The introductory section ends with a summary statement that identifies the problem, what is known, and what is needed. This summary provides the rationale for the study. This section logically concludes with a statement of the study purpose, variables, and questions and hypotheses (APA, 1995). At this point, it should be clear to the reader why the study was done and what was investigated. The next section of the research report describes what was done.

Methods

In the methods section, information about the study design, subjects, instruments or apparatus, and procedures is included, in that order. Methods are described in the past tense because they represent what was actually done. If what was done differs from what was proposed, this change is reported. Tornquist (1986), APA (1995), and Polit and Hungler (1995) are excellent resources for detailed guidelines on how to develop each method subsection, particularly when plans and outcomes differ. Additional information about describing the sample, measures, and procedures in qualitative research can be found in Knafl and Howard (1984).

Unlike the introductory section, the methods section is presented in detail. In most cases, information contained in the original proposal can be inserted directly into the article. Although original material can be used in the methods section, some information is deleted to keep within the publisher's page limitations. In a scientific paper, the author must provide sufficient information about the methods so that the reliability and validity of the quantitative investigation (APA, 1995) and the trustworthiness of a qualitative investigation (Guba, 1981; Lincoln & Guba, 1985) can be determined by the reader. Based on the methods description, other researchers should be able to evaluate its worth and replicate the study (APA, 1995).

Results

Writing the results section can seem overwhelming—so much data and so little space. Many results sections begin with a description of the sample characteristics, sample size, and information about attrition rates. However, some authors include the sample data in the methods section when the description is simple and straightforward.

QUANTITATIVE FINDINGS

The most important findings related to the study questions or hypotheses are described first. Some authors mistakenly provide interpretation and discussion material in the results section. Only statistical material should be presented. As a general rule, data on the hypothesis and main variables are presented first, even if the results are nonsignificant and disappointing (Tornquist, 1986). Once the main results are presented, both descriptively and numerically, the interesting secondary findings or analysis of subgroup data can be presented. The results are reported with the appropriate inferential and descriptive statistics. Inferential statistics include the value, degrees of freedom, probability level, and direction of effect (APA, 1995; Polit & Hungler, 1995). Descriptive statistics usually include the appropriate measure of variation (standard deviation) and dispersion (range) (Tornquist, 1986).

Results presented in tables and figures often are easier to compare and understand than numbers written in the text. They are also more interesting to readers. The disadvantage of figures and tables are that they are expensive to publish; therefore, only about three tables should be included in a manuscript. The narrative portion of the results section highlights the content of a table or figure but should not duplicate the data in the illustration (Tornquist, 1986; APA, 1995). Preparation of tables and figures requires skill. Inexperienced authors should consult style manuals such as APA (1995) or seek the advice of an experienced colleague.

QUALITATIVE FINDINGS

The results section of a qualitative study differs from that of a quantitative study. Qualitative results focus on the narrative descriptions given by the subjects concerning their perspectives and experiences. The purpose of the qualitative research, however, often influences the type of information included in the methods and results sections.

Knafl and Howard (1984) recommended the following format when reporting qualitative data:

1. When the purpose of the study is instrument development, the qualitative data are not mentioned in the procedure, results, or discussion sections.

2. For illustration purposes, the qualitative data can be included with the quantitative data to help explain the findings.

3. If the study purpose is to sensitize the reader, then categories of data concerning the subjects' views are included.

4. Larger amounts of data often are presented when the focus of the study is conceptual. Data, categories, concepts, and theoretical formulations are presented so that the reader can follow and evaluate the development of the theory.

Additional information for writing the qualitative report are included in Knafl and Howard (1984), Artinian (1988), and Polit and Hungler (1995).

Discussion

According to Fryxell (1994), endings should come full circle, back to the beginning. In the beginning of the research report, a case was made that an important problem needed to be solved. In the discussion section, the author answers the following questions: Has the situation changed? Was the plan for solving the problem a good one? What has been learned from the research?

IMPACT

The discussion section is the most important section for the reader, yet it is the section most often done superficially. Although not writing about research manuscripts per se, Fryxell's (1994) words on the importance of lasting impressions are worth noting: "A good ending can pull it all together for a reader, making the whole more than the sum of the previous parts. And a bad ending, of course, can ruin all the hard work you did in leading the reader from here to there." In bringing the reader full circle, the author discusses the major findings in relation to the study questions or hypotheses, and evaluates limitations or problems in conducting the study. The author also can use literature from the proposal or from other sources to develop an interesting and informative discussion. The literature may help confirm the findings, clarify the interpretations, or explain unusual and unexpected results.

INTERPRETING RESULTS

In a quantitative study, the discussion section begins with a statement about the support or lack of support for the original hypothesis (APA, 1995). A statement about whether the study goals were achieved or a summary of the major themes, concepts, and theory usually introduces the discussion in a qualitative study (Knafl & Howard, 1984).

If study results were not as expected, explaining why this occurred helps others with future research. Unexpected results often are caused by flawed or inadequate theory rather than problems with the methods (Polit & Hungler, 1995). Mixed results (some hypotheses are supported and some are not) are common and are usually related to problems in reliability and validity of the instruments, or to flaws in the theoretical framework (Polit & Hungler, 1995). A brief discussion of any limitations in the study should be included in the discussion section to further explain the results (Tornquist, 1986; Polit & Hungler, 1995).

IMPLICATIONS

The implications portion of the discussion section should create a good last impression and inspire the readers to apply the findings or continue with the research. The final paragraphs should be strong, positive, and persuasive (Tornquist, 1986). The writer should demonstrate to the reader, by words and examples, how the findings are applicable to practice. Changes can be recommended and new research identified. The potential for creativity and visionary leadership is at its highest in the final sentences of the research report. It is the last chance to reinforce a message and inspire readers into action.

Abstract and Title Page

Once the research report is completed, it is most satisfying to write the final submission materials. Most journals require a brief abstract and information for the title page.

ABSTRACT

Abstracts for research reports usually are limited to about 100 to 120 words. Author guidelines should be checked for variations. To describe a complete investigation in a few words, the writing style must be concise, with maximum information in each sentence. There are no sentence transitions, summaries, references, tables, figures, quotations, or literature reviews (APA, 1995). The traditional format follows the research report organization: problem and purpose statement, subject characteristics, methods (design, instruments, and procedures), findings (including statistical significance), and conclusions and implications (APA, 1995). Thus, in very few words, the author is challenged to write a comprehensive, readable, and interesting summary of the research report. It may be the author's only chance to convince the reader that the article is interesting and pertinent.

TITLE PAGE

The biggest thrill comes to the writer who finishes the manuscript and can put his or her name down as the author. The author's name usually does not include titles and degrees. It is recommended that authors use the same name format on every manuscript for consistent citation and recognition over time (APA, 1995). The affiliation usually indicates where the author conducted the study and if any financial support was received during the investigation. If the author has no affiliation, the city and state of residence are used (APA, 1995). A change in affiliation since the study was completed is handled by including the new affiliation in a sentence informing readers where the author can be contacted.

In addition to the author name and identification, the title page includes the study title and the running head. Manuscript titles are usually 12 to 15 words long with no abbreviations or extraneous words (APA, 1995). The title conveys information to the reader about the study topic by describing the study variables and their relationships (APA, 1995). Running heads and key index words are developed from the title.

Running heads are about 50 characters long including letters and punctuation. The running head captures the essence of the title and article and are used to title each page of the article (APA, 1995). Indexing services use key words from the title to categorize the content of each article.

AFTER WRITING THE RESEARCH REPORT

After the research report is finally written and a sigh of relief is issued, the manuscript goes through several revisions before publication.

Revision Before Submission

Two revisions of the manuscript are advised before it is submitted for publication. The first revision is more effective if the manuscript is put aside for a week or two. Insights concerning content and writing often occur when the author has time away from the writing process.

The second revision occurs after the manuscript has been sent to two or three colleagues for review. This review is most important because the reviewers often identify areas that are clear to the author but are confusing to the reader. Peers who give critical yet gentle suggestions for revision should be selected. If the journal guidelines are included, these reviewers can tailor their feedback to meet both the author's and publisher's needs.

Revision After Submission

After the manuscript has been submitted, it goes through an extensive review process (Litt, 1994; Morse, 1996; Oberst, 1996a, 1996b; Stern, 1996). Following review, one of four decisions is made by the publishing editor: accept as is, accept pending revision, revise and resubmit, and decline. Except for the rare manuscript that is accepted without revision, all other publication decisions require additional writing, and a few manuscripts require extensive rethinking and rewriting. The best way to facilitate the process is to seriously consider the advice of the reviewers and editors. The writer should ask himself or herself why the reviewers provided the critique that they did, and that insight should guide the revision. If something was misinterpreted, again, the writer should ask why (Morse, 1996). If suggestions cannot be incorporated, then the writer should explain the reasons when the manuscript is resubmitted; the writer knows the research better than anyone else.

Editors are usually willing to discuss the revision with the author to help facilitate the process for both author and publisher. Like authors, the editors and reviewers put considerable effort into making the published research report an important contribution to the scientific literature.

SUMMARY

Why write the research report? Why go through the hassle? At conclusion of writing the research report, the writer will clearly see the value to publishing the report. There is so much that can be done to improve health care, and through the research report, the writer provides the direction for facilitating and evaluating change. As others are inspired to continue the work, the impact grows. The writer soon forgets the hours of hard work because he or she wrote something that will make a difference. Why write the research report? Because it feels so good.

REFERENCES

American Psychological Association (APA). (1995). *Publication manual of the American Psychological Association* (4th ed.). Washington, D.C.: Author.

Artinian, B. A. (1988). Qualitative modes of inquiry. *Western Journal of Nursing Research, 10, 138–149.*

Fryxell, D. (1994). Writing full circle. *Writer's Digest,* November, 72–73, 76.

Gibaldi, J., & Achtert, W. (1988). *MLA handbook for writers of research papers.* New York, The Modern Language Association of America.

Guba, E. G. (1981). Criteria for assessing the trustworthiness of naturalistic inquires. *Educational Communication and Technology Journal, 29,* 75–91.

Johnson, S. H. (1982). Selecting a journal for your manuscript. *Nursing & Health Care, 3, 258–263.*

Killion, V. J. (1994). Information resources for nursing research: The Sigma Theta Tau International electronic library and online journal. *Medical Reference Services Quarterly, 13*(3), 1–17.

Knafl, K. A., & Howard, M. J. (1984). Interpreting and reporting qualitative research. *Research in Nursing & Health, 7, 17–24.*

Kress, N. (1993). Reeling in readers. *Writer's Digest,* August, 8, 10–11.

Lincoln, Y. S., & Guba, E. G. (1985). *Naturalistic inquiry.* Beverly Hills, CA: Sage.

Litt, I. F. (1994). Peering into the black box: The editorial process. *Journal of Adolescent Health, 15,* 358.

McElmurry, B. J., Newcomb, B. J., Barnfather, J., et al. (1981). The manuscript review process. In J. C. McCloskey, & H. K. Grace (Eds.), *Current issues in nursing* (pp. 129–143). Worcester, MA: Blackwell Scientific.

Morse, J. M. (1996). Revise and resubmit: Responding to reviewers' reports. *Qualitative Health Research, 6*(2), 149–151.

Oberst, M. T. (1996a). Behind the scenes. *Research in Nursing & Health, 19*(1), 1.

Oberst, M. T. (1996b). And still more from behind the scenes. *Research in Nursing & Health, 19*(2), 89.

Parse, R. R. (1991). Electronic publishing: Beyond browsing. *Nursing Science Quarterly, 4*(1), 1.

Polit, D. F., & Hungler, B. P. (1995). *Nursing research: Principles and methods* (5th ed.). Philadelphia: J. B. Lippincott.

Stern, P. N. (1996). Putting a manuscript to bed: Operationalizing the process. *Health Care for Women International, 17*(3), v–vii.

Strunk, W., & White, E. B. (1979). *The elements of style.* New York: Macmillan.

Swanson, E., McCloskey, J., & Bodensteiner, A. (1991). Publishing opportunities for nurses: A comparison of 92 U.S. journals. *Image, 23*(1), 33–38.

Tornquist, E. M. (1983). Strategies for publishing research. *Nursing Outlook, 31,* 180–183.

Tornquist, E. M. (1986). *From proposal to publication: An informal guide to writing about nursing research.* Reading, MA: Addison-Wesley.

Weston, A. (1992). *A rulebook for arguments* (2nd ed.). Indianapolis: Hackett Publishing.

Wydick, R. (1985). *Plain English for lawyers* (2nd ed.). Durham, NC: Carolina Academic Press.

Chapter 28

Disseminating Research: The Medium and the Message

Magdalena A. Mateo, Suzanne Smith, and Dominick L. Flarey

As the value and quality of clinical research in nursing has increased, more and more nurses are making concerted efforts to disseminate their findings through multiple channels. Because disseminating research findings is an integral part of the research process, the plan for communicating findings must be developed at the time a study is proposed.

Some funding agencies and organizations require a review of results before these are presented. Because these reviews may delay the dissemination process, it is important to be familiar with requirements of funding agencies and the organization of employment before plans for presentations or publications are initiated.

The most popular methods for disseminating research are print journals, oral presentations, and poster sessions. Although the traditional approach to publishing research findings and study outcomes is through professional journals, other publications are electronic journals, newsletters of organizations and professional societies, and newspapers. Oral and poster sessions may be conducted in formal forums such as research and clinical conferences as well as in organization-sponsored fairs, on clinical units, and through the media. Enhanced technology, such as teleconferencing, animated slide presentation software, and the Internet, provides nurse researchers with more sophisticated choices for presenting their outcomes.

This chapter examines strategies for successfully disseminating research findings. Emphasis is placed on process and the strategies to adequately develop high-quality, professional presentations. Although strategies pertinent to different types of presentations are delineated, the principles that are cited apply to most types of presentations. Chapter 27 includes information on preparing and writing the research report.

PUBLICATION

Print Journals

Even though there are close to 400 nursing journals (Citations in Nursing and Allied Health Web site, http://www.cinahl.com), only a small percentage are exclusively research journals. Publishing research reports in these research journals has the advantage of allowing nurse researchers to report the conduct of their investigation using standard, structured research report format: background, review of the literature, methods, findings, and implications (Tornquist & Funk, 1993). The primary focus of review for the research journal is scientific merit—be it quantitative or qualitative research. Publishing in a research journal is ideal for disseminating research if the writer wishes to showcase his or her methods (Waugaman, 1992).

If research outcomes and their applicability to a certain nursing audience is of interest, the writer may want to write for a non-research journal. This may be a more labor-intensive effort, because the writer cannot follow the traditional research report format. The non-research journal requires a less formal language, a process approach to the topic (what was the problem, how was it solved, and what was discovered?), and creative, interesting headings.

Editors are critically aware of the need to have a data-driven practice base and are eagerly seeking research-based information that holds the potential for transforming nursing practice. So whatever type of journal is chosen to publish research findings, editors are receptive.

CRITICAL SUCCESS FACTORS FOR PUBLISHING

Journal publication is the most frequent method for research dissemination because many nurses can be reached by one effort—writing a high-quality, focused manuscript. To increase the chance of having a manuscript accepted for publication (Blancett, 1994; Johnson, 1996), the following guidelines are recommended (Table 28–1):

Table 28–1
Critical Success Factors for Publishing

Select the appropriate audience
Select the appropriate journal
Query the editor
Conform to submission guidelines
Adhere to copyright laws
Include implications for practice
Use recent references
Maintain organization
Use tables and graphs
Determine authorship entitlement
Acknowledge appropriately
Conform to ethical practices

Select the Appropriate Audience. The first step in any writing project is to select the appropriate audience. To whom will the findings be conveyed? Who would benefit most from the research findings? The writer should be specific in the introduction as to who is the intended audience is. By focusing on a particular audience, research findings can be presented to meet that audience's needs. For example, if research findings suggest a cost-effective way to deliver nursing care, both practitioners and administrators would be interested in the topic. However, practitioners would be interested in the clinical implications, whereas administrators would be interested in the management aspects.

Select the Appropriate Journal. The most innovative, well-written manuscript will be rejected if it is submitted to the wrong journal (Blancett, 1994). Having identified the audience allows the writer to select the journals that are edited for that group. Once potential journals are selected, the writer should obtain the guidelines for authors that most journals publish in each issue. Frequently included is a short mission statement highlighting the major focus of the journal, the intended readership profile, and the types of topics that are appropriate for submission. In addition to seeking this information to make the appropriate journal choice, the writer should examine several recent issues to assess the preferred format approach of the journal.

Query the Editor. When planning a writing project, it is a good idea to first query editors of potential journals that might be appropriate for the topic. Queries can be by mail, telephone, or E-mail. Authors' guidelines often tell which approach the editor prefers.

Querying the editor can save time and effort. Although it is acceptable to query several editors at the same time, it is not acceptable to send a manuscript to more than one editor at the same time.

Editors are professionals and experts in writing for publication. Editors know the types of manuscripts they would like to obtain for publication. When querying an editor (see box), the writer should explain in detail the research and plans for writing the manuscript (Blancett, 1994). The editor may want to discuss the writer's approach for organizing the manuscript content. The editor may persuade the writer to use a different focus to increase his or her chances of acceptance of the manuscript for publication. Or, the editor may tell the writer that the particular journal is not interested in the manuscript because of its similarity to already published or soon-to-be published papers. Receiving this type of information allows the writer to tailor the manuscript to the journal whose editor has expressed the most interest in the topic.

Include Implications for Practice. Often a good manuscript is rejected for publication because the author does not discuss the implications of the research findings for the readership of the journal. Because the writer is the topic expert, readers expect a discussion of the utility of findings to practice. The length of the implications section varies depending on the purpose of the journal. The implications section in a research journal is often short compared with the focus on application in a clinical journal.

When discussing implications for the study, the writer should present findings in relation to similar studies, highlighting how the findings support as well as differ from those of others (if similar studies have been reported). Finally, the writer should suggest directions for future research to further illustrate the relation of the research to practice.

Conform to the Submission Requirements. All journals have requirements for formatting and submitting a manuscript. If these requirements are not printed in the journal, they can be obtained from the editorial office. Journal editors have a bias toward manuscripts that are correctly formatted.

➤ Sample Query Letter for Nursing Journal

(Date)
(Inside Address)
Dear *(name of editor)*:
   I wish to submit a manuscript to *(name of publication)*. Our research examined processes of change used in smoking cessation by 190 smokers and former smokers selected through random digit dialing. A mailed cross-sectional survey had an 84% response rate. Multivariate analysis of variance of 10 processes of change across five stages of smoking cessation (precontemplation, contemplation, relapse, recent, and long-term quitting) was significant, $\underline{F}$ (40,590) = 5.02, $\underline{p}$ = .0001. Post hoc analysis revealed statistically significant differences on seven of the 10 processes of change ($\underline{p}$ < .05). The readers of your journal can apply our study findings in their practice to help clients stop smoking.
   (If institutional letterhead is not used, insert here a brief paragraph indicating your qualifications to write on your topic.)
   Enclosed is an outline of the proposed manuscript, which can be submitted within 6 weeks of receiving your positive reply. I look forward to hearing from you.
Sincerely,
(Contact person)
(Address and telephone number, if not imprinted on letterhead)

An incorrectly formatted manuscript can be a "red flag." Often, editors assume that if the author of a paper was serious about its publication in the journal, the author would have made an effort to send it properly formatted. A lingering thought in the editor's mind will be, "If the author did not pay attention to simple formatting requirements, what attention has been paid to ensure the integrity of the research and the manuscript?"

Adhere to Copyright Laws. Once a manuscript is accepted for publication, authors are required by the publisher to sign an agreement that transfers copyright of the author's material to the publisher (Clegg, 1991). Once signed, the agreement renders the manuscript the copyrighted work of the publisher. The author must have the publisher's written permission to use a significant part of the article in another publication, oral, written, or electronic. When in doubt about using copyrighted work, the writer should call or write the copyright holder (Garrett & Hawkes, 1992; Blancett, 1997).

Use Recent References. References used in a manuscript should be current and relevant to the topic. The definition of current varies among editors. Generally, a 3-year range is acceptable. Obvious exceptions to this rule of thumb might be classic works related to the topic. Use of older references is also acceptable when your study is a replication. Using current references conveys to the editor and the readers that the research has been placed in the context of contemporary concerns and that a new contribution is being made to the health care literature.

Maintain Organization. A manuscript with a logical flow of ideas is easy to read and understand. Developing an organized, orderly paper, however, requires work, particularly when presenting a complex research protocol that was not necessarily linear. The writer can facilitate order and clarity by outlining the content and using headings and subheadings. A colleague should read a draft of the paper solely to check the logical progression of its content.

Use Tables and Graphs. Tables, graphs, and illustrations add significantly to the overall sophistication of the manuscript. They also serve to clarify concepts and present research findings and outcomes in a more easily understood way. The use of tables and graphs also assists in organizing the information. Before writing the paper, the writer should decide which concepts lend themselves to display in a graphic form. When discussing table or graph information in text, the writer should not restate every piece of information; rather, the writer should highlight one or two key points and refer the reader to the table or graph.

Tables should be self-explanatory using

the following guidelines (Cates, 1983; American Psychological Association, 1994):

- Keep the title clear and concise.
- Label each row and column and provide units of measure for the data.
- Include notes (general, specific, and probability note) below the table. General notes provide information applicable to the table (for example, abbreviations, symbols). Specific notes refer to an entry, column, or row. Probability notes indicate results of tests of significance.

Graphs are used to synthesize data and show the relationship between two or more variables. Effective graphs are accurate, simple, clear, neat, professional, and attractive. There are several items to consider when developing graphs (Spilker & Schoenfelder, 1990; McKinney & Burns, 1993). These include using a frame to establish a boundary between the data and other information, prominent symbols to plot data, and a scale appropriate to the data.

Determine Authorship Entitlement. Authorship implies significant involvement in writing a paper and in the work that led up to that writing. It implies "substantial intellectual contribution" (Nativio, 1993, p. 358). The reality is that authorship is often given to (or insisted on by) people with minimal involvement in the writing project—perhaps a supervisor, a data collector, or a statistician. Guidelines for authorship make it clear that "authorship credit should be based only on substantial contributions to A) conception and design, or analysis and interpretation of data; and B) drafting the article or revising it critically for important intellectual content; and on C) final approval of the version to be published. Conditions A, B, and C must all be met. Participation solely in the acquisition of funding or the collection of data does not justify authorship. General supervision of the research group is not sufficient for authorship" (Lundberg & Glass, 1996, p. 75).

In large, multisite research projects, it is becoming common to list the research group as the author, with individuals mentioned in a footnote. When this is the case, all members of the group still must meet the stringent requirements for authorship (Lundberg & Glass, 1996).

There is no rule for order of authorship. The order of authorship should be the joint decision of the authors, after analysis of each author's contribution to the work. This analysis is best done at the start of a project so that expectations are clear and conflicts are later avoided. In general, order of authorship should reflect most to smallest contribution. This order might be based on the amount of time given or on the importance of the contribution.

Acknowledge Appropriately. Even if not everyone who contributed to a research project is entitled to authorship, certainly they should be acknowledged. There is almost as much controversy about who is entitled to acknowledgment as there is about authorship entitlement (Boots, 1993). Some editors think that authors who blindly acknowledge family, friends, and colleagues are frivolous, whereas others think generous acknowledgments reflect the humanity of authors (Boots, 1993). As a rule of thumb, acknowledgments are reserved for those who have made a substantial contribution to the project being reported in a paper, including editorial and writing assistance (Flanagin & Rennie, 1995). People who might be acknowledged are data collectors, a project director, an editorial assistant, or a faculty advisor. Not everyone wishes to be acknowledged publicly. For this reason, written permission should be obtained from those named in an acknowledgment to ensure that they approve of use of their name in material that will be published and widely disseminated.

Conform to Ethical Practices. Adhering to ethical practices when publishing is vital; unethical practices can ruin a person's chances for future publication (Blancett, 1991). Two easily avoided unethical practices are (1) submitting the same manuscript to different journals at the same time and (2) plagiarism.

It is unethical to submit a manuscript to more than one journal at the same time. Every journal's authors' guidelines has a statement to the effect that the author warrants that he or she is submitting original, unpublished material, under consideration by no other publisher (Blancett, 1992). So, although it is acceptable to query as many editors as desired about interest in a manuscript, it can be submitted to only one journal at a time. If a manuscript is rejected, it is permissible then to send it to another journal.

Plagiarism is claiming someone else's ideas and work, published or unpublished, as one's own. The four common types of plagiarism are (1) verbatim lifting of passages, (2) rewording ideas from an original source into an author's own style, (3) paraphrasing an original work without attribution, and (4) noting the original source of only some of what is borrowed (American Medical Association, 1998). A writer should be acutely aware of when his or her writing reflects the ideas of others, and appropriate reference should be made to the original source. If a significant amount of material (copyright law does not define significant) is borrowed through paraphrasing or direct quotation, the copyright holder (usually the publishing company) should be contacted for written permission to republish. Likewise, any published item, no matter how large or small, that is complete unto itself, such as a table, figure, chart, graph, artwork, poem, or picture, requires that permission from the copyright holder be obtained to reproduce. For further discussion of the intricacies of copyright in order to avoid plagiarism or copyright law violation, see publications such as Clegg (1991), Garrett & Hawkes (1992), and Skiba (1997) or visit the federal government copyright office's Web site (http://www.lcweb.loc.gov/copyright/).

MANUSCRIPT REVIEW PROCESS

Peer review is the process that editors use to help ensure the professional integrity of nursing knowledge. This process has three main purposes: (1) detection of errors, (2) fair and impartial treatment of authors' ideas, and (3) identification and publication of innovative and new ideas to advance the profession (Armstrong, 1996). To accomplish these purposes, editors assume the responsibility of selecting reviewers who have demonstrated advanced knowledge or practice in a particular nursing role (administrator, researcher, educator) or patient care specialty. Manuscripts then are reviewed by at least two, often three, reviewers. Reviewers screen the manuscripts for quality, accuracy, timeliness, relevance, and appropriateness before the editor's consideration of the paper for publication.

Peer review has been criticized as not always being an effective means to ensure the validity of content published or the fairness of the manuscript selection process

(Armstrong, 1996). Despite its potential weaknesses, peer review is the most appropriate means for selecting manuscripts for publication (Fondiller, 1994). It gives readers assurance that the journal's content meets acceptable standards of scholarship, conferring validity and credibility to an author's work (Felton & Swanson, 1995).

When journals are not peer reviewed, the editor reviews manuscripts and decides which manuscripts will be published, using criteria similar to those used by peer-reviewed journals. Although the articles in such journals may be excellent, the lack of peer review lessens their credibility. Journals that are peer reviewed so state somewhere within the issue. If such a statement is not found, the journal's editorial office may be contacted for clarification.

Because of promotion and tenure criteria, faculty in institutions of higher education and some major academic health science centers receive credit only for publications in peer-reviewed journals. Although the quality of material published in a non–peer-reviewed journal may not be any different from that in a peer-reviewed journal, the choice of journal should be made in light of current job requirements as well as planned career track.

DEALING WITH REJECTION OF A MANUSCRIPT

If a manuscript is not accepted for publication by the author's first-choice journal, he or she should not give up. Many well-published authors have had their works rejected for publication. The art of writing requires practice and study. Receiving feedback about the strengths and weaknesses of a manuscript from reviewers and editors helps the writer focus on developing the skills needed to successfully publish.

If a manuscript is rejected, there are two options (neither of which is never writing again!). First, the author could call and speak to the editor personally, asking what to do to revise the work to have it published. Editors are very quick to acknowledge such requests and most recommend suggestions for revision and resubmission. A good editor is honest about the quality of the manuscript and recommends other journals that may be more appropriate for the work.

The second option is to revise and submit the manuscript to another journal. The revised content should be focused to the readership and editorial purpose of the new journal. Many excellent manuscripts are rejected because the author did not target content for journal readership or conform to its style.

There are advantages and disadvantages to publishing research findings in a print journal, with the advantages outweighing the disadvantages. Advantages include the following:

- Enhanced self-esteem
- National recognition of work
- Achievement of professional goals
- Identification as an expert in the topic area
- Ability to appropriately disseminate research
- Contribution to the nursing profession

Disadvantages include the following:

- Inability to interact with the audience
- Inability to personally answer questions
- Inability to provide clarification of content without additional effort on the part of the reader
- Limited space in which to present work
- Rare honorariums or royalties
- Transferral of copyright, and thus subsequent unlimited use, of the manuscript content to another party

Electronic Publications

Using the Internet and the World Wide Web, vast amounts of information can be "published" and retrieved. Every day, more and more businesses and people establish Web sites to promote themselves, supply information, and sell their products (Schwartz, 1996). Because of its great use and untapped potential, the Internet is an easy, quick, and inexpensive way to disseminate research findings. By visiting sites, such as a nursing journal publisher (http://www.nursingcenter.com), the Virtual Nursing College (http://langara.bc.ca/vnc), or nursing sites on the World Wide Web (http://ublib.buffalo.edu/libraries/units/hsl/internet/nsgsites.html), a person can find lists, bulletin boards, and user groups that allow a researcher to post his or her ideas. Caution should be used because what is said by one can be taken and used by another.

Numerous health care organizations

have their own Web sites, which are copyrighted and where nurse researchers may post their studies. Another possibility is to develop a dedicated Web site. To learn more about creating Web sites, consult literature (Shellenbarger & Thomas, 1996) or a computer consultant. Many commercial on-line services, such as America Online, Prodigy, and CompuServe, provide information for locating experts who can produce Web sites as well as for creating one's own Web site.

Many journal publishers are taking their originally published print journals and converting the text to an electronic format. This process gives an author who is published in the print version exposure to readers who prefer to search the Internet for information rather than use a library indexing reference. A writer can electronically search the Internet to find print journals that also have an electronic version.

Modern pioneers are those publishers who are acquiring, reviewing, editing, and publishing their journals exclusively through electronic means. A recent search of the Internet indicated that there are three such peer-reviewed journals, and more are probably in the works. The three are Sigma Theta Tau International's Online Journal for Knowledge Synthesis in Nursing (http://stti-web.iupui.edu), The Australian Electronic Journal of Nursing Education (http://www. csu.edu.au/faculty/health/nursing/nurshealth/aejne/aejnehp.htm), and Kent State University School of Nursing's Online Journal of Issues in Nursing (http://www.nursingworld.org/ojin/ojinhome.htm).

Publication in an electronic peer-reviewed journal has the advantage of almost immediate publication—material is submitted electronically to an editor, forwarded by the editor to reviewers electronically, and revised and published electronically. There is little delay between generating knowledge and disseminating it to those who can use it. Another advantage is that resources are conserved—no paper, no disks, no photocopying, no postage. In addition, content can also easily be updated with new information and hypertext links to other sites related to the topic. Readers can enter into a dialogue with the author and the editor through electronic mail, which can be appended to the electronic article.

The down side to publishing results electronically is that this medium is accessed by only a small percentage of nurses. However, this will change as electronic publication matures and gains wider acceptability. Another drawback is that promotion and tenure criteria at many institutions do not recognize electronic publications as an acceptable means of scholarship. This is, in large part, due to the fact that most of the information on the Internet is not regulated or controlled for accuracy, reliability, or validity (Murray, 1996). Again, this problem will disappear as professionals realize that scholarly oversight and rigor can be as easily maintained in an electronic journal as in a print publication. Recently, a widely disseminated report of the Rutgers University Committee on Electronic Publication and Tenure supported electronic publication as a legitimate means of scholarship (http://www.aultnis.rutgers.edu/text/ept.html).

ORAL AND POSTER PRESENTATIONS

Oral and poster presentations are effective ways to disseminate research findings. Oral presentations may be conducted at conferences, at clinical unit meetings, at organization forums, or via satellite. Although most speeches are delivered to a live audience in the same location, there are times when the audience may be in another location when a satellite teleconference or video presentation is used. Conducting face-to-face oral presentations gives the researcher the opportunity to see the audience, interact with them, and receive verbal and nonverbal feedback about the presentation. On the other hand, only a small number of people are reached.

Regardless of the medium used for presenting a paper, strategies for preparing the presentation are applicable. Poster presentations may be done at conferences, health or research fairs, or clinical unit events.

Abstract Submission

The plan to present at a clinical or research conference begins with submission of an abstract to the sponsoring organization months before the conference date; therefore, the research dissemination plan may include conference dates. The abstract, usually about 150 words in length, is used by reviewers to determine the worthiness of a study, making it vital that submission guidelines are followed. Most guidelines require the inclusion of the major aspects of the study (Evans, 1994; Dumas, Gallo, & Shurpin, 1996):

1. Title—include key variables
2. Purpose of the study
3. Brief description of sample—number of subjects, distinct characteristics such as diagnosis, age range, and gender
4. Methods—design of the study, setting, procedure for collecting data, instruments including reliability and validity
5. Findings—data and significant statistical (level of significance) or clinical differences
6. Conclusions—summary of the results in relation to the purpose of the study and meaning of the data

Criteria often used to evaluate abstracts are originality, scientific merit, clinical relevance, and congruence with the conference theme and objectives. It is important to keep these criteria in mind when writing the abstract in order to increase the likelihood of its acceptance for presentation.

Developing and Conducting the Presentation

Acceptance of an abstract for paper or poster presentation triggers the need to start preparing for a successful event. The preparation starts with a review of the guidelines for presentation, which are usually included in the letter informing the researcher of the acceptance of the abstract for presentation. Although guidelines vary, most paper presentations are scheduled for 20 minutes, with 15 minutes for the delivery of the presentation and 5 minutes for questions. Poster presentations may occur over several days, with designated times when presenters need to be at the poster to interact with conference participants.

ORAL OR PAPER

Things to keep in mind when developing a paper presentation are the target audience—researchers, clinicians, laypeople; setting—size of the room; and time. Language should be adapted to the audience: for example, research language is used when the audience is primarily researchers. If the presentation room is large enough to hold more than 100 people, slides should be used; in smaller rooms, transparencies are sufficient. Presentations such as those scheduled after lunch, late in the afternoon or evening, and at the end of a conference are more challenging because the audience may be at a low energy time. The presenter may include humor so that the presentation is lively or develop strategies that frequently encourage audience participation (Gigliotti, 1995).

Because oral presentations usually precede publications, an outline of the paper presentation may be developed with the categories used for the abstract—purpose of the study, sample, methods, findings, and conclusions. Following an oral presentation sequence that is similar to the headings used in a research manuscript, that is, background, literature, and so on, facilitates development of a manuscript from the presentation. During the presentation, the questions from the audience should be noted, and these questions should be considered when writing the manuscript.

A detailed outline serves as a roadmap for writing the script for the presentation. Also, the script can be used in writing the first draft of a manuscript or an audio tape of the presentation. When slides are developed for a presentation, these can be used in the development of manuscript. Because each slide contains a key concept, it can be used to develop a paragraph for the manuscript (Klopovich, 1986).

As the presentation is developed, the writer should determine the types of slides that will be used— word, pictorial, or a combination. There are numerous computer software programs (for example, Harvard Graphics, PowerPoint, Presentation) that can be used for making slides. Using the computer to develop slides allows easy preview and reordering of the slides. Also, the color combinations can be previewed before producing the slide. The choice of colors is vital for readability; for example, light pink when used for words on a light blue background is difficult to read. Using a computer to develop a slide presentation saves money because a large number of slides do not have to be physically produced. If the slide presentation is saved to a floppy disk to be used on another computer, the writer should make sure that the slide program is compatible with the host computer system. More than one version of the file may need to be saved. If possible, slides should be previewed using the equipment that will be used during the presentation.

Legibility of text slides is vital. Things to keep in mind for a legible slide are (1) the type of font (for example, Helvetica and bold) and (2) format (for example, bullets highlight main points; number of words limited to seven per line and each slide to seven lines; left justify text) (Wells & Reynolds, 1997).

POSTER

Like the paper, the poster includes the major categories included in the abstract. Because the primary purpose of a poster is to visually communicate research in a simple way, it is necessary to be concise and clear in presenting the information (Sherbinski & Stroup, 1992). A poster should be easily understood within 5 minutes. Readability is enhanced when the text is concise, the flow of the segments is logical, left to right in the Western world, and font is readable from a distance of at least 4 to 6 feet. Several authors have suggested methods for preparing for poster presentations (Bushy, 1991; Sherbinski & Stroup, 1992; McDaniel, Bach, & Poole, 1993; McCann, Sramac, & Rudy, 1994; Turner, 1995).

1. Information gathering
   - Conference date and location
   - Length of time for poster session and requirement for being present at poster
   - Type of display—table or board usually 4 × 8 feet. When a table is provided, a stand-alone table-top display can be used. A stand-alone display can be constructed by using a foam board or a portable commercial stand in which Velcro fasteners can be used to mount segments of the poster. A cork board requires a method for mounting the poster (such as using pins).
2. Types of information to be included
   - Title, author names, and affiliations
   - Problem and a brief background
   - Method—design, sample, setting, data collection process
   - Data analysis
   - Results and implications
   - Acknowledgment—sources of funds

3. Marketability of the poster
   - Layout of poster—consider the sequence of ideas; use headings, arrows, or broken lines to guide the reader
   - Use of color—pictures, title of sections
   - Self-explanatory graphs or tables
4. Poster assembly
   - Resources—audiovisual department or self-assembly
   - Use of poster boards in separate pieces for portability as a hand carry
   - Personal computer to print texts of sections
5. Other considerations
   - Availability of handouts (for example, abstract that includes authors, affiliations, addresses, and telephone numbers)
   - Use of display items such as data collection tools marked "for display only"
6. Poster session
   - Set up the poster and take down at designated times
   - Be at the poster and interact with participants—introduce self and ask attendees their research interests
   - Note participant requests for information by requesting individuals to write their request on the back of their business cards or on a clipboard at the poster
   - Look at other posters and seek permission from authors to take a picture of posters you find attractive
7. Evaluation
   - Immediately following the presentation, jot down things that might be done differently—format, colors, written content, type and number of handouts
   - Consider the following criteria when evaluating other posters: (1) overall appearance—attractiveness, accuracy of information, color combination, readability, inclusion of only necessary information, uncluttered appearance; (2) content—current, logical, words and grammar correct, inclusion of components of the research; (3) presentation—author knowledge of the study, professional appearance of the presenter, and availability of presenter to participants.

➤ Guidelines for Developing a Well-Designed Poster

1. Adhere to sponsoring agency guidelines.
2. Keep it simple, concise, and uncluttered.
3. Use simple letters that are readable from 3 to 5 feet.
4. Make it interesting by using color, graphs, and pictures.
5. Highlight significant points by using bullets or asterisks.
6. Design a poster that is easily understood within 5 minutes.
7. Guide the reader by using directional lines, headings, and subheadings in bold print.

Poster presentations have distinct advantages over oral presentations or publications when disseminating research (Sherbinski & Stroup, 1992). In a poster presentation, findings are communicated by authors to participants in an informal way. The informal exchange of ideas between the author and the participant promotes immediate feedback to the author, which may be useful in future presentations and preparation of manuscripts, clarification of unclear or confusing aspects of the study, and networking.

Posters are excellent vehicles for disseminating research findings to the community as well as to the profession. They can easily be used at community health fairs and at local professional meetings and seminars and can be developed for display in shopping malls, physicians' offices, and community and social service agencies. When the plan is to use a poster for different types of audience, it is helpful if the entire poster is not developed as a whole piece. Separate segments can be developed for sections, such as the research methods and conclusions, so that these sections could be adapted to the audience (see box).

Strategies for Public Speaking

Despite the anxiety that is provoked by public speaking, the experience can be most rewarding and exciting. Public speaking, like any skill, requires learning and practice.

Nurses have much to say that will positively impact health care delivery (Jimenez, 1991). Public speaking by nurses will surely escalate in the coming years. This will occur secondary to the vast amount of research that is currently underway in clinical and administrative practice. Another factor that will contribute to presenting research publicly is the move to community health, to wellness and prevention models of care. Even though nurses have always played important roles in teaching self-care to patients, the demand is increasing in a capitated, managed care environment. It is necessary that nurses engage in research and seek out appropriate opportunities to present their findings publicly.

Preparation for public speaking is vital. There are many strategies that can be used to help make this experience exciting and worthwhile (Miracle & King, 1994; Dumas, Gallo, & Shurpin, 1996; Wachs, 1996).

- Know the audience. Speak their language and present the material in a way that is meaningful to them.
- Organize your thoughts.
- Use audiovisual aids.
- Use charts and graphs—most often, research findings can best be displayed with the use of tables, charts, graphs, and figures. These tools help to organize the findings for the audience.
- Speak to the audience and maintain eye contact.
- Rehearse the presentation and know the time it takes so that it fits the schedule.
- Dress appropriately—if the presentation is given during working hours, on-site at an organization, a uniform may be appropriate. In other instances, when presenting off-site, business clothing is the appropriate attire.
- Elicit audience participation by asking questions or presenting a concept, idea, or finding, and then ask, "What does this mean to you?" or "What do you think about this study result?"
- Vary your tone of voice.
- Provide time for questions and always repeat the question asked. The nature of research stimulates inquiry, so people are likely to have questions.
- Use tact in responding to criticism and keep an open mind.

- Recognize people who have made significant contributions to the research.
- Thank the audience and provide a telephone number, address, or business card.

DISSEMINATING RESEARCH FINDINGS THROUGH THE MEDIA

The media—newspapers, newsletters, television, and radio—are powerful vehicles for the dissemination of nursing research (Diers, 1992; Meade, 1992). Before considering the media as an outlet for disseminating information, the researcher should check with his or her employer about existing policies. There may be staff charged with assisting those who wish to communicate research findings to the media. Some organizations submit press releases of events, a written overview of what is occurring. If this is being done, researchers should find out how to submit their research findings.

When professional organizations invite local television channels to conferences, there is an increased chance that research that may be interesting to the public is identified. Because of this possibility, some acceptance of abstract forms include a section in which an author indicates willingness to share the study with the media.

Another outlet for research findings is the lay literature. The focus of articles published in consumer magazines related to nursing research includes topics such as acquiring a healthy lifestyle, exercise, and how to avoid various diseases. One of the best resources for finding magazine editors and publishers who accept unsolicited material is the *Writer's Guide to Magazine Editors and Publishers* (Mandell, 1996). A query letter (see box) should be sent to ascertain editor interest in your topic. Note the increased emphasis on highlighting the benefits of a topic to the readers when compared with the nursing journal query letter (see previous box).

Newspapers

Nurses participating in research are in an ideal position to make the work and contribution of nursing visible to the public by publishing their findings in local newspapers. Cultivation of a relationship with a local newspaper's health editor is a way to

➤ **Sample Query Letter for Consumer Magazine**

(Date)
(Inside Address)
Dear *(name of editor)*:
   Smoking is an addiction with severe consequences—cancer, emphysema, and circulatory problems, to name a few. Despite the widely known negative effects of smoking, people have great difficulty quitting, spending millions to beat their addiction.

   As a nurse expert with years of helping people stop smoking, I would like to write a manuscript for *(insert magazine name)*. The manuscript will present 10 significant strategies shown in a recent nursing research study to assist people to advance successfully through the five stages of smoking cessation.

   This practical manuscript to assist your readers to stop smoking can be mailed to you now. I will call you in a few days to discuss this project. Thank you.
Sincerely,

(Contact person)
(Address and telephone number, if not imprinted on letterhead)

---

establish oneself as a credible source for health care information (Gordon & Buresh, 1996). Editors are eager to have professionals who are willing to share their knowledge. When a newspaper article is written to discuss a finding from research, the writer should keep it simple and concise, focusing on what consumers need to know about the topic and what actions they should take (Laizner, 1992).

In addition to one-on-one relationship building with a local newspaper editor, the researcher can contact local chapters of large nursing organizations such as the American Nurses Association, Sigma Theta Tau International, and the American Association of Critical-Care Nurses (to name a few). They have sophisticated media programs to disseminate contributions of their organizations and their members. By obtaining a media kit and joining the publicity committee, the researcher can gain invaluable tools to do personal publication in a variety of media, particularly newspapers.

Newsletters

Most professional, community, health care, and service organizations publish newsletters. Nurses must tap these resources and inquire about submitting manuscripts of their research findings. Although the format and style of writing for newsletters differ from that of a professional journal, the critical success factors for publishing are applicable. It is vital to use terms and the language that are understood by the target audience.

Television and Radio

Television is another powerful medium. Studies show that people spend an inordinate amount of time watching television, and most homes have at least two television sets. Nurses must seek out this medium by contacting local television stations and meeting with the producers. Before contacting the local station, the researcher should ensure that his or her institution is supportive of the effort. The researcher should have a clear idea of the type of local show that might broadcast the findings, know the type of people who watch particular shows, determine the fit between the topic and the show, and maintain confidentiality of study participants. If an interview is granted, the researcher should inquire whether the interview will be live or taped and whether he or she is the only person being interviewed. If there are other participants, the researcher should find out the background of each participant. The researcher should start preparing by doing an outline, a script, and practicing with a colleague or by videotaping the presentation and reviewing the tape. Considerations for preparing for an oral presentation and public speaking strategies presented in this chapter are useful.

Carefully preparing for an interview with the media is important. There are several strategies for a successful interview (Sevel,

1986; Alward & Camuñas, 1990; St. James & Spiro, 1996):

1. Be clear on ground rules related to topics that will and will not be addressed and the opportunity to review and correct misstatements.
2. Identify possible questions that support and do not support the study and formulate a 10- to 30-second response.
3. Respond directly to a question, use citations, and do not predict when hypothetical situations are presented and an answer is being sought.
4. Determine the key points of the interview and emphasize the points each time there is an opportunity.
5. Look at the interviewer during the taping or when not being interviewed. Look above the camera when speaking.
6. Use terms that laypeople will understand.
7. Limit movements during the interview.
8. Immediately correct the interviewer when something that is said is incorrect.
9. Communicate enthusiasm and smile.
10. Wear a solid-color outfit.
11. Write a thank-you note to the host and the producer.

A local news channel is likely to be open to allowing a short segment presentation when the topic is one that is of great interest to its viewers. Also, consider a national channel. If research findings have major implications for the health of society, this may not be so far-reaching an idea. By reading newspapers and magazines that the public reads, a researcher will acquire an idea of topics that are relevant and interesting to the public as well as how information is presented.

The radio is a powerful medium for research dissemination. Most people invest daily time in radio listening. Hence, the audience potential is vast. Many local stations host special interest shows and talk shows and invite people to participate. It is wise to invest time in searching out these likely opportunities.

There are advantages and disadvantages to the use of the media in disseminating research findings. Distinct advantages are that television and radio have a greater potential for reaching a larger audience and influencing the perception of the public of nurses' contributions to their health. On the other hand, television and radio are likely to allot only a short time for the presentation, thereby increasing the possibility of misinterpretation of the message. Thus, researchers are challenged in providing a comprehensive presentation of the research methodology, findings, and implications in an understandable and concise manner. To help counter the simplicity and brevity of the research findings, the researcher should provide his or her name and a telephone number or address so that the community may have further access to learn more about the studies. This is also a helpful way to solicit participants for future studies.

Videotape

Videotapes are popular vehicles for obtaining information and can be used in effectively disseminating research findings. Some of the most popular include fitness programs or health-related teaching. Videos of a research presentation can be made and given to colleagues, patient care units in the hospital, television stations, community agencies, and professional organizations.

There are advantages and disadvantages to using videotapes (Alward & Camuñas, 1990). The advantages are that videotapes enable the researcher to reach a large number of people, and if creatively done, they are an exciting and interesting way to present content. Disadvantages include the cost, technical difficulty, and length of time needed for production. The right physical setting is required—lighting, reduction in noise level, and staging scenes (Sternberger & Freiburger, 1996).

When planning the videotape, the researcher must include the target audience, the desired outcomes, and the content, identifying the most effective ways to communicate the message—using visual aids that support the script or photography.

Videotaping could be intimidating to presenters, especially when taping is done without a live audience; therefore, writing a script is important to ensure that the message is succinct and is delivered within the allotted time. During the taping, it is helpful to consider the camera as the audience and to pretend to be in a living room speak-

ing to guests. A researcher could market a videotape by giving a copy to professional organizations who may find utility for its members.

SUMMARY

Nursing research contributes positively to the health care delivery system. As more nurses are prepared at the graduate and doctoral levels, more and more nursing research is being conducted in clinical, administrative, and education settings. Nurses who conduct research have a professional obligation to share their findings. This is how a profession grows and matures. In the past, nurses have been shy about presenting their findings (Winslow, 1996), but this is changing. Nurses are making outstanding contributions to the future health state of the world.

It is vital that nurses use various approaches for disseminating research findings. Nursing, other colleagues, and the public benefit from advances in nursing science when formal and informal paper presentations, posters, and print and electronic publications are used to disseminate findings. Technology continues to play a major role in providing more opportunities and vehicles by which nurses can further disseminate research. Connecting to the Internet, the new information highway of the world, allows transfer of vast amounts of knowledge through new and sophisticated means. This new means of knowledge transfer is rapidly and radically transforming the way nurses disseminate knowledge and influence the health of the nation. Whatever method is chosen, effective communication with the target audience is crucial and conforming with the guidelines set by the journal or organization that is sponsoring a publication or an event is essential for success.

REFERENCES

Alward, R. R., & Camuñas, C. (1990). Public relations. Part II, Strategies and tactics. *Journal of Nursing Administration, 20*(11), 31–42.

American Medical Association. (1998). *Manual of style* (9th ed.). Baltimore: Williams & Wilkins.

American Psychological Association. (1994). *Publication manual of the American Psychological Association* (4th ed.). Washington, DC: Author.

Armstrong, J. S. (1996). The editorial role of peer reviewers. *The Chronicle of Higher Education*, October 25, B3–4.

Blancett, S. S. (1991). The ethics of writing and publishing. *The Journal of Nursing Administration, 21*(5), 31–36.

Blancett, S. S. (1992). Plagiarism revisited. *Nurse Educator, 17*(6), 4.

Blancett, S. S. (1994). Advancing nursing management through writing. In T. Porter-O'Grady (Ed.), *The nurse manager's problem solver* (pp. 283–291). St. Louis: Mosby–Year Book.

Blancett, S. S. (1997). The manager as published author: Tips on writing for publication. In M. D. Harris (Ed.), *Handbook of home health care administration* (2nd ed., pp. 795–807). Gaithersburg, MD: Aspen.

Boots, S. (1993). Who should be acknowledged in a journal article? *CBE Views, 16*(3), 57.

Bushy, A. (1991). A rating scale to evaluate research posters. *Nurse Educator, 16*(1), 11–15.

Cates, W. (1983). Tricks of the trade in displaying data. *Contemporary OB/GYN, 22*, 87–103.

Clegg, R. L. (1991). Copyright law and the nursing professor. *Nurse Educator, 16*(6), 28–31.

Diers, D. (1992). On the good news. *IMAGE: Journal of Nursing Scholarship, 24*, 252.

Dumas, M. A. S., Gallo, K., & Shurpin, K. M. (1996). Search and research. Research presentations: Disseminating knowledge for practice. *Journal of the American Academy of Nurse Practitioners, 8*, 277–281.

Evans, J. C. (1994). The art of writing successful research abstracts. *Neonatal-Network, 13*(5), 49–52.

Felton, G., & Swanson, E. A. (1995). Peer review. *Journal of Professional Nursing, 11*(1), 16–23.

Flanagin, A., & Rennie, D. (1995). Acknowledging ghosts. *Journal of the American Medical Association, 273*(1), 73.

Fondiller, S. H. (1994). Editorial peer review: Is nursing at risk? *Nursing and Healthcare, 15*(3), 142–148.

Garrett, B., & Hawkes, W. G. (1992). Copyright—what's right? *Journal of Continuing Education in Nursing, 23*, 101–104.

Gigliotti, E. (1995). Let me entertain . . . er . . . teach you: Gaining attention through the use of slide shows. *Journal of Continuing Education in Nursing, 26*(1), 31–34.

Gordon, J. S., & Buresh, B. (1996). Speak up speak out: Publicizing nursing research. *American Journal of Nursing, 96*(10), 62, 64.

Jimenez, S. L. (1991). Consumer journalism: A unique nursing opportunity. *Image: Journal of Nursing Scholarship, 23*, 47–49.

Johnson, S. H. (1996). Adapting a thesis to publication style: Meeting editors' expectations. *Dimensions of Critical Care Nursing, 15*(3), 160–167.

Klopovich, P. A. (1986). A personal experience . . . turning a speech or lecture into a manuscript: Part 2. *Oncology Nursing Forum, 13*(4), 74–75.

Laizner, A. M. (1992). Surveillance of news media: A nursing responsibility. *Imprint, 39*(3), 37, 39–40, 43.

Lundberg, G. D., & Glass, M. (1996). What does author-ship mean in a peer-reviewed medical journal. *Journal of the American Medical Association, 276*(1), 75.

Mandell, J. (1996). *The writer's guide to magazine editors and publishers*. Rocklin, CA: Prima Publishers.

McCann, S. A., Sramac, R. S., & Rudy, S. J. (1994). The poster exhibit: Planning, development, and presentation. *Orthopaedic Nursing, 13*(3), 43–49.

McDaniel, R. W., Bach, C. A., & Poole, M. J. (1993). Poster update: Getting their attention. *Nursing Research, 42*, 302–304.

McKinney, V., & Burns, N. (1993). The effective presentation of graphs. *Nursing Research, 42*, 250–252.

Meade, C. D. (1992). Approaching the media with confidence. *Public Health Nursing, 9*, 209–214.

Miracle, V. A., & King, K. C. (1994). Presenting research: Effective paper presentations and impressive poster presentations. *Applied Nursing Research, 7*, 147–151.

Murray, P. J. (1996). Connecting points: Web sites. Click here—and be disappointed? Evaluating web sites. *Computers in Nursing, 14*, 260–261.

Nativio, D. G. (1993). Authorship. *IMAGE: Journal of Nursing Scholarship, 25*, 358.

Schwartz, A. P. S. (1996). Nursing resources on the net expand at a rapid rate. *Internet Medicine, 3*(1), 6.

Sevel, F. (1986). Are you prepared to meet the media? *Journal of Nursing Administration, 16*(3), 21–24.

Shellenbarger, T., & Thomas, S. (1996). Creating a nursing home page on the World Wide Web. *Computers in Nursing, 14*, 239–245.

Sherbinski, L. A., & Stroup, D. R. (1992). Developing a poster for disseminating research findings. *Journal of the American Association of Nurse Anesthetists, 60*, 567–572.

Skiba, D. J. (1997). Intellectual property issues in the digital health care world. *Nursing Administration Quarterly, 21* (3), 11–20.

Spilker, B., & Schoenfelder, J. (1990). *Presentation of clinical data*. New York: Raven.

Sternberger, C. S., & Freiburger, O. A. (1996). Faculty-produced videos. *Journal of Nursing Staff Development, 12*(4), 173–178.

St. James, D., & Spiro, H. (1996). Writing and speaking for excellence: A guide for physicians. Boston: Jones and Bartlett.

Tornquist, E., & Funk, S. G. (1993). How to report research with clarity, coherence, and grace. *Journal of Emergency Nursing, 19*, 498–502.

Turner, B. S. (1995). Posters: Getting your message across. *Tar Heel Nurse, 57*(3), 22–24.

Wachs, J. E. (1996). From idea to publication: The secrets of publishing. *American Association of Occupational Health Nursing Journal, 44*, 273–777.

Waugaman, W. R. (1992). Publish your thesis as an article or a book. *Nurse Anesthesia, 3*, 183–187.

Wells, S. E., & Reynolds, W. J. (1997). Computer generated slides—Cheap! *The Journal of Continuing Education in Nursing, 28*, 83–87.

Winslow, E. H. (1996). Failure to publish research: A form of scientific misconduct? *Heart and Lung: The Journal of Acute and Critical-Care, 25*, 169–171.

Glossary

Abstract Brief summary of the main ideas of a study, including the purpose, methods (sample, instruments, procedure), and findings

ASCII (American Standard Code for Information Interchange)—computer representation used in the transfer of information between different software packages

Bias Prejudice that influences research and can cause distortions in all phases of a study, including observation, recall, and response

Central tendency Indication of the center of data in a distribution (mean, median, and mode)

Chi-square A nonparametric statistical test based on comparing actual observed frequencies and theoretical expected frequencies. A statistical test used to test for independence between two characteristics or to compare groups on the distribution of a single characteristic

Clinical significance A judgment about the interpretation of the statistical results (that the difference or relationship has meaning for patient care)

Code book Record of value definitions and column location of each variable

Collaboration Working together to achieve joint goals

Conceptual or theoretical framework Concepts that provide structure for the research questions, method, and interpretation of findings

Control group Research participants who do not receive experimental treatment and whose data are used for comparison with the experimental group

Data Information gathered for research

Deductive reasoning Thought proceeding from the application of general principles to the particular instance

Definition of terms
 Conceptual The real meaning of the word
 Operational The meaning used in *this* study

Demographics Background variables (age, sex, education, and so forth) that define the sample or participants

Double-blind Experimental research method in which neither researcher nor participants know which group is experimental and which is control

Experimental group Research participants who receive experimental treatment

Frequency Number of times a value of a variable occurs

Frequency distribution Tally of frequencies of all of the values of a variable

Halo effect Observer's bias of positivity or negativity toward a subject (usually affects the measurement taken)

Hard disk Fixed storage disk usually inside the computer

Hardware Basic tangible computer equipment (including computer, keyboard, monitor, printer, and modem)

Hawthorne effect Behavior change caused by knowledge of being observed

Histogram Bar chart used to display frequencies of data

Hypothesis Statement of relationship between two or more variables
 Null hypothesis The statistical hypothesis of no relationship or difference between groups or variables

Directional   Relationship in one direction only

Nondirectional   Relationship in either direction, positive or negative

Research   Statement of the predicted relationship between two or more variables or difference between two or more groups

Inductive approach   Thought proceeding from particular instances to generalization of the instances into a theory or concept

Informed consent   Voluntary agreement of a person to participate in a research program after being informed of the purpose, type, and extent of participation (as well as the risks and benefits of the study)

Instrument   Device used to collect data (such as a questionnaire or a thermometer)

Levels of measurement

Nominal   Categories that have no order, the numbers represent labels (sex, diagnosis)

Ordinal   Categories where numbers reflect an order (class rank, degree of agreement)

Interval   Numerical scale with equal distance between scale points (body temperature)

Ratio   Interval scale with a true zero (age, weight)

Longitudinal study   Research in which the same variables are measured over time

Mean   Average; sum of all scores divided by the number of scores

Median   Number in a data set at which one half of scores are higher and the other half lower

Meta-analysis   Mathematical summary of results of several studies

Method   Sample, instrument, and procedures used for a study

Mode   Value of a variable in a data set that occurs most frequently

Multivariate statistics   Simultaneous study of multiple variables

Normal curve   Frequency distribution that is a symmetrical bell-shaped curve (mean, median, and mode are all the same and are located at the center)

Nurse researcher   Usually used to mean a nurse with a doctorate who is conducting research

Parameter   The actual value (such as the mean) for the entire population that is being estimated based on a sample from that population

Phenomena   Observable data

Pilot study   Small-scale version of the research study used as a trial to make decisions about the best way to conduct the major study

Population (N)   Total possible number (of participants, objects, and so forth) meeting the qualification of the study (usually a sample of the population is studied)

Posttest   Test following an intervention

Power analysis   Statistical procedure for estimating the number of subjects needed to show the desired difference between groups at predetermined (and acceptable) Type I and Type II error rates

Pretest   Test preceding an intervention

Problem statement   Description of the research focus including variables and population

Proposal   Written plan that summarizes the research

Qualitative analysis   Procedures for categorical or nonnumerical data (such as words or statements from subjects)

Quantitative analysis   Statistical procedures for numerical data

Range   Technically a single number—the distance between the lowest and highest values of a variable; however, sometimes the lowest and highest values are given in a table

Ranking   Ordering data according to an increasing amount of a quality

Reliability   Measure of consistent test results with repeated use of an instrument or tool

Internal consistency   Measure of consistency of each test item to the whole

Interrater   Measure of agreement between two or more independent observers who are rating the same attribute

Test-retest   Measure of the stability of a tool to consistently measure an attribute

Research

Descriptive   Collected data define or describe a population or phenomenon

Experimental   Design includes hypothesis testing, random sampling and random assignment to groups, control group, and manipulation of the independent variable

Quasi-experimental Design does not meet all of experimental design characteristics but does include manipulation of the independent variable

Replication Repetition of previous research

Research question Statement of the relationship between variables stated as a question

Risk-benefit ratio Comparison of personal risk to benefits from participating in research

Sample Subset (n) of the total population (N)

Sampling

Convenience sampling Choosing the most readily available subjects

Random sampling Each person in the population has a known and equal nonzero chance of being selected

Stratified random sampling Random sampling within strata after the population has been categorized into strata

Systematic A random start with subsequent selection occurring at a fixed interval

Time sampling Collection of data at predetermined points of time

Sampling error Differences between sample means because of different sample selections

Scales (characteristics)

Likert An ordinal scale that is usually rating agreement

Semantic differential Bipolar scale rating word meanings

Scatterplot Diagram of plotted points of two variables depicting their relationship

Software Programs that instruct a computer what to do

Standard deviation Measure of dispersion of individual values around the mean (square root of the variance)

Standard error of the mean Estimate of the precision of the mean (standard deviation divided by the square root of n)

Statistics

Parametric For interval or ratio data having normal distribution

Nonparametric For nominal or ordinal data that do not meet requirements for parametric statistics

Statistical significance Likelihood that results are caused by chance

Statistical test Procedures used to test the research hypothesis

Theory Organization of concepts for explaining a phenomenon

t-Test

Pooled or independent Parametric test that determines significant differences between means of two independent groups

Paired Tests differences between two measurements on the same group

Type I error Rejection of a true null hypothesis

Type II error Acceptance of a false null hypothesis

Validity

External Measure of appropriateness for generalization

Internal Measure of independent variable being responsible for observed effect

Variable A characteristic, attribute, or outcome

Dependent Variable affected by the independent variable

Extraneous or confounding Variable that can affect the relationship between the dependent and independent variables

Independent Variable that is manipulated or is the presumed cause

Dichotomous Variable with only two values

Variance Measure of dispersion derived by taking the average of squared deviations from the mean

Index

Page numbers in *italics* refer to figures; page numbers followed by b refer to
text in boxes; page numbers followed by t refer to tables.